RESEARCHING
Health

QUALITATIVE, QUANTITATIVE AND MIXED METHODS

Edited by

Mike Saks and Judith Allsop

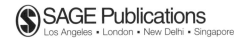

SAGE Publications
Los Angeles ▪ London ▪ New Delhi ▪ Singapore

SAGE Publications Ltd
1 Oliver's Yard
55 City Road
London EC1Y 1SP

SAGE Publications Inc.
2455 Teller Road
Thousand Oaks, California 91320

SAGE Publications India Pvt Ltd
B 1/I 1 Mohan Cooperative Industrial Area
Mathura Road, New Delhi 110 044
India

SAGE Publications Asia-Pacific Pte Ltd
33 Pekin Street #02-01
Far East Square
Singapore 048763

British Library Cataloguing in Publication data

A catalogue record for this book is available
from the British Library

ISBN 978-1-4129-0363-9
ISBN 978-1-4129-0364-6 (pbk)

Library of Congress Control Number: 2006933954

Typeset by C&M Digitals (P) Ltd, Chennai, India
Printed in Great Britain by The Alden Press, Witney
Printed on paper from sustainable resources

Contents

List of Contributors

Andy Alaszewski
Professor of Health Studies and Director of the Centre for Health Services Studies at the University of Kent, UK

Priscilla Alderson
Professor of Childhood Studies in the Social Sciences Research Unit at the Institute of Education, University of London, UK

Judith Allsop
Professor of Health Policy at the University of Lincoln, UK

George Argyrous
Senior Lecturer in the School of Social Science and Policy at the University of New South Wales, Australia

Alex Broom
Postdoctoral Research Fellow in the School of Healthcare at the University of Leeds, UK

Viola Burau
Associate Professor in the Department of Political Science at the University of Aarhus, Denmark

Michael Calnan
Professor of Medical Sociology in the Medical Research Council HSRC in the Department of Social Medicine at the University of Bristol, UK

Peter Davis
Professor and Head of Department of Sociology at the University of Auckland, New Zealand

Judith Green
Senior Lecturer in Sociology at the London School of Hygiene and Tropical Medicine, UK

Sophie Hill
Coordinating Editor of the Cochrane Consumers and Communication Review Group in the Faculty of Health Sciences at La Trobe University, Australia

David Hughes
Professor of Health Policy in the School of Health Science at the University of Wales, UK

Mark R.D. Johnson
Professor of Diversity in Health and Social Care in the School of Nursing and Midwifery at De Montfort University, UK

Kathryn Jones
Senior Research Fellow in the Department of Public Policy at De Montfort University, UK

George Lewith
Reader in the Complementary Medicine Research Unit, University of Southampton, UK

Paul Little
Professor in the School of Medicine at the University of Southampton, UK

Jacqueline Low
Associate Professor in the Department of Sociology at the University of New Brunswick, Canada

Alan Maynard
Professor of Health Economics at the University of York, UK

Janet Richardson
Reader in the Faculty of Health and Social Work at the University of Plymouth, UK

Mike Saks
Professor and Pro Vice Chancellor (Research and Academic Affairs) at the University of Lincoln, UK

Alastair Scott
Professor in the Department of Sociology at the University of Auckland, New Zealand

A. Niroshan Siriwardena
Visiting Professor of Primary Care at the University of Lincoln, UK

Jonathan Tritter
Executive Director of the NHS Resource Centre for Patient and Public Involvement and Senior Lecturer in Sociology at the University of Warwick, UK

Heather Waterman
Professor of Nursing and Ophthalmology in the School of Nursing, Midwifery and Social Work at the University of Manchester, UK

Evan Willis
Professor of Sociology in the Faculty of Humanities and Social Sciences at La Trobe University, Australia

Guided Tour

4

Using Documents in Health Research

ANDY ALASZEWSKI

INTRODUCTION

Documents, especially personal documents such as diaries and letters, provide a relatively neglected resource for health service researchers. They can be used to access data that are difficult to obtain in other ways. For example, such documents can tell us about individuals who died several centuries ago; people from marginalized and stigmatized groups who are often reluctant to participate in research; or activities, such as gay sex, that are otherwise concealed. In this respect, the overall aim of this chapter is to examine the ways in which documents have been and can be used for health research. This includes describing documentary research, identifying the type of resources it requires, and examining the research issues for which it is appropriate. The chapter will also, amongst other things, outline the strengths and weaknesses of documentary research and consider how documentary data can be coded, analysed and presented.

DEFINING DOCUMENTARY RESEARCH

Health-related documentary research involves the use of any 'records relating to individuals or groups of individuals that have been generated in the course

Chapter Introductions: An introduction to orient the reader is provided at the start of each chapter.

CASE STUDY

Case study: Exploring accounts of food risks using focus groups

As part of a large European study of the public perceptions of the risks associated with bovine spongiform encephalopathy (BSE), we wanted to explore public concerns about food risks in general, and to identify what kinds of information on food safety were trusted (Green et al. 2003; Green et al. 2005). The aim was to include people from four European countries, which had been chosen to represent a range of 'food cultures' (Germany, Italy, the United Kingdom and Finland), and to include people from different stages in the life cycle theoretically associated with different approaches to food choice (adolescents, young single people, those responsible for shopping for young children and older citizens). In addition to providing detailed data on how these population groups talked about their food choices, we also aimed to compare findings across the four countries and the four life cycle stage groups. An international study presents particular challenges (see Chapter 20), but many are typical of the kinds of decisions researchers in any focus group study have to take. The first is selecting an appropriate sample of groups.

Given our comparative aim, we wanted a similar range of groups in each of the four countries. However, within each country, of course, the meaning of the life cycle groups and other population groups is rather different. As an example, young single men in Italy had rather less experience of choosing their own food than those of similar age in other countries. In some countries, regional or rural/urban differences were more pronounced than in others. Second, focus group methodologies have to resonate with local cultural norms about interaction. In some countries, it became clear it would not be productive to run single-gender groups, as there are few situations in which men would interact normally in this way and the focus group setting simply would not reproduce 'natural' talk in the way that it might for other groups. We therefore created a sampling grid, which aimed to select a range of life cycle groups in each country, but to also select within each country a range representing other factors theoretically linked to food cultures, such as geographical location or social class. A total of 36 groups were sampled to generate a data set that would enable us to compare countries and life cycle groups, and within each country to take account of differences in location or social class, as illustrated in Table 7.1.

The aim was to recruit natural groups wherever possible, to maximize the methodological advantages discussed above. Research teams used a mixture of methods to do this, including contacting community groups such as church-based or local associations, and working with schools to recruit friendship groups of adolescents. However, for the 'young single' groups, which may consist of relatively mobile individuals with few

Case Studies: Case studies by the contributors are given in the text of each chapter to bring the subject to life.

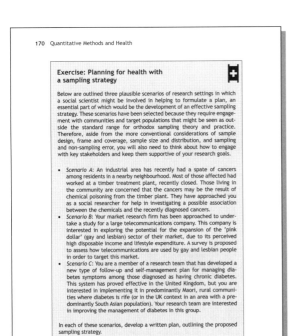

Exercise: Planning for health with a sampling strategy

Below are outlined three plausible scenarios of research settings in which a social scientist might be involved in helping to formulate a plan, an essential part of which would be the development of an effective sampling strategy. These scenarios have been selected because they require engagement with communities and target populations that might be seen as outside the standard range for orthodox sampling theory and practice. Therefore, aside from the more conventional considerations of sample design, frame and coverage, sample size and distribution, and sampling and non-sampling error, you will also need to think about how to engage with key stakeholders and keep them supportive of your research goals.

- **Scenario A:** An industrial area has recently had a spate of cancers among residents in a nearby neighbourhood. Most of those affected had worked at a timber treatment plant, recently closed. Those living in the community are concerned that the cancers may be the result of chemical poisoning from the timber plant. They have approached you as a social researcher for help in investigating a possible association between the chemicals and the recently diagnosed cancers.
- **Scenario B:** Your market research firm has been approached to undertake a study for a large telecommunications company. This company is interested in exploring the potential for the expansion of the 'pink dollar' (gay and lesbian) sector of their market, due to its perceived high disposable income and lifestyle expenditure. A survey is proposed to assess how telecommunications are used by gay and lesbian people in order to target this market.
- **Scenario C:** You are a member of a research team that has developed a new type of follow-up and self-management plan for managing diabetes symptoms among those diagnosed as having chronic diabetes. This system has proved effective in the United Kingdom, but you are interested in implementing it in predominantly Maori, rural communities where diabetes is rife (or in the UK context in an area with a predominantly South Asian population). Your research team are interested in improving the management of diabetes in this group.

In each of these scenarios, develop a written plan, outlining the proposed sampling strategy.

Exercises: An exercise is included at the end of each chapter to enable readers to test their skills.

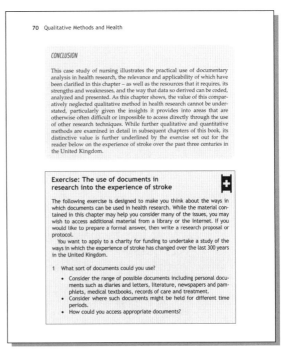

CONCLUSION

This case study of nursing illustrates the practical use of documentary analysis in health research, the relevance and applicability of which have been clarified in this chapter – as well as the resources that it requires, its strengths and weaknesses, and the way that data so derived can be coded, analyzed and presented. As this chapter shows, the value of this comparatively neglected qualitative method in health research cannot be understated, particularly given the insights it provides into areas that are otherwise often difficult or impossible to access directly through the use of other research techniques. While further qualitative and quantitative methods are examined in detail in subsequent chapters of this book, its distinctive value is further underlined by the exercise set out for the reader below on the experience of stroke over the past three centuries in the United Kingdom.

Exercise: The use of documents in research into the experience of stroke

The following exercise is designed to make you think about the ways in which documents can be used in health research. While the material contained in this chapter may help you consider many of the issues, you may wish to access additional material from a library or the Internet. If you would like to prepare a formal answer, then write a research proposal or protocol.

You want to apply to a charity for funding to undertake a study of the ways in which the experience of stroke has changed over the last 300 years in the United Kingdom.

1 What sort of documents could you use?
- Consider the range of possible documents including personal documents such as diaries and letters, literature, newspapers and pamphlets, medical textbooks, records of care and treatment.
- Consider where such documents might be held for different time periods.
- How could you access appropriate documents?

Chapter Overviews: An overview of the key issues contained in each chapter is provided on the website.

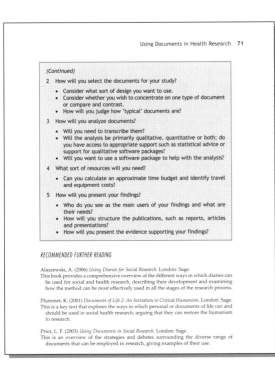

(Continued)

2 How will you select the documents for your study?
- Consider what sort of design you want to use.
- Consider whether you wish to concentrate on one type of document or compare and contrast.
- How will you judge how 'typical' documents are?

3 How will you analyze documents?
- Will you need to transcribe them?
- Will the analysis be primarily qualitative, quantitative or both; do you have access to appropriate support such as statistical advice or support for qualitative software packages?
- Will you want to use a software package to help with the analysis?

4 What sort of resources will you need?
- Can you calculate an approximate time budget and identify travel and equipment costs?

5 How will you present your findings?
- Who do you see as the main users of your findings and what are their needs?
- How will you structure the publications, such as reports, articles and presentations?
- How will you present the evidence supporting your findings?

RECOMMENDED FURTHER READING

Alaszewski, A. (2006) *Using Diaries for Social Research*. London: Sage.
This book provides a comprehensive overview of the different ways in which diaries can be used for social and health research, describing their development and examining how the method can be most effectively used in all the stages of the research process.

Plummer, K. (2001) *Documents of Life 2: An Invitation to Critical Humanism*. London: Sage.
This is a key text that explores the ways in which personal or documents of life can and should be used in social health research, arguing that they can restore the humanism to research.

Prior, L. F. (2003) *Using Documents in Social Research*. London: Sage.
This is an overview of the strategies and debates surrounding the diverse range of documents that can be employed in research, giving examples of their use.

Annotated Further Reading: Further readings are recommended at the end of each chapter and on the website.

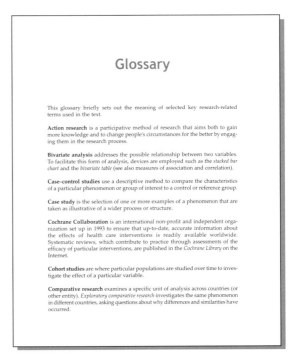

Glossary

This glossary briefly sets out the meaning of selected key research-related terms used in the text.

Action research is a participative method of research that aims both to gain more knowledge and to change people's circumstances for the better by engaging them in the research process.

Bivariate analysis addresses the possible relationship between two variables. To facilitate this form of analysis, devices are employed such as the *stacked bar chart* and the *bivariate table* (see also measures of association and correlation).

Case–control studies use a descriptive method to compare the characteristics of a particular phenomenon or group of interest to a control or reference group.

Case study is the selection of one or more examples of a phenomenon that are taken as illustrative of a wider process or structure.

Cochrane Collaboration is an international non-profit and independent organization set up in 1993 to ensure that up-to-date, accurate information about the effects of health care interventions is readily available worldwide. Systematic reviews, which contribute to practice through assessments of the efficacy of particular interventions, are published in the *Cochrane Library* on the Internet.

Cohort studies are where particular populations are studied over time to investigate the effect of a particular variable.

Comparative research examines a specific unit of analysis across countries (or other entity). *Exploratory comparative research* investigates the same phenomenon in different countries, asking questions about why differences and similarities have occurred.

A Glossary of Key Concepts: Definitions of key terms derived from the text are provided at the end of the book and on the website.

Companion Website

Visit the companion website at http://www.sagepub.co.uk/saks_allsop to find a range of teaching and learning material for lecturers and students including the following:

For instructors:
— Instructor's Notes: A password protected Instructors' Manual is provided on the website with teaching notes indicating how the subject might best be taught.
— PowerPoint Slides: PowerPoint slides for each chapter for use in teaching are also provided in the Instructors' Manual on the website.

For students:
— SAGE Online Readings: Access is provided to up to three Sage journal articles related to each chapter, summaries of which are given on the website.
— Links to Relevant Websites: Links to related websites for each chapter are provided as appropriate.
— Online Glossary: The glossary of key concepts in the text is also available to students online.

The editors wish to thank Dr Katherine Jones and Katherine Hooper for their assistance in compiling this website.

PART I
Conducting Health Research

1

Introduction

The Context for Researching Health

MIKE SAKS AND JUDITH ALLSOP

INTRODUCTION

This specially commissioned, edited book aims to provide a guide to the range of ways in which readers may approach researching health in practice. After the opening chapters on conducting health research (Chapter 1 to Chapter 3), each of the mainstream chapters on qualitative and quantitative methods and health (Chapter 4 to Chapter 14) gives an account of a specific research method in health and/or how to research a particularly significant specialized area of health care. In the case of research methods, the type of questions that the method is intended to address and its strengths and weaknesses are described, followed by a consideration of the challenges likely to be encountered in carrying out research. The book then turns to consider selected contemporary debates about the best ways of researching the health field which also to varying degrees draw attention to the use of mixed methods (Chapter 15 to Chapter 20). In so doing, each chapter in the book provides examples of health research in practice to aid readers in carrying out their own research project or in using the research of others in their work. These examples include those from the authors' own research, as appropriate. Such illustrations are also provided in the concluding chapter by the editors on the dissemination of health research (Chapter 21).

We take the view as editors that two principles underlie all research. First, research is about producing new insights and new knowledge by setting answerable research questions, collecting data in a systematic way, analyzing these intelligently and rigorously, as well as identifying patterns and establishing associations. In this way, researchers may contribute, amongst other things, to a greater understanding of individual health and collective health behaviour, the role and impact of health providers and the options for delivering health services to communities. In putting together the book, we believe that:

> Research is about illumination. If we don't succeed in that we have failed. If a person reads something and doesn't feel any wiser, then why was it done? Research should fire curiosity and the imagination ... If people feel research illuminates their understanding and gets into their thinking, then it's of use. (Quoted in Richardson et al. 1990: 75)

The second principle is that the findings produced by research are always contingent on the context in which the research is carried out, the methods used and how the data have been analyzed and interpreted. We therefore think that it is incumbent upon the researcher to be as explicit and transparent as possible about these elements in the research process. New knowledge or insights occur in small steps. Often, studies need to be replicated and/or reanalyzed and revisited before findings can be said to be soundly based. All research results are subject to reinterpretation and review. In this sense, the production of new knowledge is a collective enterprise and each researcher, even if working alone, is part of a wider research community. Although there is no single organization that covers all researchers in health and/or other fields, there are both formal and informal rules that govern research. These are outlined and assessed in the various chapters in this volume.

WHAT IS HEALTH RESEARCH?

What, though, is 'research' in the health context? At its most general level the conventions of health research can be viewed as work conducted to develop knowledge based on available evidence, following certain rules and procedures. However, as Henn et al. (2006) point out, what is to count as knowledge and how we acquire that knowledge is a contested area. Most significantly, there are different paradigms or clusters of beliefs and assumptions that shape what is studied, how research is conducted, what methods are used to ground knowledge and how results are interpreted. These frame how we view the world and lead to many different types of research. They are more fully discussed in the next chapter and also by Brown et al. (2003).

At a macro level, there is a division between research in the natural sciences (including, for example, physics, chemistry and biology), on which the more clinical areas of health research tend to be based, and the social sciences (such as policy, politics, history and sociology) that explore patterns of health and illness and the social meanings surrounding these. At a micro level, there are also distinctive approaches both between, and within, such disciplines and sub-disciplines (Daly et al. 1992). There are distinctions too between the various methods used in health research that are divided broadly between qualitative and quantitative research. Classically, these are based on the paradigms that provide a philosophical and methodological context for such work in the health field (Dyson and Brown 2006). However, as some of the chapters in this book illustrate, many research projects are now carried out using a mixture of methods. In these circumstances, it is vital for the researcher to understand what kind of knowledge each type of method produces, what kind of evidence supports the interpretation of findings from research data and how different kinds of evidence may or may not be linked together to determine how a particular piece of research adds to knowledge.

According to Richardson et al. (1990), within the broader frame of reference delineated by paradigms, health research itself can take many different forms based on the purpose of the research and its subject matter. These principally include the following types: contextual/descriptive, diagnostic/analytical, strategic, evaluative, developmental and methodological (see Box 1.1).

These types of research have different audiences. To illustrate this, contextual research has broad appeal to academic and other communities, while strategic research is of most interest to those concerned with policy and practice. The varying forms of research also relate to various stages of a research project. Thus, for example, methodological research is usually involved in establishing the foundations for further research, while evaluative research typically looks back on programmes already developed. In the health sphere, the methods employed to collect data within these various types of research are wide ranging – from surveys to observational techniques. A fuller account can be found, amongst others, in Jenkinson (1997).

The notion of 'health' itself has been conceptualized in many ways. Turner (2003) charts the manner in which the concepts of health and illness have changed historically, from primitive societies where they were linked to spiritual notions of purity and danger, to the dominant biomedical, scientific and professional definitions that focus on disease and pathology. In the modern context, though, as he notes, there are still many debates about interpretation. Typically, social scientists view health as a moral norm defining a socially

---

Box 1.1 *Different types of research: a summary*

Contextual or descriptive: Providing current information or intelligence on a problem — for example, the prevalence of Alzheimer's disease

Diagnostic or analytical: Attempting an explanation of phenomena based on a notion of cause and effect — such as accounting for changes in the birth rate

Strategic: Discovering implications, assessing alternatives and finding solutions — as, for instance, in the analysis of those at risk from a universal vaccination programme

Evaluative: Assessing the benefits and costs of a specific programme or course of action to those directly concerned or the wider community — as illustrated by the testing of a new drug

Developmental: Studying the implementation of programmes to feed back information to enable change — for example, on an anti-smoking campaign

Methodological: Assessing methods and techniques and developing new ones — as in the case of finding new means to diagnose particular diseases

---

Source: Richardson et al. (1990)

constructed, prescriptive standard that tends towards an ideal of well-being or social functioning – although people in different social groups also define health very differently depending on such variables as social class, gender, ethnic group and age. Within this perspective, illness is usually conceptualized as the obverse of health, and as a socially sanctioned, but legitimated role – which may be further socially patterned through the interpretations of the individuals themselves and significant others, such as family, friends and health providers.

Within the natural scientific viewpoint, there has been a greater emphasis on the identification and classification of disease categories, and on the causes of mortality and morbidity, based on objective clinical pathology. This has led to considerations of how particular interventions can best treat diseases in individuals and to the epidemiological study of the incidence and prevalence of particular diseases in groups and communities – although epidemiology itself is a highly specialized area not covered in this book.

This latter point highlights that research on health, illness and disease can be focused at many different levels in the contemporary context: from the individual to the community, from the activities of patients as health producers to the contribution of informal carers, and from health care assistants with a short training to fully fledged health professionals in the labour force. Those concerned with health care may also operate at a local, national or international level. This is reflected in the range of research undertaken in the health field, as well as its differential applicability to aspects of government policy.

RESEARCH FOR POLICY

From this viewpoint, we would emphasize that health research using a range of methods may be undertaken not only to gain an understanding of health, illness and disease in contemporary society, but also to contribute to policy development. In this regard, there has been a major change in the culture of health services in the developed world. Not only have clinical interventions become more evidence based, but policy makers too aim to base their policies on the interventions that are most efficacious. Recently, clinical science centred on a biomedical model of disease has made a considerable contribution to developing evidence for treatments based on clinical trials and experimental methods. This is witnessed by the establishment of the Cochrane Collaboration, for example, which has driven the growth of international centres for preparing, maintaining and disseminating systematic reviews in health care, typically based on randomized controlled trials (Lancaster et al. 1997).

In the United Kingdom specifically, since the 1997 general election, Labour governments have put an emphasis on the maxim 'what counts is what works' (Rawnsley 2001). In the clinical care arena, this is illustrated by such developments as the National Institute for Clinical Excellence (NICE) that produces clinical guidelines based on research evidence and National Service Frameworks (NSFs) that seek to develop a firmer foundation for clinical interventions (Brown et al. 2003). NICE includes a remit to reconsider the funding of interventions that are not effective. For balance, it also has a Patients' Council with representatives of consumers and there is a network to support health consumer groups to submit evidence. NSFs, on the other hand, have set the parameters for a framework of policy priorities, in terms of which diseases and illnesses should have priority for funding, and what are considered to be the most efficacious interventions.

Both clinical and policy research have benefited from hitherto unprecedented levels of research funding to evaluate interventions and to carry out pilot projects. The Research and Development Programme directed by the Department of Health in particular has made substantial research funds available for work on policy priorities. However, there has been considerable debate and controversy about the validity and utility of the evidence base for clinical and policy guidelines on the efficacy of treatments and the appropriateness of the services provided; evolution has been fast and not all of these have been based on sound research evidence (Brown et al. 2003). There have also been differences of opinion about the balance between clinical and more social scientifically oriented research and the role of lay people in providing a perspective and form of knowledge distinct from those of health professionals, as well as about the ethical issues raised in health research (Gabe et al. 2006).

THE READERSHIP, AIMS AND FOCUS OF THE BOOK

In this context, the main readership of this book is intended to be health researchers, academics working in the health field, health care managers, and health practitioners from doctors, nurses and midwives to pharmacists and physiotherapists – together with students on health programmes. In this latter regard, it is designed especially to appeal to those working on courses at a higher undergraduate and postgraduate level who are interested in health research. Although based predominantly on research undertaken in the United Kingdom, the aim has been to give the book an international dimension with contributors from other English-speaking countries such as Australia, New Zealand and Canada, as well as from a wider European context. This provides the reader with access to examples of health research undertaken in other countries. It also underlines the trend towards the globalization of health research, which has developed across national boundaries. We have acknowledged this as editors by including Chapter 20 that is dedicated to exploring how to conduct comparative health research by looking at single issues across countries. Although the comparative method presents many challenges, there is much to be learnt from policy and practice in other countries – not least in the health area where research can reveal that what appears immutable in any one country may be context specific and far from best practice.

The book has been planned to be clear, accessible and oriented to practice. It provides a distinctive overview in a critical, but constructive, manner of the research methods commonly used in health. This overview differentiates it from many recent books pitched at a variety of levels published on research methods both generally and more specifically (as exemplified by Argyrous 2005; Punch 2005; Silverman 2004). Unlike many texts in the health research field, the book also does not focus on a closely defined set of qualitative or quantitative research methods (see, for instance, Scott and Mazhindu 2005; Green and Thorogood 2004); specific groups of health practitioners (see, for example, Ernst 2001; McSherry et al. 2001); or particular practice contexts such as clinical hospital-based medicine or primary care (as illustrated by Earl-Slater 2002; Wilson et al. 2000). Instead, it discusses more expansively how health research methods can be applied and the issues that they raise. In appealing to a wider audience, this book also addresses a number of topical areas, some of which have become of increasing importance such as research ethics, using mixed methods in research, researching ethnic minorities, and comparative international research.

Despite its length, no single book can of course cover in detail all areas of health research. The references in each chapter, therefore, act as a guide to additional study, complementing the focused recommended further reading lists for each chapter. Contributors not only cover the technical issues related to their areas, but also illustrate their accounts with reference to their own personal experience of conducting health research, highlighting its pleasures and pitfalls. Each of the subsequent chapters contains case studies and concludes with a problem-solving exercise to encourage readers to demonstrate how theory, methods and data interrelate. In addition, chapters are cross-referenced to each other to assist readers in navigating the text.

As an edited collection with a consistent format, the book has the advantage of drawing on a range of contributions from leading experts in the field without losing coherence. It therefore provides a contribution distinct from, but complementary to, the widely used text by Bowling (2002) on *Research Methods in Health: Investigating Health and Health Services,* and its recently published companion volume edited by Bowling and Ebrahim (2005) entitled the *Handbook of Health Research Methods* which is designed specifically to enable researchers from different disciplinary backgrounds to work together.

In putting this volume together, the editors bring much experience of both writing and editing books on many aspects of health, applying research methods to health and receiving funding from bodies such as the Department of Health, the Economic and Social Research Council and the European Union. Recent projects include studies of using research methods in primary care, professional regulation, orthodox and alternative medicine, consumers in health care, and quality assurance in medical care (see, for example, Saks et al. 2000; Allsop and Saks 2002; Saks 2003; Baggott et al. 2005; Allsop and Jones 2006). They also bring experience of commissioning research and reviewing research protocols as well as evaluating research reports through their membership of a range of government policy and research committees. Their experience is complemented by that of the wide range of nationally/internationally recognized specialists in different forms of health research who have written the specific chapters that make up this text.

THE ORGANIZATION OF THE BOOK

The book has been organized into Parts and starts with Part I on conducting health research. Aside from Chapter 1 on the context for researching health by the editors, Mike Saks and Judith Allsop, it also contains two further building block chapters relevant to conducting all health research. Chapter 2 is written by Alex Broom and Evan Willis on competing paradigms and health research, which examines different methodological paradigms in the process of production of research knowledge – with a focus on outlining and evaluating the various dimensions of the more quantitative positivist and more qualitative interpretivist approaches. Chapter 3 is by Kathryn Jones on undertaking literature reviews in health, who considers the two main types of literature review – the narrative and the systematic review – before going on to describe techniques for undertaking a comprehensive search, and giving guidance on how best to present an analysis of the literature.

Authors in the next two parts on qualitative and quantitative research methods were asked to give attention to why the specific research methods concerned should be employed, what kind of research questions could be addressed by the methods and how the data would be gathered using them – including data coding, analysis and presentation. The main areas that authors were requested to address in each chapter on research methods were as follows:

- Definition/elaboration of the research method to be considered.
- The rationale for employing the type of research method concerned.
- Examples of employing the research method in practice.
- Strengths and weaknesses of the research method in question.
- Resources required to apply the method in practice.
- Issues involved in the coding/analysis of data using the research method.
- The identification, writing up and presentation of the findings.

Within this framework, Part II on qualitative methods and health covers a broad span of chapters on research methods written by seasoned qualitative researchers in the field. Andy Alaszewski starts this part by examining in Chapter 4 the ways in which documents have been and can be used for health research – not least by describing the nature of documentary research, identifying the resource base needed, assessing the research issues for which it is most appropriate and considering how documentary data can best be analyzed. In Chapter 5, Jacqueline Low looks at parallel issues related to the increasing use of unstructured interviews including their advantages and disadvantages, the recruitment of participants and the techniques of both carrying them out and assessing and presenting the data that they produce. While a range of observational methods, including unobtrusive measures, are used in researching health, David Hughes in Chapter 6 provides a specific outline of, and justification for, the extensive use of participant observation in health research. Judith Green in Chapter 7 then considers the use of focus groups in research into health, examining various aspects of the employment of such groups, from their strengths and weaknesses to the resources they require and the ethical issues that they raise. The more general theme of action research in health is addressed by Heather Waterman in Chapter 8, who discusses some of the challenges of action research and how these difficulties can be overcome with positive effects on health and health care.

Part III on quantitative methods and health also draws on the experience of a range of well-established authors, this time in the quantitative area. It begins with Chapter 9 from Peter Davis and Alastair Scott, which sets out the fundamental aspects of health sampling methods, with primary reference to probability sampling, drawing on a number of examples from the health field. Michael Calnan in Chapter 10 explains the nature of quantitative survey methods in health research, and describes how to go about using such methods. This chapter is linked to the previous one in so far as sampling is usually employed in conducting large-scale questionnaire surveys. George Argyrous in Chapter 11 clearly describes and evaluates a range of basic statistical methods to analyze the quantitative data deriving from these and other sources in researching health. The basic concepts and principles related to randomized controlled trials are then outlined by George Lewith and Paul Little in Chapter 12. Niro Siriwardena complements this contribution in Chapter 13 by selectively providing insights into experimental and quasi-experimental methods, which offer alternatives to the randomized controlled trial in health research. Alan Maynard in Chapter 14 completes this section by writing on the use of economics in health research, in which he sets out a research framework for appraising evidence on cost and effectiveness to inform difficult rationing choices in health care.

The next part of the book deals with a selection of topical issues in health research. Contributors consider a number of contemporary challenges to researchers working in the health field. In the context of the wide range of research methods discussed, they were asked to:

- Define the issues involved.
- Consider the advantages and disadvantages of different approaches.
- Outline how the issues can best be addressed.
- Illustrate these points with examples of their own work in the area concerned.
- Discuss the politics of the process of applying research methods in health in their field.

Accordingly, Part IV on contemporary issues in researching health begins with a discussion in Chapter 15 of the increasingly important area of governance and ethics in health research by Priscilla Alderson, who considers the merits of various approaches to ethics review and governance, including how ethical issues can best be addressed in health research. Jonathan Tritter in Chapter 16 then examines the advantages and disadvantages of mixed methods and multidisciplinary research in the health context, and also assesses their implications for research design and project management. Janet Richardson and Mike Saks in Chapter 17 go on to explore some of the issues involved in researching complementary and alternative medicine, as opposed to orthodox medicine, in which there is fast-rising public interest. In Chapter 18 Mark Johnson discusses in their wake the issues of health research involving minority groups – who span from women to marginal religious groups – by writing on the illustrative case of ethnic minorities in a multicultural society. In such areas the participation of users in lobbying for particular causes can be very significant, so it is most appropriate that Sophie Hill next examines the nature and characteristics of consumer engagement in health research in Chapter 19. This part of the text ends with Chapter 20 by Viola Burau on comparative health research, which points up the range of international challenges to health research and how these can be tackled.

Finally, the book finishes with Part V on disseminating research in health. This consists of a single but substantial chapter on writing up research and getting published in the health field by the editors, Judith Allsop and Mike Saks. The initial section of this chapter emphasizes the importance of selecting an appropriate research question and method(s) to match and showing due sensitivity to the issues raised by the changing research environment for the effective dissemination as well as conduct of research in health. The chapter then highlights the range of skills involved in writing up health research, as well as the benefits and pitfalls of publication of this research. However, given the energy and resources necessary to disseminate work in the health area, this concluding contribution – together with the other chapters – raises the crucial question of why we should research health in the first place.

CONTEMPORARY THEMES IN RESEARCHING HEALTH

In this volume, two strong substantive and interlinked contemporary themes emerge across a number of chapters. These are, first, the role of consumers or users in contributing to the research process and, second, the ethics of research in health. Consumers can contribute at all stages of the research process, from helping to determine topics for research to contributing to the publication and dissemination of research findings. Consumers are drawn into research in different ways in different projects. There are now usually both institutions and rules to ensure that patients give their informed consent to taking part in research and that they understand what will be involved, as well as rules to protect confidentiality. Nevertheless, there are still underlying issues about power relationships in the research process and debates about whether research is done 'on' or 'for' consumers. There are therefore powerful arguments in favour of trying to ensure that consumers are active participants in health research, although their involvement poses a range of ethical, scientific and administrative problems that are discussed at different points in this book.

One major methodological theme that runs through this text is that many current research projects use a mixture of methods and research is consequently often interdisciplinary. This raises issues of how data collected using different methods can be analyzed and integrated into the whole. In many respects, this kind of approach sits uneasily with the traditional model of lone researchers pursuing their own interest and making a career and reputation based on individual publications. The final chapter of the text will assist singleton researchers, amongst others, in developing and presenting their work. However, there is no doubt that the form of research based on the work of teams – that often poses considerable management problems – is now a more typical setting for the career researcher. The concluding chapter and a number of other chapters in the book comment on this more collective way of working.

CONCLUSION

Research in principle, with some caveats, benefits those involved with health whether as provider, producer or consumer. This is a very good reason in its own right for conducting research into health. So too is the sheer exhilaration of engaging in health research that can further disciplinary and interdisciplinary knowledge, even where there is no obvious application. However, we note that the contribution of research has developed unevenly in practice. The prime beneficiary of funds for evidence-based research in the health service in the United Kingdom at least has been conventional hospital-based acute care, following the establishment and expansion of scientific medicine (Le Fanu 1999). In contrast, many areas from nursing (Witz and Annandale 2006) and primary care (Saks et al. 2000) to complementary and alternative medicine (Saks 2005) have until recently been Cinderella areas. Nonetheless, this balance in the United Kingdom and elsewhere is beginning to change as governments worldwide invest more extensively in health research and associated health policies.

We trust that this book will contribute in future to growth in both hitherto under-resourced areas of health research and health research more generally in this context. While opportunities for research are increasing, it is significant that the onus on researchers to produce robust results based on sound methods has never been greater. This will also be vital if researchers are to make a positive input to policy formation in the fast-changing health field locally, nationally and internationally. We hope that this book on researching health will assist in this critical process too, in shaping the health strategies and activities that lie ahead.

RECOMMENDED FURTHER READING

Bowling, A. (2002) *Research Methods in Health: Investigating Health and Health Services*, 2nd edition. Buckingham: Open University Press.
This gives a clear description of a range of selected research methods and has been produced in a second edition to reflect new methodological developments.

Bowling, A. and Ebrahim, S. (eds) (2005) *Handbook of Health Research Methods: Investigation, Measurement and Analysis*. Maidenhead: Open University Press.
This book contains a useful set of further readings, with the main aim of helping researchers from different disciplines work collaboratively in health research.

Dyson, S. and Brown, B. (2006) *Social Theory and Applied Health Research*. Maidenhead: Open University Press.
This introductory book highlights in an accessible manner the theoretical context underpinning applied research in the health care field.

REFERENCES

Allsop, J. and Jones, K. (2006) *Quality Assurance in Medical Regulation in an International Context.* Available at: http://www.lincoln.ac.uk/policystudies/Research/docs/CMO Report. pdf
Allsop, J. and Saks, M. (eds) (2002) *Regulating the Health Professions*. London: Sage.
Argyrous, G. (2005) *Statistics for Research*, 2nd edition. London: Sage.
Baggott, R., Allsop, J. and Jones, K. (2005) *Speaking for Patients and Carers: Health Consumer Groups and the Policy Process*. Basingstoke: Palgrave.
Bowling, A. (2002) *Research Methods in Health: Investigating Health and Health Services*, 2nd edition. Buckingham: Open University Press.
Bowling, A. and Ebrahim, S. (eds) (2005) *Handbook of Health Research Methods: Investigation, Measurement and Analysis*. Maidenhead: Open University Press.
Brown, B., Crawford, P. and Hicks, C. (2003) *Evidence-based Research: Dilemmas and Debates in Health Care*. Maidenhead: Open University Press.
Daly, J., McDonald, I. and Willis, E. (eds) (1992) *Researching Health Care: Designs, Dilemma, Disciplines*. London: Routledge.
Dyson, S. and Brown, B. (2006) *Social Theory and Applied Health Research*. Maidenhead: Open University Press.
Earl-Slater, A. (2002) *The Handbook of Clinical Trials and Other Research*. Abingdon: Radcliffe Medical Press.
Ernst, E. (2001) *The Desktop Guide to Complementary and Alternative Medicine: An Evidence-based Approach*. London: Mosby.
Gabe, J., Kelleher, D. and Williams, G. (2006) 'Understanding medical dominance in the modern world', in J. Gabe, D. Kelleher and G. Williams (eds), *Challenging Medicine*, 2nd edition. London: Routledge.

Green, J. and Thorogood, N. (2004) *Qualitative Methods for Health Research*. London: Sage.

Henn, M., Weinstein, M. and Foard, N. (2006) *A Short Introduction to Social Research*. London: Sage.

Jenkinson, C. (1997) 'Assessment and evaluation of health and medical care: an introduction and overview', in C. Jenkinson (ed.), *Assessment and Evaluation of Health and Medical Care: A Methods Text*. Buckingham: Open University Press.

Lancaster, T., Shepperd, S. and Silagy, C. (1997) 'Systematic reviews and meta-analysis', in C. Jenkinson (ed.), *Assessment and Evaluation of Health and Medical Care: A Methods Text*. Buckingham: Open University Press.

Le Fanu, J. (1999) *The Rise and Fall of Modern Medicine*. London: Abacus.

McSherry, R., Simmons, M. and Abbott, P. (eds) (2001) *Evidence-informed Nursing*. London: Routledge.

Punch, K.F. (2005) *Introduction to Social Research: Quantitative and Qualitative Approaches*, 2nd edition. London: Sage.

Rawnsley, A. (2001) *Servants of the People: The Inside of New Labour*, 2nd edition. London: Hamish Hamilton.

Richardson, A., Jackson, C. and Sykes, W. (1990) *Taking Research Seriously: Means of Improving and Assessing the Use and Dissemination of Research*. London: HMSO.

Saks, M. (2000) 'Introduction', in M. Saks, M. Williams and B. Hancock (eds), *Developing Research in Primary Care*. Abingdon: Radcliffe Medical Press.

Saks, M. (2003) *Orthodox and Alternative Medicine: Politics, Professionalization and Health Care*. London: Sage.

Saks, M. (2005) 'Improving the research base of complementary and alternative medicine', Editorial, *Complementary Therapies in Clinical Practice*, 11: 1–3.

Saks, M., Williams, M. and Hancock, B. (eds) (2000) *Developing Research in Primary Care*. Abingdon: Radcliffe Medical Press.

Scott, I. and Mazhindu, D. (2005) *Statistics for Health Care Professionals*. London: Sage.

Silverman, D. (2004) *Qualitative Research: Theory, Method and Practice*, 2nd edition. London: Sage.

Turner, B.S. (2003) 'The history of the changing concepts of health and illness: outline of a general model of illness categories', in G.L. Albrecht, R. Fitzpatrick and S.C. Scrimshaw (eds), *The Handbook of Social Studies in Health and Medicine*. London: Sage.

Wilson, A., Williams, M. and Hancock, B. (eds) (2000) *Research Approaches to Primary Care*. Abingdon: Radcliffe Medical Press.

Witz, A. and Annandale, E. (2006) 'The challenge of nursing', in J. Gabe, D. Kelleher and G. Williams (eds), *Challenging Medicine*, 2nd edition. London: Routledge.

2

Competing Paradigms and Health Research

ALEX BROOM AND EVAN WILLIS

INTRODUCTION

From newspaper and television documentaries to web sources and academic journals, research on health abounds. As indicated in Chapter 1, the broad area of 'health research' uses a plurality of research methodologies and related methods, from documentary analysis and unstructured interviews to randomized controlled trials and experimental methods. However, there are differences between particular methodological approaches that are systematic rather than idiosyncratic. In this chapter we make use of the sociological concept of 'paradigms' to illustrate the way in which research methodologies are embedded in particular political and ideological positions. This chapter aims to provide a critical overview of what we might broadly call research paradigms. We explore the nature of a paradigm, examining different types of paradigms in health research, and the implications of using a particular paradigm for knowledge production. Furthermore, by giving the reader a critical understanding of the nature of particular research methodologies and associated methods, we aim to provide a means to establish the most effective way of answering research questions about health and health care.

In order to do this, we need to have a clear understanding of the epistemological foundations and philosophical roots of particular forms or styles of research. Epistemology in this context refers to the nature of knowledge or how we come to know certain things about the world. In the context of health care, an understanding is necessary of how certain research methods and certain approaches to data collection have emerged from vastly different traditions, and, importantly, how they produce different understandings of the social world.

Within this discussion we examine broad traditions in health research, from positivism to interpretivism, exploring the implications of these traditions and the various methodological approaches derived from them for health research. We seek not to make an argument about which methodological paradigm is best, but rather to provide the reader with a critical understanding of how the methodologies presented in the following chapters have emerged from, and contribute to, the reproduction of particular understandings of the social and natural world. We propose the view, also reflected in subsequent chapters, that certain phenomena, and thus certain research questions, are best explored by drawing on one particular paradigm rather than another. We present the reader with a critical view of each, and how this can be used to inform research design and analysis.

In this chapter, we draw on a particular research study to illustrate the difference. The research study examined the impact of the Internet on health care services, using men and medical specialists' experiences of prostate cancer as a case study. It was conducted by one of the authors for purposes of a higher degree under the supervision of the other (see Broom 2004).

DEFINING TERMS: WHAT IS A PARADIGM?

A paradigm can be defined as an overarching philosophical or ideological stance, a system of beliefs about the nature of the world, and ultimately, when applied in the research setting, the assumptive base from which we go about producing knowledge (Rubin and Rubin 2005). In the context of health care research, a researcher's paradigmatic positioning relates to their understanding of the nature of knowledge (their epistemological standpoint) and of reality (their ontological standpoint). An interpretivist researcher will maintain that knowledge is socially constructed and reality is ultimately subjective. A positivist paradigm, however, will maintain that reality is fixed and that objective knowledge can be produced through rigorous methodology. Methodologies utilized by the former are referred to as qualitative and those by the latter as quantitative.

Health researchers vary greatly in their epistemological and ontological standpoints, and these paradigmatic differences have an important influence on their study objective and design, and thus on the type of knowledge they produce from their research. Nonetheless, researchers may actually draw on a number of different paradigmatic positions to achieve the best possible outcome in terms of knowledge production. In fact, the separation of particular ontological and epistemological positions can come across as a somewhat artificial dichotomy, in that health researchers are increasingly pragmatic. They choose the best means to answer a research question and use a mixed-method approach, rather than being explicitly philosophically driven. However, although researchers may embrace disparate methodologies and methods within a single research project, there is a tendency for the actual analysis, including the conceptualization of results, to be derived from one distinct philosophical standpoint and to take a positivist or constructivist/interpretivist approach.

Nevertheless, it is necessary to confront the issue of the extent to which quantitative and qualitative paradigms of research are metaphysically incommensurable. By this we mean the extent to which they are logically inconsistent or mutually exclusive. For example, ontologically speaking, social reality cannot be both objectivist in nature and also a social construction. It is either one or the other. This is another way of saying that these two paradigms of research are in fact incommensurable and that health research cannot be simultaneously quantitative and qualitative. However, it is possible to have separate quantitative and qualitative components, or, as we sometimes say, there may be different 'arms' to a research project.

Traditionally, health researchers have tended to embrace one particular paradigm. The commonest split has been between the positivists and the constructivists. It is these schools of thought that will be examined closely in this chapter. As suggested by Wolfe (1997), this positivist/constructivist split can be seen as the 'two faces of the social sciences'. As such, most of the methods outlined in this book can broadly be seen as philosophically congruent to one of these traditions. In saying this, we argue that positivism and constructivism should be viewed as 'ideal types' in the Weberian sense. An ideal type, according to Weber, is formed by the one-sided accentuation of one or more points of view. Hence although the distinction between positivism and constructivism is useful and important, in practice the boundaries between different paradigms are blurred (De Vaus 1995).

As reflected in the structure of this book, a paradigmatic difference exists between what we call qualitative and quantitative research methods. This is not a matter of study design such as the use of observational methods (for instance, case–control study or survey) versus experimental methods (for example, the randomized controlled trial). Rather, the distinction between qualitative and quantitative approaches lies in the assumptive base that underpins the research design and thus data collection. A general distinction is made between these two methodological traditions based broadly on either an *inductive* or a *deductive* approach to research. In the case of induction, the researcher gathers qualitative data (such as on patients' experiences of pain) and then establishes patterns drawing on theory, thereby, for example, establishing how things may be improved for those patients in a health care setting. However, a deductive, quantitative approach involves the researcher testing an existing theory or hypothesis. A hypothesis might, for instance, be that patients who are given pain killers two days after treatment will report no different experiences than those who are not. The research then aims to prove or disprove the hypothesis.

Quantitative and qualitative methodologies are different strategies used by health researchers with quite different visions of the social world. These are the product of a number of very important Western philosophical traditions that have been developing for centuries. As such, social scientists have for long challenged one another – as well as scientists in the natural sciences. Some argue that quantification using a positivist paradigm is essential for an objective and rigorous investigation. Others argue from an interpretivist approach that no description could be complete without a qualitative understanding of the subjective meanings of social actors involved in social interactions (Glassner and Moreno 1989).

Our view is that such arguments are ideological and neither quantitative nor qualitative methods should be viewed as superior. Rather, each serves a particular purpose. Methodologies are not neutral tools and health researchers need to be able to think critically about the ways in which certain methods produce certain types of knowledge. In the twentieth century health research was dominated by positivist approaches to knowledge production epitomized by the randomized controlled trial. This involves randomization of patients into at least two different intervention groups (normally usual care versus experimental treatment) discussed in detail in Chapter 12. However, in recent decades there has been greater scepticism about the positivist methods associated with modern medicine. The aim of the rest of this chapter is to highlight the political and ideological nature of health research by outlining the philosophical underpinnings and paradigmatic bases of the research methods discussed in the following chapters.

POSITIVIST PARADIGM

Roots of positivism

Positivism is a somewhat ambiguous and loaded philosophical idea, but it continues to form the paradigmatic basis for much health research today. The term positivism has represented a means to critique the natural sciences and researchers espousing a scientific model within the social sciences. By default, a positivist assumes that reality is concrete and objectivity is achievable – therefore the notion of science being ideologically driven is supplanted by the notion of science as transcending ideology – a rather circular logic. Rather than defining a clear set of practices, positivism represents a broad tradition of thought that assumes that reality is constant. It can be measured, and thus the concepts and methods employed in the natural sciences can be applied to form a 'science of man' (Giddens 1987).

Of course, the immediate dilemma is that what constitutes 'science' within the natural sciences is not an entirely coherent and consistent entity, with a number of internal differences in the conceptual base of each method. Thus, the notion of 'positivism' within the social sciences as the imposition of a natural 'science' model imposed on the social world is at best problematic. Rather, positivism in the social sciences should be seen as a tradition followed by certain social scientists who aim to follow the basic premises of scientific enquiry. This includes the assumption that the researcher is able to collect and interpret social facts objectively; produce laws and models of behaviour from these social facts (Bryman 2001); and view 'scientifically' produced data as ultimately neutral and unbiased (Rubin and Rubin 2005).

Positivism has its roots in a long history of Western philosophy and the agenda for early Enlightenment thinkers was to 'enlighten' the masses. The belief was that human reason could be used to combat ignorance, superstition and tyranny, and, ultimately, be used to build a better world. Gradually scientific method and quantification would come to be seen as the means to improve both the natural and the social worlds (Glassner and Moreno 1989).

The actual notion of positivism per se was first coined by Auguste Comte. Comte saw sociology as the very culmination of positivism: a science of man that would complete the historical evolution of the hierarchy of the scientific disciplines (Giddens 1987). Positivism was thus cemented in sociology through Comte's idea of transforming society on the basis of science. Herbert Spencer's organic theory of society built on this. Spencer conceived of society as an organism and held that human society reflects the same evolutionary principles in its development as biological organisms. The dominance of positivism in the social sciences came to a peak in the post-war United States with the structural functionalist work of Talcott Parsons and Robert Merton, only then to wane in the late twentieth century with the emergence of post-structuralist and postmodernist paradigmatic – a shift discussed later in this chapter.

These philosophical ideas have evolved considerably since Comte and Spencer and still form the basis for much health research today. Of course, there are now much more effective and systematic tools that are used to achieve the so-called 'truth' or produce a 'scientific fact'. However, the basic premise of a reality that can be objectively measured, given the right instruments and conditions, still dominates health research in the clinical and social sciences.

Positivism in health research: From randomized controlled trials to social surveys

As we will see in the following chapters on quantitative methods, there are many different methods for advancing our knowledge of health and illness within a positivist framework. Trial designs, and particularly randomized controlled trials, are the most commonly used designs in medical research, although medical researchers are increasingly incorporating social science methods in their studies. Retrospective cohort and cross-sectional designs are also based on a positivist assumptive base and are used to map out such things as aetiology (the characteristics of disease), prognosis (the predicted course of a disease) and prevalence of disease (the extent of spread of a disease within a population), as well as other factors that may influence health outcomes or health behaviour.

These types of approaches have emerged from, and contribute to, the reproduction of the positivist paradigm, focusing on establishing objective scientific facts about disease and the body, through scientific method and quantification. Based on the biomedical model of disease, such studies approach the patient as a physical/mechanistic entity that can be measured, controlled and ultimately manipulated. Assumptions about the objectivity, neutrality and generalizability of data place most biomedical research methods squarely within the realms of a positivist paradigm.

Likewise, quantitative methods commonly used by social scientists – such as structured interviews, surveys and self-completion questionnaires – also seek to test hypotheses by quantifying human behaviour (Bryman 2001), with the objective of creating models that can predict behaviour (De Vaus 1995). An example of this was the pilot research the authors undertook on online communities. This embraced a positivist paradigm in that it sought to establish and quantify patterns in men's experiences of online support groups as opposed to face-to-face support groups. As can be seen below, the knowledge produced through this paradigm is very different from the findings that emerged from more qualitative frames of reference. We will return to this theme later in the chapter.

Although randomized controlled trials and quantitative surveys may have very different foci (for example, disease reoccurrence versus feelings of autonomy), and may utilize different tools for testing their hypotheses (for instance, blood tests versus anxiety scales), they are ultimately commensurable within this broad paradigm. The methods and features associated with this paradigm are as follows:

- Methods utilizing a positivist paradigm:

  — Epidemiological/analytical design strategies (for example, randomized controlled trials, before and after studies, cohort/incidence studies, cross-sectional studies)
  — Survey research
  — Secondary document analysis (for instance, content analysis)
  — Structured interviewing
  — Systematic reviews (meta-analysis).

- Features of a positivist paradigm:

  — *Determinism*: Phenomena can be predicted from a knowledge of scientific laws.
  — *Objectivity*: The researcher is separate and detached from the patient/participant, maintaining objectivity, assisted by scientific evidence.
  — *Quantification*: Information is derived from what can be quantified.
  — *Reliability*: Through randomization we can know that our findings support or negate the hypothesis in the study and can be extrapolated to a larger population.
  — *Generalizability*: Data are reliable and unbiased and we can therefore generalize our findings to the rest of the population.

There are considerable advantages to using methods that are based on a positivist paradigm, and which seek to use the scientific method to answer important questions about the effectiveness of health care. For example, randomization is an effective means of reducing bias in the assessment of how effective an intervention is as it guarantees, assuming it is carried out properly, that treatment assignment will not be based on patients' prognostic factors. This prevents the investigators from assigning, consciously or unconsciously, patients with a greater likelihood of responding well to a treatment that they hope will be superior. It increases confidence that the study has identified the most effective treatment. Blinding the researchers and their clients is also a method of eliminating bias (Altman 2000). Randomized trials that have not used appropriate levels of blinding tend to show significantly larger treatment effects than blinded studies (Schulz et al. 1995). Thus, although in the process of randomization the patient is effectively reduced to a number, and thus to some degree their individuality is lost, this process has the benefit, amongst other things, of increasing our knowledge of the effects of a drug on an organ, or the effect of a psycho-social intervention when a course of treatment is followed.

Another benefit of a randomized controlled trial design is that consistent and relatively concrete outcome measures are used (as, for instance, pain, recovery time or anxiety). In this way, we know that the study is assessing, albeit in a restricted way, the actual effects of the intervention or the disease process, and not merely recording people's subjective feelings about how they have improved over the course of treatment. We can thus be confident, if we ever get ill and need treatment, that we are not merely being treated according to an individual doctor's preference, or on the basis of the outcomes from a group of atypical patients, but as a result of a well-conducted trial. In a similar way, surveys and structured interviews can be extremely useful for assessing such issues as patients' views on the quality of treatment information provided and their experiences of treatment for a particular illness.

   Despite the potential benefits of drawing on a positivist paradigm, and utilizing study designs such as clinical trials and surveys, there are also potentially negative implications of which health researchers should be aware.

A critique of positivist approaches to social research

While trial designs and other positivistic research methods have much to offer in health research, their promotion – which is approached with great zeal in some quarters – can be misplaced. Many questions about health care are not amenable to randomized controlled trials. For example, a randomized trial could not research the question of the number of people who die every year as a result of waiting too long with severe chest pain before calling an ambulance for ethical and practical reasons. A randomized controlled trial design cannot answer the question of why – it cannot explore what is going on in a person's life and relationships that may have influenced them to delay seeking help. Herein lies one of the weaknesses of utilizing a positivist, quantitative methodology.

   To be more specific, there has been considerable concern, within both academic and lay communities, about the epistemological assumptions that inform the process of categorization in quantitative research. For example, some have argued that positivist quantitative research designs give insufficient attention to a person's lived experience (Rubin and Rubin 2005; Bryman 2001). Sociologists are increasingly arguing that people's experiences are complex, subjective and embedded in specific social and historical contexts (Silverman 2001). Take for example the research undertaken by one of the authors on Australian men with prostate cancer and their use of the Internet (see Broom 2005a; 2005b). Results from the pilot survey showed the numbers of men who were more comfortable expressing their concerns and fears in an online environment. Although useful, this did not give any indication of why this was the case. We needed to know the systems of meaning and cultural understandings that actually shaped these men's perceptions of face-to-face versus online support groups that might influence their use. This was only achievable with a qualitative methodology.

   The difficulty is that it is not possible to dissect and categorize social life objectively, through blinding and randomization procedures (Rubin and Rubin 2005). Furthermore, many qualitative social scientists reject the claims of natural scientists and quantitative social sciences to objectivity; the mechanisms they use for measuring validity; and their desire for generalizability. They argue that it is impossible to talk about, understand or communicate social phenomena without employing a particular language or conceptual scheme and this is not neutral (De Vaus 1995). It can be argued that all representations, like data from a survey, clinical trial or interview-based study, are socially and culturally constructed (Rubin and Rubin 2005). Researchers choose the questions and interpret the results. Ultimately, therefore, all knowledge produced by research is subjective, interpreted, political and, in part, ideologically driven. This leads to the consideration of an alternative frame of reference – that of interpretivism or, as it is sometimes called, the constructivist tradition.

INTERPRETIVIST PARADIGM

The constructivist traditions: Dislodging the positivist canon

Although positivist approaches within medicine and the social sciences have maintained their dominance for a significant part of the twentieth century, a strong qualitative or interpretive tradition emerged in the social sciences in the 1960s and 1970s. Grounded theory, symbolic interactionalism and phenomenology, and more recently poststructuralism and postmodernism are part of the interpretivist or constructivist tradition. This is associated with such authors as Glaser and Strauss (1967), Berger and Luckmann (1967), Geertz (1973), Lofland and Lofland (1984) and Rubin and Rubin (2005).

Originating at the Chicago School in the 1920s and 1930s, and gathering momentum in the late 1960s, factions within the social sciences were beginning to diverge from the positivist and deterministic approaches of the classical social scientists, refocusing social science on the ways in which meanings are constructed, negotiated and managed by different individuals and groups within various social and historical contexts. Before this movement, research methods were largely quantitative and firmly based on a positivist paradigm. The interpretive paradigm precipitated the development of the tools we now know as qualitative methods.

The qualitative methodologies, emerging from methods such as in-depth interviewing and observation, sought to establish an understanding of people's lives, experiences and the subjective meanings that could explain the process of decision making and action. Rather than seeking to measure or categorize behaviour or attitudes, interpretivist researchers focused on the understandings of research respondents, pursuing an analysis based on the constructivist ontological position that individuals actively negotiate meaning. As ontology refers to the study of the nature of reality, a constructivist ontological view is that reality is constructed rather than 'set in stone'. It is not objectively measurable, and, furthermore, individuals construct their reality by associating 'meaning' with certain events or actions (Bryman 2001).

By approaching an issue from this position, a researcher can establish regular patterns and irregularities in the meanings associated with particular life events. For example, there may be social patterning in terms of whether or not particular signs and symptoms are interpreted as an illness, whether professional help is sought, and how the chance of a cure is perceived. As Rubin and Rubin (2005) suggest, interpretive social research is about figuring out what events mean to research subjects: how people adapt and how they view what has happened to them and around them (see also Bryman 2001). It is identifying this complexity and subjectivity that Ezzy (2002) and others argue should underpin qualitative research projects.

Interpretivist approaches to health research

Researchers who have positioned themselves within an interpretivist, constructivist paradigm tend to use qualitative methods, such as in-depth interviews, focus groups and ethnographic observation. These types of methods are consistent with the interpretivist paradigm, in that they aim to record the types of data that will enable the researcher to reflect on subjective meanings and interpretations; the social and culturally embedded nature of individual experiences; and the relationship between the researcher and the researched (Rubin and Rubin 2005). What we see is a shift in focus from a position where the researcher seeks to observe patterns in group behaviour to a position that seeks to understand individual experiences of interactions, events and social processes and identify patterns in these subjective experiences. The methods and features associated with this paradigm are as follows:

- Methods utilizing an interpretivist/constructivist paradigm:
  - In-depth, semi-structured or unstructured interviews
  - Observation (participatory or non-participatory)
  - Focus groups
  - Secondary discourse analysis.

- Features of an interpretivist/constructivist paradigm:
  - *Interpretivist*: Seeks 'understanding' with a focus on subjective meanings and interpretation.
  - *Naturalistic*: Data are collected in the setting of everyday life.

  - *Subjectivity*: Research practice and knowledge production is not objective or neutral — rather it is gendered and partial.
  - *Complexity*: Not so concerned with inference but rather with the depth of analysis.
  - *Political*: The position of value neutrality is viewed as misleading as it makes the focus on the research seem independent from social relations.
  - *Validity*: High on validity as it draws on the understandings of research subjects, but not necessarily generalizable as it relies on the interpretation of the researcher.

Overall, the advantage of a flexible, descriptive and qualitative approach is that researchers are less likely to become stuck in conventional ways of thinking or particular sets of assumptions – as the qualitative chapters in this book highlight. Rather than merely testing pre-existing ideas, they can make observations that demand the creation of new ideas and categories that might not emerge in quantitative designs (Ezzy 2002; Strauss and Corbin 1998). Good qualitative researchers will adjust their approach in response to data which may contradict their initial assumptions or theories. Within a positivist paradigm, by insisting on a strict protocol for the study design and parameters, based on fixed hypotheses, only those events considered relevant are recorded. Conversely, qualitative studies may begin to uncover the complexity of social processes (Strauss and Corbin 1998).

A qualitative, interpretive approach allows acknowledgement of conflict, ongoing struggle, tension and subjectivity, as well as the situated and co-produced nature of accounts (Rubin and Rubin 2005). Interpretive research is about subjectivity and complexity. It seeks not necessarily to count or reduce, but to represent rich, subjective experience in such a way as to reflect on consistencies and parallels, while retaining the various nuances of the data. As Ezzy (2002) argues, qualitative research is biased to a degree, but all research contains a degree of bias and is thus inherently political. To suggest that something can be biased is by default to suggest that there is an unbiased 'truth' that we could access. The view taken here is that all research is driven by political interests and theoretical models, and qualitative research is no different.

As suggested earlier, qualitative researchers tend to espouse a constructivist ontological view of the world. As a result they are focused less on generalizability or external validity and more on reliability and internal validation – that is, the degree to which the data accurately represent attitudes, perceptions and views of the population being studied. Rather than establishing universal truths about the world, a qualitative study is about gaining an understanding of how some differently positioned actors talk about their experiences and the meanings they associate with particular events, actions and claims. This is a valuable approach because so often the cost of attempting to generalize is that we do not see and investigate those aspects of a process that do not fit our presuppositions about a particular phenomenon.

A critique of interpretivist approaches

However, there are a number of problems with interpretivist or constructivist approaches when applied to health research, some of which are paradigmatic and some of which relate to methods. As Bryman (2001) notes, first, there is no real consensus among qualitative researchers on appropriate methods for data collection and analysis. Second, qualitative researchers do sometimes attempt to make unjustified generalizations from the accounts of a small number of individuals. It could be argued that there is little value in funding research that cannot be generalized to the larger population. Furthermore, qualitative researchers often adopt convenience sampling strategies, resulting in samples that could be seen to be 'biased' through researcher assumptions and respondent self-selection strategies (Bryman 2001). It has also been argued that informants' accounts are not so much uncovered as created by the researcher (Silverman 2001). If the method adopted is to facilitate an open discussion, for example through unstructured interviews or focus groups, how can the researcher determine which aspect of an account is what a person actually thinks, and which part simply reflects what the researcher prompted the research subject to say?

There are also issues that arise when the constructivist ontological position is taken in researching health and disease. What can be more 'real' than cancer, pain or diabetes? How can it be argued that these phenomena are socially and culturally determined rather than purely physiological conditions? Of course, we come back to the 'ideal type' mentioned earlier. In practice sociologists of health and illness will usually take the middle ground, sometimes called the 'soft constructivist position', and acknowledge that there are both subjective and purely physical aspects to disease and treatment processes.

In terms of the qualitative arm of the Internet study, the objective was to explore the experiences of a specific group of men regarding their use of online communities for social support for prostate cancer. Rather than claiming to map out the experiences of all men with prostate cancer, this study aimed to provide a set of indications as to the possible experiences of other men and the potential benefits of the online support groups as sources of information and support. As such, an in-depth exploratory approach to data collection was taken to document the complex, subjective experiences of the respondents, instead of merely reflecting on, for instance, the frequency of Internet usage, existing sources of information and the type of information and support retrieved. The study focused on understanding the ways in which the online support groups had impacted on the lives of the respondents, building theory from their accounts rather than imposing it on them. What emerged was a process by which men with prostate cancer attempt to negotiate cultural constructions of masculinity and prostate disease, along with particular understandings about the nature of cyberspace. Such subjective processes were analyzed by using positivist designs through quantification and abstraction.

CONCLUSION

The argument made in this chapter is that health researchers should take a pragmatic approach to research design and data collection. From a methodological perspective, we advocate what could be called a 'horses for courses' approach. However, before such an approach can be taken, researchers must gain a critical understanding of the different kinds of paradigms that inform health research. They should have an appreciation of the complex epistemological and ontological differences between qualitative and quantitative research methods. Previously quantitative, positivist research methodologies have been seen by many stakeholders within the health care community as the only useful way of generating knowledge. Indeed, it is still the case that research funding is more likely to be forthcoming for grant applications demonstrating a quantitative rather than a qualitative methodological approach. However, qualitative research has grown in importance and indeed legitimacy, and increasingly qualitative approaches are being used to inform health care policy and practice. Moreover, some questions can only be answered – or at least will be answered more effectively – by a qualitative design. Ultimately, therefore, we argue that the appropriateness and usefulness of a particular paradigm is inextricably tied to the nature of the research question. This point is tested out in the exercise for the reader below on research into prostate cancer.

Exercise: Different methodological approaches to researching the use of the Internet in the case of men with prostate cancer

Based on what you have read in this chapter, what different sorts of information are yielded by the data sources set out in Boxes 2.1 and 2.2 based on the work conducted by the authors in Australia in the study of men with prostate cancer? Which do you think are the most important? Give reasons for your answer.

Box 2.1 *A quantitative pilot survey design and example of output*

Selected interview themes:

1 = strongly disagree 2 = disagree 3 = neutral 4 = agree 5 = strongly agree					
1	It would be easier to share my personal experiences in an anonymous environment like an online (Internet) support group.	1	2	3	4	5
2	In face-to-face support groups, the threat of embarrassment stops some men from sharing concerns about fears, emotional distress, symptoms or complications of treatments.	1	2	3	4	5

Example of data:

- Of the 50 men surveyed 46 per cent agreed that it would be easier to share experiences online.
- Approximately 30 per cent of respondents agreed that face-to-face support groups can deter self-expression.

Box 2.2 *A qualitative in-depth interview study and example of output*

Selected interview themes:

Patients' reasons for decisions over whether or not to use online support groups.
Patients' perceptions regarding the benefits and limitations of online support.

Example of data:

Andrew: 'One of the things you find is an amazing openness and frankness about these sort of matters that I'm sure men if they were meeting face-to-face would not talk about ... we're doing it through this medium [the Internet] and we can be a lot more frank ... There's the anonymity, there's the disembodiment ... you're able to project in a way that isn't having any comeback on you.' (Six months' post-treatment, organ-confined disease, Internet user/online support, 40–50 years)

David: 'Some men don't want to be face-to-face. Maybe they're frightened of it; maybe they don't want to travel the distances. Maybe they're scared of being ridiculed or something ... all sorts of reasons like that. Maybe they're a bit anxious about having the problem [prostate cancer] and not wanting to share it with other people. I think that's men for you. Some will find it easier to talk online.' (Three years' post-treatment, organ-confined disease, Internet user/online support, 61–70 years)

RECOMMENDED FURTHER READING

Brown, B., Crawford, P. and Hicks, C. (2003) *Evidence-based Research: Dilemmas and Debates in Health Care*. Maidenhead: Open University Press.
This book focuses on charting the philosophical background and debates surrounding the use of health research methods, including the importance of paradigms.

Daly, J., MacDonald, I. and Willis, E. (eds) (1992) *Researching Health Care: Dilemmas, Designs and Disciplines*. London: Routledge.
This is an older, but now classic, reference with relevant contributions by many leading researchers in the field internationally.

Rice, P. and Ezzy, D. (1999) *Qualitative Research Methods: A Health Focus*. Melbourne: Oxford University Press.
This is an excellent introductory textbook on the use of qualitative methods in researching health.

REFERENCES

Altman, D. (2000) 'Blinding in clinical trials and other studies', *British Medical Journal*, 321: 504.
Berger, P. and Luckmann, T. (1967) *The Social Construction of Reality: A Treatise in the Sociology of Knowledge*. London: Allen Lane.
Broom, A. (2004) 'Virtually he@lthy: the impact of Internet use, by Australian men with prostate cancer, on patient/medical specialist interaction and disease experiences'. PhD thesis, La Trobe University, Australia.
Broom, A. (2005a) 'The eMale: prostate cancer, masculinity and online support as a challenge to medical expertise', *Journal of Sociology*, 41(1): 87–104.
Broom, A. (2005b) 'Virtually he@lthy: a study into the impact of Internet use on disease experience and the doctor/patient relationship', *Qualitative Health Research*, 15(3): 325–45.
Bryman, A. (2001) *Social Research Method*. Oxford: Oxford University Press.
De Vaus, D.A. (1995) *Surveys in Social Research*. Crows Nest, NSW: Allen & Unwin.
Ezzy, D. (2002) *Qualitative Analysis: Practice and Innovation*. Crows Nest, NSW: Allen & Unwin.
Geertz, C. (1973) *The Interpretation of Cultures: Selected Essays*. New York: Basic Books.
Giddens, A. (1987) *Positivism and Sociology*. London: Heinemann.
Glaser, B. and Strauss, A. (1967) *The Discovery of Grounded Theory: Strategies for Qualitative Research*. Chicago: Aldine.
Glassner, B. and Moreno, J. (1989) 'Introduction: quantification and enlightenment', in B. Glassner and J. Moreno (eds), *The Qualitative–Quantitative Distinction in the Social Sciences*. Boston: Kluwer Academic.
Lofland, J. and Lofland, L. (1984) *Analyzing Social Settings: A Guide to Qualitative Observation and Analysis*, 2nd edition. Belmont, CA: Wadsworth.

Rubin, H. and Rubin, I. (2005) *Qualitative Interviewing: The Art of Hearing Data*, 2nd edition. London: Sage.

Schulz, F., Chalmers, I., Hayes, R. and Airman, D. (1995) 'Empirical evidence of bias: dimensions of methodological quality associated with estimates of treatment effects in controlled trials', *Journal of the American Medical Association*, 273: 408–12.

Silverman, D. (2001) *Interpreting Qualitative Data*. London: Sage.

Strauss, A. and Corbin, J. (1998) *Basics of Qualitative Research*, 2nd edition. London: Sage.

Wolfe, A. (1997) 'The two faces of social science', in K. Erickson (ed.), *Sociological Visions*. Oxford: Rowman and Littlefield.

3

Doing a Literature Review in Health[1]

KATHRYN JONES

INTRODUCTION

The literature review aims to identify, analyze, assess and interpret a body of knowledge related to a particular topic and is normally required as part of a dissertation or thesis. In this case, it sets a context for a research study and provides a rationale for addressing a particular research question in the light of an existing body of literature. Research proposals to funding bodies also typically include a literature review. Here the purpose is to justify the proposal in terms of a gap in existing knowledge. Some literature reviews are substantive, stand-alone studies in their own right that serve to assess what is known and what is not known on an area of study. The aim in both cases is to show how a particular topic has been approached by other scholars. Within the health field, the literature review can also aim to assess existing knowledge on the efficacy of an intervention such as the evidence base for the preferred treatment of a particular disease or the response to a social problem.

This chapter describes how to undertake a rigorous and thorough review of the literature and is divided into three sections. The first section examines the two main types of review: the narrative and the systematic review. The second section describes some techniques for undertaking a comprehensive search, while the third gives guidance on how an analysis of the literature can be presented. It is assumed in the chapter that those undertaking a review will have access to college or university library resources and to the Internet. The majority of sources can now be accessed electronically. Those who have not previously searched using an online catalogue or database are advised to seek assistance prior to starting out. Most college and university libraries offer courses, publish guidelines or make help available online. Throughout the chapter, examples are drawn from recent studies undertaken by the author and others.

TYPES OF LITERATURE REVIEW

All reviews aim to provide an overview of what is known about a particular phenomenon and what the gaps in knowledge are. However, narrative reviews, which are used widely in social scientific research, place an emphasis on identifying the key concepts or specific terms used in the literature and the particular theoretical approaches adopted by different authors to understanding a phenomenon. Concepts and theories may be employed implicitly or explicitly in an investigation of a topic. A review of the literature will identify the range of approaches and offer a critique of their contribution to understanding.

The systematic review of the literature in health and social care has a different focus. It aims to contribute to clinical practice through an assessment of the efficacy of a particular health care intervention and, with the emphasis on evidence-based practice, has become increasingly important. A basic overview is given here but the researcher should seek advice from a trained information specialist prior to undertaking a search. Specialized statistical skills are also necessary (see Egger et al. 2001).

The narrative review

The narrative review is the commonest form of literature review. It aims to show how concepts, theories and methods have developed within particular subject areas. The key differences between concepts, theories and methods are:

- *Concepts*: Terms and ideas used to describe a particular phenomenon.
- *Theories*: Ideas that have been developed to explain a specific phenomenon.
- *Empirical research*: Research that has already been undertaken to observe the phenomena.

- *Methodology*: The philosophical approach adopted by a researcher to study a particular phenomenon and not to be confused with methods.
- *Methods*: Techniques such as questionnaires, observation or interviewing used to collect data.

In a narrative review the reviewer offers a critique in order to assess, analyze and synthesize previous research, and place it in its current context. The review can take a number of forms: a chapter within a dissertation showing the context of the research; a section of a proposal justifying the work; or a stand-alone summation of thinking around a particular subject area. In each, the reviewer draws on and critiques the conceptual and theoretical approach of different authors and offers an assessment and interpretation.

When reading the item concerned, the reviewer seeks to identify the particular conceptual and theoretical approach taken by the author. This is likely to be influenced by the author's background and discipline. So, for example, a political scientist interested in public involvement in health policy making is likely to draw on theories relating to interest groups in the policy process, participation and representation. A sociologist of health and illness writing on the same topic might place their work in the context of people's experience of illness and how this may affect their wish to participate in decisions and policy making. Identifying the conceptual and theoretical approaches taken by different authors is the first step to understanding the literature and, in the writing up stage, will influence the structure of the report, another vital component of the narrative review as will be seen below.

The systematic review

Over the past few decades, evidence-based practice has achieved growing recognition as a means of increasing the efficacy of health care interventions. Initiatives such as the international Cochrane Collaboration (see Chapter 19 for a fuller description) and organizations such as the National Institute for Health and Clinical Excellence in the United Kingdom assess available evidence to inform guidelines, policy and practice. A systematic review enables the reader to appraise critically the most robust evidence available in an attempt to synthesize what is known, and not known, about the efficacy of particular interventions. According to Petticrew (2001), systematic reviews can be characterized by the following criteria:

- They aim to answer a particular question or test a hypothesis — usually in relation to a particular health care intervention on a particular population group.
- They attempt to be as exhaustive as possible, identifying all known references.
- Studies included in the review are chosen as a result of explicit inclusion and exclusion criteria. The assessment of the evidence and the synthesis of results are based on the thoroughness of a study's research method.

Systematic reviews place an emphasis on judging the quality of evidence. Here, the priority is to utilize studies where the research design minimizes bias – as highlighted by the list below showing the traditional hierarchy of evidence for reviews assessing the effectiveness of a particular intervention. Street (2001) notes that the quality levels of evidence in systematic reviews of health care interventions can be categorized as follows:

- *Level I*: Evidence obtained from a systematic review of all relevant randomized controlled trials.
- *Level II*: Evidence obtained from at least one properly designed randomly controlled trial.
- *Level III.1*: Evidence obtained from a well-designed controlled trial without randomization.
- *Level III.2*: Evidence obtained from a well-designed cohort or case-control analytic study, preferably from more than one centre or research group.
- *Level III.3*: Evidence obtained from multiple time series with or without the intervention, or dramatic results in an uncontrolled experiment.
- *Level IV*: Opinion of respected authorities based on clinical experience, descriptive studies or a report from an expert committee.

However, researchers have been criticized for assuming this hierarchy is relevant to all systematic reviews (Petticrew and Roberts 2006). If a review is attempting to understand *why* a particular intervention works, rather than *what* interventions work, then other research designs, including qualitative studies, are likely to provide more relevant data (Dixon-Woods et al. 2001; Petticrew 2001). The key thing is to make sure that the quality of study designs is addressed in any analysis. Petticrew and Roberts (2006) provide a useful overview of the value of systematic reviews in the social sciences. Guidelines on judging the quality of qualitative studies in systematic reviews are now available (NHS CRD 2001; Thomas et al. 2004).

A specialized technique in systematic reviews is the use of a meta-analysis where the results from studies identified in a literature search are reanalyzed and reinterpreted. The use of statistical techniques can account for differences in quantitative methods and enables the researcher to pull together the findings of numerous studies to offer a more substantive assessment of the available evidence. This is particularly useful when studies are based on a small sample. However, meta-analysis is a highly sophisticated tool and should only be undertaken by researchers with statistical skills. The NHS Centre for Reviews and Dissemination at York (www.york.ac.uk/inst/crd) provides useful guidelines for those wishing to undertake a systematic review. It explains the various statistical techniques that should be utilized.

The key source for identifying systematic reviews is via the Cochrane Collaboration, an international network of those working on systematic reviews (www.cochrane.co.uk). Its website includes a searchable database. The National

Research Register also provides information on ongoing systematic reviews (www.nrr.nhs.uk). The TRIP (Turning Research into Practice) Database of evidence-based articles covering medical science may also be searched (www.trip-database. com). In addition, specialist publications such as *Bandolier* are indexed by the major abstract and indexing journals.

CARRYING OUT A LITERATURE SEARCH

This section outlines good practice in how to undertake a literature search: that is, how to set search parameters; identify appropriate databases; write the search strategy; and record the results (for further guidance see Gash 2000). In a sense, literature searching is like detective work – the aim is to identify the most appropriate sources to answer a question within a field of study. The key sources used by information specialists are listed below:

- *Bibliography*: A bibliography is a list of publications relating to a particular subject area. Various types of bibliography are:

  - *General bibliographies*: The *British National Bibliography* is a weekly publication from the British Library of all new books published in the United Kingdom and should be checked regularly.
  - *Specialist subject bibliographies*: Produced by research centres, scholars or specialist information services such as the US National Library of Medicine. This publishes *Current Bibliographies in Medicine* bringing together references on specific issues, such as health literacy (Zorn et al. 2004).
  - *Publications*: Journal articles note the works the author has quoted in a list of references at the end. Research monographs and textbooks will also provide a list of sources but will often include all items read by the author rather than just those quoted in the text.

- *Catalogues*: Most academic libraries and specialist institutions maintain a catalogue that shows the details and location of all items in stock. This is the most obvious place to start any search. COPAC (www.copac.ac.uk) is the merged catalogue of a number of university libraries and the British Library and national libraries of Scotland and Wales. Most other libraries make their catalogues available over the Internet and all academic libraries have reciprocal access arrangements for students.

- *Abstracting and indexing journals*: An abstract is a short summary of an academic journal article. This is an aid to assessing relevance without reading the full article:

  - *Abstracting journals* provide details of articles drawn from a range of journals within a particular subject area. They tend to be arranged alphabetically by author, with a subject index to locate relevant papers.
  - *Indexing journals* are usually arranged in subject order and provide basic bibliographic details of articles (title, author, journal, date, volume, page number).

  Most abstracting and indexing journals are now available electronically on specialist databases.

The Internet and electronic sources have made the search process quicker and broadened the range of sources that can be accessed. This can be a problem as an overwhelming number of potentially useful articles may be retrieved. It is imperative, therefore, to plan a search effectively, and to review the strategy as the search progresses.

Library catalogues allow searches based on author, title, subject classification and keyword. Subject codes are assigned to books and other publications using classification schemes such as the Dewey Decimal System. The majority of classifications systems are based on numeric codes. For example, in the Dewey System, books on the medical sciences are located at 610. In addition, most cataloguers apply keywords to publications. The classification of articles in electronic databases is more sophisticated and has a higher degree of specificity than items in library catalogues. In other words, database searching can be more precise and retrieve more items of relevance as they are coded in more depth. A number of subject headings are assigned to summarize the coverage of each article. For example, the US National Library of Medicine uses MeSH (Medical Subject Headings) in the Medline database. In addition, databases assign keywords to each item drawn from the abstract or provided by the author. Some databases also make abstracts searchable. A keyword or abstract search can be a useful way to narrow down the focus of a search.

The reviewer may use various sources to identify the best database to search. Most academic libraries produce guides to the subject areas they cover and list the databases they subscribe to. It is usually possible to check where journals are abstracted and indexed on the publishers' websites, although no one database will cover all journals within a subject area. Databases are generally free at the point of use for students. If a library does not subscribe to a particular database, it may be possible to gain access on a pay-as-you-go basis. Table 3.1 summarizes some of the main subject databases covering health care. In addition there are numerous specialist databases such as AgeInfo, PsycINFO and Alternative Medicine which focus on particular sub-specialities in the health care field.

How to set the search profile

While it might be tempting to start immediately entering search terms into databases, an effective literature search requires careful planning. The reviewer should begin by setting down on paper a brief title for the review; a summary of the areas of interest, including the type of evidence and publications required; and any parameters for the search such as the date or language of publication. A search profile serves two key purposes. First, it requires the researcher to clarify the scope and parameters of the study and, second, it acts as an *aide-memoire* throughout the search process. In this way, the searcher is encouraged to remain focused and not be side-tracked down interesting but irrelevant byways. Narrative reviews offer

Table 3.1 *Key databases in health care*

Database	Scope	Content	Years
General:			
Applied Social Sciences Index and Abstracts	Health, social services, psychology, sociology, economics, politics, race relations and education. International in scope	Indexes and abstracts 650 journals	1987–
International Bibliography of Social Sciences	Anthropology, economics, politics and sociology. International in scope	Bibliographic references to journal articles. Abstracts and some full-text access are provided. Includes research notes, responses and short essays, book reviews and book chapters	1951–
ScienceDirect	Science, technology and medicine full text and bibliographic information. International in scope	Bibliographic details and abstracts from the 2,000 journals published by Elsevier. Includes access to full text	
Health:			
Cumulative Index to Nursing and Allied Health Literature	Nursing, allied health, biomedicine, alternative/complementary medicine, consumer health and health sciences librarianship. International in scope	Bibliographic references from 2,593 journals of which 1,831 are currently indexed. Abstracts are also provided for about 1,000 journals. Includes a citation index from 1994	1982–
Health Management Information Consortium	Clinical medicine, behavioural and social sciences, management and hospital administration. International in scope	Bibliographic references and abstracts from three institutions: the United Kingdom Department of Health and Nuffield Institute for Health (Leeds University Library) and King's Fund Library	1983–
Medline	Medicine and health policy. International in scope	Bibliographic references and abstracts. Some links to full text	1950s–

more temptations to the unwary researcher. Systematic reviews usually set explicit inclusion and exclusion criteria. The search profile in Box 3.1 below for a study funded by the Office of the Deputy Prime Minister in the United Kingdom on the effects of overcrowding on health and education (Brown et al. 2004) was adapted from guidelines provided by Gash (2000). The profile was also uded as a structure for describing the literature search process in the final report of this project.

Box 3.1   *Search profile for the effects of overcrowded housing on health and education*

Scope:
Health impacts: For example, mental health and infectious disease.
Educational consequences: For example, attainment and child development.
Empirical and conceptual studies: The academic literature, excluding publications that merely report on levels of overcrowding in particular areas.
Adopt a snowball technique: Read reference lists in articles and books for follow up. Citation search of key articles to identify other potential sources of data.

Date: 1970s onwards —

Language: English

Type: Academic literature — excluding newspaper articles and policy reports.

Sources: Academic and policy databases, websites of key research organisations, charities and government departments.

Country: OECD countries.

Key words: 'Overcrowding', crowding', 'houses in multiple occupation', 'health', 'physical health', 'mental health', 'child development', 'academic achievement', 'educational attainment' and 'deprivation'.

Source: Marsh, A. et al, (1999) *Home Sweet Home*, Bristol: The Policy Press; Thomson, H. et al. (2001) 'Health effects of housing improvement', *British Medical Journal*, 323: 187—90.

Writing the search strategy

While the search profile provides an overview of the scope and parameters of the search, it is the search strategy that is actually used to retrieve journal articles and books from databases. The strategy requires the identification of the terms that best describe the area of interest. These can be found in the definitions provided in subject-specific dictionaries and encyclopaedias. This list should include synonyms, abbreviations and related terms. As most databases have an international scope, researchers should allow for possible variations in language. For example, while United Kingdom authors use the word 'overcrowding' in relation to overcrowded housing, North American authors tend to use 'crowding' to describe the same phenomenon. Browsing the subject index of the database can ensure that the most appropriate words are searched for. It may also be worth checking how a key reference has been indexed in the database to see what subject terms and keywords were used to catalogue the article.

Once a list of search terms is identified, a search strategy must be written by deciding how these terms should be entered into the computer. It is rare that a search can be completed by inputting one or two words. Often the search strategy is built using Boolean operators – 'and', 'or', 'not' – which can be used to combine search terms to retrieve the most relevant articles. These three simple words can be used to broaden or narrow the search. For example, using the 'or' operator ensures that synonyms for the chosen term can be searched; the 'and' operator provides a narrower focus; and the 'not' operator ensures that records with this term are not retrieved. Prior to entering the strategy in the database, it is important to check how the Boolean operators should be entered. Some databases use symbols rather than words. Table 3.2 provides working examples of how Boolean operators were used in the overcrowding and health review.

Refining the literature search

Always be prepared to rethink the search strategy in light of the results. The search may retrieve too many results. A useful technique is to download or print out the complete references (or a sample of them) – together with the abstract and subject classifications – and use these to identify the relevant articles. The enquirer should look to see how these have been catalogued and refine the search strategy. If this does nothing to reduce the numbers, then limits such as date, language or place of publication should be applied. Most, if not all, databases offer on-screen help or prompts for this. More recent articles are likely to give a summary of previous research, and from these it should be possible to judge how far back the search needs to be taken. With luck, the search may identify an earlier review article which can be updated. If there are still too many references, then the focus of study will need rethinking in order to narrow the search further.

Conversely, searches may end with no results, or very few. This could be because little has been written on the subject, or may be due to inconsistencies in cataloguing and indexing on different databases. Each database will have its own house style so differences may occur in subject and keyword classification or in the logging of bibliographic details such as the author name. For example, in any database the name of the author could be indexed as *Jones, K*; *Jones, K.L.*; *Jones, Kathryn* or *Jones, Kathryn L.* So an author search for *Jones, K.L.* in one database may come back as having no hits, because papers are listed in the author index under *Jones, K.* Most databases offer the possibility of browsing the author index or to search for the surname alone. In the case of a common name such as Jones, this should be combined with a subject term to narrow the search focus.

Table 3.2   *The use of 'and', 'or', 'not' in a search strategy*

	Search	Outcomes	Uses
	Using the **AND** operator:		
#1	Overcrowding		
#2	Asthma		
#3	#1 and #2	Records that contain both 'overcrowding' and 'asthma'	Narrowing the focus of the search by including particular terms
	Using the **OR** operator:		
#1	Overcrowding		
#2	Crowding		
#3	#1 or #2	Records that contain either 'overcrowding' or 'crowding' or both terms	Ensuring synonyms are included in search strategy
	Using the **NOT** operator:		
#1	Overcrowding		
#2	Trains		
#3	#1 not #2	Records that contain 'overcrowding', but not 'overcrowding' in 'trains'	Narrowing focus of search by excluding particular variables

Keyword searching may not retrieve results because different authors may assign different words for the same phenomena. For example, some academics may use 'patient group', 'self-help group' or 'health consumer group' to describe similar types of organization. Or cataloguers could use the same word to describe different phenomena. For example, 'complaint' may mean an illness or an allegation that something has gone wrong. In addition, different cataloguers may code the same article under different subject headings. Most databases give the option of truncating search terms, by using a particular symbol (usually $) to retrieve more references. For example, a search on 'consum$' would retrieve articles on consumers, consumerism and consumption. It is essential to browse both subject and keyword indexes in databases. Recognizing that inconsistencies can occur ensures a healthy scepticism of retrieved results. A quick way of testing the results is to look at a journal reference list on a topic to see if at least some of the same articles are cited.

Another technique is to search for who has quoted an important journal article as this can help to snowball the search to ensure a comprehensive coverage. The *Science* or *Social Science Citation Index* allows the researcher to identify articles, and, increasingly, also books and book chapters that have cited a particular reference. This provides access to further work on the subject, and gives an indication of how others view this work.

The literature within a particular subject area is never static, so it is essential to build in a mechanism for keeping a search up to date. Some databases will save searches that can be rerun later. Many libraries and institutions produce a current awareness service of publications. For example, the King's Fund Information and Library Service (www.kingsfund.org.uk) specializes in health policy and economics and publishes a bimonthly current awareness service. The latest versions of journal content pages are produced by zetoc Alert email service (www.zetoc.mimas.ac.uk).

Searching for grey literature

Grey literature refers to literature published independently by, for example, specialist research units rather than mainstream publishers. The *Aslib Directory of Information Sources in the UK* is a useful starting point for identifying specialist collections. Grey literature may be difficult to obtain, but can be extremely valuable as it can include cutting-edge research. Some research bodies such as the King's Fund or the Institute of Health Services Management Research in the United Kingdom have websites that list, and increasingly provide, their publications online. It is also worth looking at the websites of research funding bodies such as the Economic and Social Research Council (www.esrc.ac.uk), the Medical Research Council (www.mrc.ac.uk) or the Department of Health (www.dh.gov.uk). Some research reports are available electronically. There are also various specialist indexes that cover particular types of publication such as conference papers, dissertations and official documents. These may provide access to information that has not been formally published. In the overcrowding study, grey literature was identified through hand searching specialist journals, specialist indexes and the websites of key research units and housing charities.

Although it is tempting to rely on Internet search engines to locate information in relation to grey literature and other material, it is important to remember that this does not substitute for properly constructed search strategies using specialist databases. First, a search engine will not search with the same degree of rigour as an online database. Second, some literature found on the Internet may look official but it may be inaccurate and unverified by external experts.

Recording the search

The type and extent of information provided on the results of the database search will vary according to the database publisher. Most databases provide options for how results can be viewed online. At a minimum, the bibliographic details (such as author, date, title, journal, volume/issue number and page number(s)) will be provided for each item. The majority of databases will also provide the abstract and subject classification. An increasing number now offer access to the full article. It is worth downloading or saving the bibliographic and abstract details of the search into an email account or some form of specialist software, so they can be looked at more comprehensively at a later stage. The database will generally offer prompts to achieve this. It is vital to keep track by noting the databases searched, the years covered, the number of retrieved articles and the search strategy used, to ensure that the search is undertaken as systematically as possible. This record will also be useful if the search strategy needs to be revised.

The bibliographic details and abstract of each item retrieved should provide a good indication of whether the full article is worth reading. If a journal or book is not available locally, it can be obtained via interlibrary loans. For each item read, the reviewer should complete a data extraction form and this is used to summarize key details from the item, as set out in Box 3.2. The type of information logged will depend on the purpose of the review, but keeping a record is essential. In the example given at the end of the chapter, the bibliographic details necessary for referencing are noted as well as information on definitions of keywords; the concepts that make up the conceptual framework; the findings or results of the study; the argument put forward; and the conclusions drawn. The form also provides space for personal comment, and a prompt for a rating of the quality and relevance of the paper.

For the literature review on overcrowding, a more complex form was devised that recorded details about the type of study and the methods used. It also included stricter guidelines for judging the quality of the papers (see Brown et al. 2004). Completing a form for each item may seem cumbersome, but is essential. A number of sources are likely to be identified and it will be impossible to remember everything that has been read. When planning and writing the review, it is less time consuming to read through one-page summaries than to reread every article. A useful tip in completing the form is to put the page number beside each new sentence. This is an aid to checking information or obtaining a page number if a direct quote is used. Some people suggest that this process should be computerized. However, unless the researcher is working at PhD level, or it is a long-term project, or a large amount of material is identified, a paper-based method should suffice.

Box 3.2 *A data extraction form*

Article no:		Review date:		
Title:				
Author(s):		Publication date:		
Publisher:		Place of publication:		
Journal:		Volume:	Number:	Page no:
Keywords/definitions:				
Conceptual framework:				
Findings/argument:				
Author conclusions:				
Own notes:				

Rating: quality of research			Rating: relevance to study		
A	High quality		1	Extremely relevant	
B	Medium quality		2	Quite relevant	
C	Low quality		3	Marginal relevance	

Assessing relevance and quality in a literature review

A major part of the literature review will involve making a judgement on the relevance of what is being read. The significance of the findings to a project should be assessed as well as the effect of the research design on the outcome of the study. Once a number of studies have been read, it should be possible to make an accurate assessment of the importance of each item extracted.

Even within a narrative review an attempt must be made to judge the relative merits of the methods employed in each study. For example, a study rated as highly relevant may be based on only a small sample. A researcher may use this to make a case for a larger study. Alternatively, a search may identify issues that were explored using quantitative methods but there may be a benefit in further investigation using qualitative methods, and vice versa. The reviewer should comment on the reliability and validity of the methods used, and the extent to which they can be generalized to a larger population. It is also important to note whether findings support or contradict previous research.

A number of guides are available which describe approaches to evaluating different types of research in the clinical and social sciences. These have been developed for researchers wishing to undertake a systematic review. However, they raise questions pertinent for any review (see for example Greenhalgh 1997; NHS CRD 2001). The key questions for assessing the quality of studies in a literature review are summarized as follows:

- Conceptual framework:

  — Are the aims clearly stated and research questions clearly identified?
  — Does the author link the work to an existing body of knowledge?

- Study design:

  — Are the methods appropriate and clearly described?
  — Is the context of the study well set out? Did the research design account for possible bias?
  — Are the limitations of research explicitly identified?

- Research analysis:

  — Are the results clearly described, valid and reliable?
  — Is the analysis clearly described?

- Conclusions:

  — Are all possible influences on the observed outcomes considered?
  — Are conclusions linked to aims of study?
  — Are conclusions linked to analysis and interpretation of data?

WRITING THE LITERATURE REVIEW

A literature review is not simply a regurgitation of who said what on a particular subject. A successful review is an interpretive piece of work that offers an assessment of the quality and scope of existing studies in a particular subject area. It brings together what is known in order to state what further research or analysis is required. In essence, a review acknowledges what has come before and how this can be built upon and expanded.

The review should define the key concepts to be used in the research and how these will be used within the reviewer's own work. It is good practice to draw attention to different definitions of key terms and why the researcher has decided to follow one definition rather than another. For example, the term 'consumer' is contested; different authors attach different meanings. In a study undertaken by the author and others of health consumer groups, attention was paid to explaining why this term was used rather than 'patients' group' or 'patients' association' or 'health user group' by discussing debates in the literature (Baggott et al. 2005).

In discussing the theoretical framework for a study, the researcher must justify why a certain theory has been adopted and spell out what research questions are raised by this approach. Some studies use a number of theories, a strategy termed by Sabatier (1999) as a 'multiple-lens' approach. For example, in the health consumer group study, the research team drew on a number of different theoretical perspectives that raised different questions to assess the influence and impact of health consumer groups on the policy process. These included theories about the configuration, and relative power, of various structural interests in health care; explanations of the power and influence of particular pressure groups; and theories about issue networks and policy communities within the policy process. Theories of representative and participative democracy were also reviewed in the context of questions about how health consumer groups represented their members, and how representatives were seen by health care stakeholders. These theories informed the questionnaire design, the semi-structured interviews with health consumer group leaders and contributed to developing a theoretical framework for subsequent analysis of the qualitative data.

A literature review should also report on previous empirical work undertaken, what methods have been adopted and relevant findings. In the study of health consumer groups, previous work on patient groups and patient and public involvement in policy making at local and national level provided the basis for identifying gaps in the research. In addition, factors that limited the validity or generalizability of previous research findings were noted.

Deciding a structure for the literature review

One challenge for the researcher is to select the most relevant articles for inclusion from a large quantity of material. The basis for inclusion in the narrative review is the relevance of the conceptual, theoretical and methodological approach taken by different authors to the study in question. A second challenge is to find a logical structure in writing the review. This will depend on its purpose. A review that seeks to assess the evidence base for a particular health care intervention will be structured differently from a review for a dissertation, thesis or project. Thus, for example, the overcrowding review took a themed approach. In the introduction, issues relating to definitions and methods were discussed. Subsequent chapters reported evidence on the impact of overcrowding on various aspects of health (such as the higher incidence of respiratory illness) and education (like the effect of overcrowding on educational attainment).

It would be unusual to follow a simple chronological arrangement in the literature review, by for instance starting a discussion with the earliest work on the subject and ending with the latest. A review is more likely to be arranged according to themes drawn from the literature or framed around certain research questions. Within a narrative review, the reviewer should take care to ensure that the structure follows the logic of their argument. In effect, the reviewer aims to establish that a gap in knowledge exists and suggests a way forward, through further research (see Hart 1998).

Effective planning is essential in order to identify the most logical structure. Before writing, an outline or plan of the review should be written. This will involve jotting down the key themes identified from the reading and making links between them to establish an appropriate order. It is helpful to identify headings and subheadings. These may not be used in the final review but can help to ensure a logical flow to the argument.

Style and referencing in a literature review

The writing style adopted in a review will depend on what is being reviewed. One benefit from reading widely around a subject area is to gain a feel for scholarly writing. Sentences commonly used to develop an argument are summarized below:

- *Where there is agreement and disagreement on particular issues*: 'While there is general agreement that this has occurred (references), there has been some debate about whether this is due to x (references) or y (references).'
- *On the criticisms levelled at particular studies*: 'Jones's work has been criticized because of a, b, c (references), but it is of relevance to this study because it suggests x, y, z.'
- *Offering suggestions of what can be surmised or understood from the literature*: 'In summary, it is possible to suggest that x is related to y; however, what is still not known is how z fits into this, which is the purpose of the study.'

A review will go through several drafts. Early drafts are likely to be more descriptive than analytical as the reviewer must first decide how the literature fits together before they can present a coherent argument. As the argument develops, the literature can be revisited. The extraction forms will be invaluable at this point to identify key findings. Articles that contradict findings, or question theoretical or conceptual frameworks, are also important. A good review offers a balanced perspective.

It is not necessary to cite or quote every reference retrieved, only those that are relevant to the question. The primary aim is to construct a clear narrative and to distinguish the author's argument from the works referenced. In deciding what to include, the researcher should bear in mind the intended audience. For example, a supervisor or external examiner will already have general background in the subject area. The literature should be analyzed with reference to the research aims or questions. A common mistake is simply to describe the literature – the approach must be analytic and critical.

Correct attribution is also important. Failure to acknowledge a source can lead to an allegation of plagiarism. For dissertation or research students, a preferred citation style may be recommended. One common style is the Harvard system – as used in this volume – based on an author and year system, with fuller details listed in alphabetical order at the end of the work. Another style is the Oxford system where numbers for each source are used in the text and then full bibliographic details are given in a footnote or endnote. Legal or historical texts tend to favour page footnoting as readers may wish to see precise amplification as they read. If guidelines are provided by a book publisher or editors of a journal, they should be followed to the letter and consistently applied. Moreover, if a source is quoted directly, it should always be cited and the page number given. If particular ideas or arguments are summarized, this should also be acknowledged. Chapter 21 discusses writing style further.

Case study   The Black Report

In 1977 the Secretary of State for Health and Social Security requested a review of existing knowledge on the differences in health status between social classes, their causes and implications for policy and future research. The review was chaired by Sir Douglas Black (then Chief Scientist at the Department of Health and Social Security, and later President of the Royal College of Physicians). This hard-hitting report on the evidence of inequalities in health (Department of Health and Social Security 1980) was finally made more widely available by Townsend and Davidson (1988) and subsequently has been updated in the light of further evidence. The aim was to provide evidence of the extent of inequality in health and offer an assessment of its implications. The report reviewed the following:

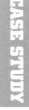

- *Concepts of health*: How is health, ill-health and inequality defined?
- *Concepts of health and inequality*: Definitions of health, indicators of health and illness including disablement, inequality indicators based on occupational group, income and expenditure.
- *Theoretical debates*: What theoretical approaches can explain why health inequalities occur?
- *Empirical evidence*: The sources of evidence on health inequalities, for example the statistical returns from the General Household Survey, birth cohort studies and published reviews of data.
- *The pattern of present inequalities*: Mortality by gender, race, region, occupational class, incidence of common illnesses.
- *Trends in inequality of health; inequality in the availability and use of the health service*: A review of published studies and critique of methods.
- *International comparisons*: Comparison with developed countries, particularly European countries.
- *Towards an explanation of health inequalities*: Theoretical approaches to understanding health inequalities were assessed against the human life cycle.
- *Recommendations*: These outlined (a) the need for further primary and secondary research on particular issues and in policy terms; and (b) the need for a comprehensive anti-poverty strategy covering a range of social services based on a broader concept of inequalities in health.

Case study	Carrying out a literature review for a short paper: Health consumer networks and alliances

This review was undertaken for a chapter in a book by Baggott et al. (2005), entitled *Speaking for Patients and Carers*, on health consumer groups in the national policy process and was funded by the Economic and Social Research Council (R000237888). The chapter formed a link between the early part of the book, which had set out research into the general conceptual, theoretical and policy context and explored the characteristics and social and political resources of health consumer groups, and the later chapters which dealt with the relationships between such groups and other actors/institutions in the policy process. The aim of the chapter was to explore how and why contacts and links

(Continued)

(Continued)

between health consumer groups formed; how these alliances supported these groups' role in policy; and the factors that encouraged collaboration rather than competition. The issues were identified as:

- *Conceptual issues*: How are networks and alliances defined?
- *Theoretical debates*: How can alliance working in the policy process be understood and explained?
- *Empirical evidence*: What evidence exists on current patterns of alliances and networking within the health consumer group and the voluntary health sector?

CONCLUSION

This chapter has emphasized the importance of the literature review in identifying concepts, theories and existing empirical studies on a particular phenomenon in the early stages of developing a research proposal or project. This enables a researcher to build on the basis of existing knowledge and on what other scholars have achieved, but also to identify gaps in the literature and to identify interesting new questions. While systematic reviews are a specialized form of study, narrative reviews are fundamental to any project.

The Internet has brought access to a vast range of electronic sources for the researcher. A well-written review will provide enough background to bring the reader up to speed in the subject area and give them a framework within which to assess the evidence. In order to navigate a way through the quantity of sources available, two strategies may be employed. First, it is important to plan a search strategy carefully and to record sources and their content meticulously. The chapter outlines ways in which this can be done, so that with practice, the researcher can be quick and efficient at finding the sources most likely to be relevant to their research question. Second, the expansion of the Internet has led to the increase of information specialists who are employed by many organizations, and not only higher education institutions, to assist people in gaining access to information and what they need to know. This is particularly the case in the health field where a wide range of people, both professionals and the lay public, now wish to inform themselves better using both national and international sources. An exercise now follows for readers further to develop their understanding of this chapter.

Exercise: A literature search on New Labour's expert patients agenda from a consumer/citizen perspective

The following exercise provides an opportunity to think through the process of developing a search strategy and a structure for a literature review. While the subject area may not be one you are familiar with, the process described in this chapter should give you a framework to plan a successful search.

Think about the type of literature review that you would undertake for a dissertation entitled 'A critical analysis of New Labour's expert patients agenda in the United Kingdom from a consumer/citizen perspective'.

1   What conceptual and theoretical issues will you need to consider?

- Consider what definitional issues you will need to address.
- How will perspectives on consumerism/citizenship influence the analysis of the literature?

2   Which electronic databases will you need to search?

- Consider the scope and coverage of the database. How important is it that it is international in scope?
- Are you going to attempt to identify primary research studies, secondary policy analysis or both?

3   What search strategy will you build?

- Consider what keywords and phrases you will need to use.
- Consider what the most appropriate limits might be for your search — for example, language and date of publication.
- Are there any terms that can be truncated to broaden the search?

4   What will be the most relevant sources of grey literature?

- Which key research organizations may have an interest in the Expert Patients Programme?
- What information will you need to obtain from the Department of Health website?

(Continued)

> *(Continued)*
>
> 5   What key data will you need to log from the literature?
>
> - Consider how these may change according to the type of information — for example, policy documents, policy critiques and policy analyses that draw on field research.
>
> 6   How will you structure the review?
>
> - What information will the reader require on the Expert Patients Programme?
> - What information will the reader require on the theoretical and conceptual issues underpinning your review?
> - Will you tackle the advantages/disadvantages of the Expert Patients Programme separately or by theme?
> - Will you discuss primary and secondary research together or separately?

NOTE

1   The author would like to thank the following for permission to draw on projects undertaken while part of a larger research team: Judith Allsop, University of Lincoln; Rob Baggott, Health Policy Research Unit, De Montfort University; and Tim Brown and Ros Hunt, Centre for Comparative Housing Research, De Montfort University.

RECOMMENDED FURTHER READING

Gash, S. (2000) *Effective Literature Searching for Research.* Aldershot: Gower.
This is an excellent, easy-to-understand guide for students and other researchers on the process of planning, executing and recording a literature search, covering both print and electronic sources.

Hart, C. (1998) *Doing a Literature Review: Releasing the Social Science Research Imagination.* London: Sage.
This book provides a comprehensive guide to the process of accessing, analyzing and understanding the arguments presented in academic texts, giving useful advice on how the literature review fits into undergraduate and postgraduate dissertations.

Petticrew, M. and Roberts, H. (2006) *Systematic Reviews in the Social Sciences*. Malden, MA: Blackwell.
  This highlights how systematic reviews of research evidence are becoming increasingly important in the social sciences, much of which is also relevant to narrative reviews as well.

REFERENCES

Baggott, R., Allsop, J. and Jones, K. (2005) *Speaking for Patients and Carers: Health Consumer Groups and the National Policy Process*. Basingstoke: Palgrave.

Brown, T., Baggott, R., Jones, K. and Hunt, R. (2004) *The Impact of Overcrowding on Health and Education: A Review of the Research Evidence and Literature*. London: The Office of the Deputy Prime Minister.

Department of Health and Social Security (1980) *Inequalities in Health: A Report of a Research Working Group* (Chair: Sir Douglas Black). London: DHSS.

Dixon-Woods, M., Fitzpatrick, R. and Roberts, K. (2001) 'Including qualitative research in systematic reviews: problems and opportunities', *Journal of Evaluative Clinical Practice*, 7: 125–33.

Egger, M., Smith, G.D. and Altman, D.G. (2001) *Systematic Reviews in Healthcare. Meta-analysis in Context*. London: BMJ.

Gash, S. (2000) *Effective Literature Searching for Research*. Aldershot: Gower.

Greenhalgh, T. (1997) *How to Read a Paper: The Basics of Evidence Based Medicine*. London: BMJ.

Hart, C. (1998) *Doing a Literature Review: Releasing the Social Science Research Imagination*. London: Sage.

NHS CRD (2001) *Undertaking Systematic Reviews of Research on Effectiveness: CRDs Guidelines for Those Carrying Out or Commissioning Reviews*. York: CRD.

Petticrew, M. (2001) 'Systematic reviews from astronomy to zoology: myths and misconceptions', *British Medical Journal*, 322: 98–101.

Petticrew, M. and Roberts, H. (2006) *Systematic Reviews in the Social Sciences*. Malden, MA: Blackwell.

Sabatier, P.A. (1999) 'The need for better theories', in P.A. Sabatier (ed.), *Theories of the Policy Process*. Boulder, CO: Westview Press.

Street, A. (2001) 'How can we argue for evidence in nursing?', *Contemporary Nurse*, 11(1): 5–9.

Thomas, J., Harden, A., Oakley, A., Oliver, S., Sutcliffe, K., Rees, R., Brunton, G. and Kavanagh, J. (2004) 'Integrating qualitative research with trials in systematic reviews', *British Medical Journal*, 328: 1010–12.

Townsend, P. and Davidson, N. (1988) *Inequalities in Health*. London: Penguin.

Zorn, M., Allen, M.P. and Horowitz, A.M. (2004) *Understanding Health Literacy and Its Barriers, January 1998 through November 2003, Plus Selected Earlier and Later Citations*. Bethesda, MD: National Library of Medicine.

PART II
Qualitative Methods and Health

Using Documents in Health Research

ANDY ALASZEWSKI

INTRODUCTION

Documents, especially personal documents such as diaries and letters, provide a relatively neglected resource for health service researchers. They can be used to access data that are difficult to obtain in other ways. For example, such documents can tell us about individuals who died several centuries ago; people from marginalized and stigmatized groups who are often reluctant to participate in research; or activities, such as gay sex, that are otherwise concealed. In this respect, the overall aim of this chapter is to examine the ways in which documents have been and can be used for health research. This includes describing documentary research, identifying the type of resources it requires, and examining the research issues for which it is appropriate. The chapter will also, amongst other things, outline the strengths and weaknesses of documentary research and consider how documentary data can be coded, analyzed and presented.

DEFINING DOCUMENTARY RESEARCH

Health-related documentary research involves the use of any 'records relating to individuals or groups of individuals that have been generated in the course of their daily life' (Clarkson 2003: 80). Such records may be created by a third party, for example a hospital will over time build up a store of records including patients' notes, letters of complaint and minutes of meetings. Documentary research can also include personal and family records such as letters or diaries. Such 'documents of life' (Plummer 2001) can be used as the basis of biographical case studies or life stories (Clarkson 2003).

Documentary evidence can take a variety of forms. The traditional form of such evidence – and the one that tends to predominate and is the easiest to use for research – is written text, such as hospital records, letters and diaries. These may be stored in archives or published in collected works or as memoirs, biographies and institutional histories. However, with the development of other media, written text can be supplemented, or even replaced, by photographs, film, and audio and video recordings.

Documentary research is not restricted to the use of unsolicited material but the researcher can also solicit the creation of documents specifically for the purposes of the research (Alaszewski 2006). In particular, diaries – which can be seen as the 'document of life' *par excellence* (Plummer 2001) – can be used in a range of health-related research. These may have been used to keep a record of the symptoms experienced by individuals who have relapsing–remitting multiple sclerosis (Parkin et al. 2004), the sexual activities of men who have sex with men (Coxon 1996) or illness behaviour and decisions to seek expert advice (Robinson 1971).

While the documents used may take a variety of forms, the defining characteristic of documentary research is that the researcher draws on documents created by others. This is self-evident when the researcher is accessing unsolicited documents that are stored in archives and created by individuals who died long before the research started. However, when researchers solicit documents for the purposes of a research project then they can influence the way in which the document is created. This influence should fall short of control. The key feature of documentary research is that the record creator has ultimate control and ownership of the document. They can choose to destroy it or give others access. For example, Elliott (1997) undertook a study of the help-seeking behaviour of eight people who were aware of having musculoskeletal problems and invited them to keep a health diary. Diarists were asked to record their personal details and the time period covered by the diary on the first page, and on subsequent pages to keep a daily record. To help them to structure their records, they were invited to respond to a set of questions about their health. Elliott held that the documents created by these diaries and follow-up interviews were texts mainly authored by informants and used informants' own words and ideas, rather than those of the researcher.

WHY USE DOCUMENTARY RESEARCH?

Documentary sources are especially important when the researcher wishes to access individuals' own accounts and there are no alternative sources. This is the case in historical research on health and health-related issues where the researcher does not have the facility to supplement documents with interviews or observation. Pollock (1983) used documents to examine the ways in which child rearing changed between 1500 and 1900. From a variety of bibliographic sources she identified 496 documents of which 416 contained information on childrearing practices: 114 were American diaries, 236 were British diaries and 36 were autobiographies. The study included 98 diaries written by children or at least started during childhood. Pollock was able to use these sources to challenge the received wisdom that childcare had become more liberal and less violent over the period concerned.

Even when researchers can access other sources of data, documentary sources are important where a researcher needs to minimize memory or recall problems. Documents are often based on records that were made shortly after the actual events. Stone et al. (2003: 182) in a review of medical research diaries noted the value of diaries in 'capturing experience close to the time of its occurrence', especially medical symptoms which are 'subjective and/or variable'. They estimated that these types of documents feature prominently in drug trials and have been used in nearly 25 per cent of clinical trials.

Documentary sources also provide a way of collecting data that minimizes the intrusiveness associated with much social research. This is self-evident when the researcher uses unsolicited documents. Solicited documents may also minimize intrusion. The researcher specifies what sort of information is wanted. Participants are then free to decide when, and how, they record this information. Minimizing intrusion is important when a researcher wants to address sensitive issues or work where groups or individuals want to avoid scrutiny of their activities. In a Hong Kong study of men who have sex with men, Jones and his colleagues recruited 16 men to keep a daily record of their activities, relationships and feelings. The researchers asked participants to submit their records weekly and offered a variety of media for doing so including mail, fax, anonymous email, tape recording or face-to-face interviews (Jones et al. 2000; Jones and Candlin 2003).

RESOURCES NEEDED FOR DOCUMENTARY RESEARCH

The resources required for documentary research depend on the type of documents the researcher wants to use. Researchers who wish to use unsolicited documents need to locate and access relevant documents and sources, while researchers who use solicited documents must invest resources in creating, collecting and analyzing these documents.

Unsolicited documents

Researchers using unsolicited documents need to identify where such documents are held. Historic documents are likely to be stored in archives and the researcher will need to ensure resources are available to identify and access appropriate archives. Until relatively recently this involved using published bibliographies and other sources to identify possible archives and then physically visiting each place to access suitable documents (see Jordanova 2000; Corti 2003). This required resources to cover travel costs as well as photocopying, where that was permitted, and the costs of subsequent analysis. The development of electronic and Internet resources has increased access to, and reduced the costs of using, archives. Bibliographies and other resources can increasingly be accessed through the Internet. For example, Penn Library (2004) has specifically produced a research guide to finding diaries. Some archives are also available on the Internet. In the United Kingdom the DIPEx website (www.primarycare.ox.ac.uk/research.dipex) is an online archive of personal experiences of health and illness. The Mass Observation archive maintains a website that provides information both on the diaries archived and on publications based on the diaries. Mass Observation recruited 500 men and women to develop an 'anthropology of ourselves' (Sheridan, 1991: 1). Most recruits kept a diary from 1939 until 1945 and some continued until 1965.

Researchers dealing with recent documents may need to identify who is holding the documents and who can provide access. Searching for such individuals can be a difficult and time-consuming activity and generally researchers use intermediaries. Miller (1985) in his study of Irish migrants in the United States followed the approach pioneered by Thomas and Znaniecki (1958) in their classic study of the Polish migration that drew on unsolicited personal documents, such as letters and diaries. Miller used institutions, and individuals with contacts in the Irish migrant community, to access documents. Researchers can also advertise through media such as newspapers and the Internet. For example, the British Broadcasting Corporation used public interest in the Second World War, stimulated by 60th anniversary events, to promote an Internet archive of personal stories. Individuals were encouraged to contribute to a rapidly growing archive of personal documents by sending their stories and associated photographs electronically (WW2 People's War Team 2004). While setting up and promoting a website is expensive, it may be possible for researchers to use established websites. For example, there is a range of websites for users of health services, such as the different stroke website for stroke survivors (www.differentstroke.co.uk) which could be used to contact document holders.

Solicited documents

The resources needed by researchers who are using solicited documents specifically created for a research project will be determined by the purposes of the study and its design. The study may be based on experimental, survey or other methods. The major resource implications are those normally associated with using such designs. For a survey design resources are needed:

- To identify the population.
- To select and recruit a sample.
- To collect data from the subjects or units in the sample.
- To code and enter the data into a database.
- To analyze the data statistically.
- To write a report.

The additional resources needed for a survey of documents are those associated with the creation of suitable documents. For example, when monitoring the impact of different treatment regimes on chronic illnesses such as diabetes or multiple sclerosis, the researcher may need the research subject to record not only compliance with the prescribed treatment regime, but also relevant clinical data such as blood sugar levels or level of pain. In this context, the researcher will wish to recruit subjects who can be trusted to follow the instructions and keep an honest and accurate record. The researcher will also need to provide appropriate recording equipment. Traditional record keeping requires basic competence in literacy (Corti 2003), although subjects can now use audio and video recorders as well. The chances of creating documents suitable for research purposes are increased when adequate resources are provided for:

- The initial recruitment process.
- Training and support for diarists.
- Checking the reliability of entries and providing feedback.

The use of incentives, such as the payment of modest sums of money, is controversial but not uncommon in research soliciting documents from subjects (Coxon 1996; Jones et al. 2000).

THE STRENGTH AND WEAKNESS OF DOCUMENTARY SOURCES

Authenticity

Documents offer an authenticity which is difficult to gain through other methods. Documents such as diaries capture the richness of everyday life as it happens. Plummer noted that 'each diary entry – unlike life histories – is sedimented into a particular moment in time' (2001: 48). Bolger et al. (2003: 580) have argued that such documents facilitate 'the examination of reported events and experiences in their natural, spontaneous context'.

The authenticity of unsolicited documents makes them a particularly valuable resource for social or ethnographic histories. For example, MacFarlane (1970: 11) used Ralph Josselin's diary to 'step back 300 years and to look out through the eyes of an Essex vicar of the mid seventeenth century'. He used the diary to examine demographic and social issues, such as Josselin's relationship with his kin, godparents, servants and neighbours. He was interested in the cultural dimensions of these relationships and other aspects of Josselin's life. MacFarlane (1970: 3) noted that such a document 'enables us to probe a long-vanished mental world, as well as to describe the social characteristics of a previous civilization'.

If the researcher is careful not to impose an over-rigid structure then solicited documents can also be used as a means of obtaining authentic accounts of contemporary social events and experiences. Coxon (1996), in discussion of the use of diaries in Project SIGMA which studied gay men, noted that the diary method arose out of the researchers' experience as sexually active gay men. This use of solicited documents was 'natural' as it was not imposed on, or alien to, individuals who participated in the research. Diary keeping was common amongst gay men and several of the researchers had kept sexual diaries for a number of years before the research. Thus, the researchers drew on their own experience in developing the method and encouraged the diarists to describe their experiences in their own words.

Nonetheless, the authenticity of such documents is problematic. Documents such as letters and diaries are created to perform a particular function and achieve this using specific structures and forms. As Thomas and Znaniecki (1958) commented in their study of Polish migration in the early part of the twentieth century, the existence of extensive family correspondence is fairly remarkable, as in the peasant community literacy skills were not highly developed. The letters were the product of a social duty and written by, or to, an absent family member, including those who had migrated to the United States. They tended to follow certain well-established conventions. As Clarkson (2003: 82) has noted, documents need to be treated with caution as they 'are tricky; they tell us what the author wants us to know, which is not necessarily what the researcher is really interested in'.

Flexibility

Data from letters or diaries can be used in combination with other sources of data in a range of research designs. In historical research different types of documents can be used to triangulate findings, since convergent views from multiple sources can help to overcome potential weaknesses arising from a single source. Sahlins (1995) in his analysis of how Hawaiian Islanders made sense of an unprecedented event – their first encounter with Europeans – used a variety of diaries and other documents kept by Captain Cook and his crew and compared them with oral traditions and histories from the Islands. Sahlins argued that the comparison of these interpretations helped better to explain Cook's death.

Various methods can also be combined in research on contemporary issues. For example, Zimmerman and Wieder (1977) have developed a diary–interview approach that has three components:

- An initial interview
- The research diary
- A debriefing interview.

The initial interview is to provide participants with a briefing about how they should use their diaries and answer their questions. The participants maintain their diary for a specified period and at an agreed time they return their diaries. Zimmerman and Wieder developed their approach as an alternative to participant observation to access settings and activities that they could not directly observe. Elliott (1997) also used this approach in her diary study of illness and help-seeking behaviours. She maintained close contact with the participants in the research, visiting them at least three times: once to brief them and give them their diary; a second time to give them another diary and to have an initial 'conversation' about the diary; and a third and final visit to conduct an in-depth interview. She used both the conversations and interviews to explore themes identified in the diaries. For example, in the interviews, participants discussed not only actions which they had recorded in their diaries, but also actions they had considered but did not take, as well as actions they intended to take at some time in the future.

ANALYZING DOCUMENTARY MATERIAL

Statistical analysis

Researchers using experimental or survey methods will see the entries in such documents as recording specific forms of social reality that are reflected in recurring themes in the data. These can be coded within each case and organized into categories or variables. The data relevant to each variable for each case can then be expressed as a number (Moser and Kalton 1971). Such coding creates a data set which can be analyzed using statistical techniques. The aim of the analysis is to identify relationships between variables and demonstrate that they are unlikely to be a product of chance.

Parkin et al. (2004) used a statistical analysis of their diary data to examine the ways in which the symptoms of individuals with relapsing–remitting multiple sclerosis varied over time. The cross-sectional time series data enabled them to analyze the stability and variability of their main measuring instrument, the Euroqol Visual Analogue Scale.

Content analysis

Documents that have not been created within a closely defined structure tend to produce qualitative data, which in written documents take the form of written text. Data may take other forms, such as audio or video recordings, which are usually transcribed to form written text. One approach to such text is to analyze it to identify and isolate the information that it contains. This approach to analyzing text usually involves some form of content analysis (Brewer 2003). While the term content analysis may be used to refer to all forms of textual analysis, it can also refer more narrowly to the identification of specific information.

The starting point for such an analysis is the identification of constituent units in the text. If the researcher does not start with a clear idea of the specific characteristics that they are interested in, then the categories and overall scheme will develop following further investigation and comparison. Such an approach has been formalized as part of grounded theory, following a set of analytical strategies that can be applied to a variety of data collection techniques (Charmaz 2003). In this approach, which is considered further in Chapter 5, researchers develop their coding categories through a process of constant comparison. As they collect data, so they identify emerging themes and issues – and, as new themes emerge, they reconsider previously analyzed texts in the light of the developing categories.

Griffiths and Jordan (1998) used this approach in their exploratory diary/interview study of the patients' experiences during recovery from a lower limb fracture. The study was based on a convenience sample of nine patients who were recovering from emergency surgery following a lower limb trauma. The researchers developed a grounded theory by each reading the texts and identifying categories. From their analysis, they found three major themes which were concordant with a theoretical model evident in the literature. The patients went through three stages during their recovery: first, stress and uncertainty, then seeking control and finally returning to normal.

Structural analysis

An alternative approach to analyzing texts is to treat each text as an entity in its own right as a form of social reality which is the product of, and provides information on, the social processes that shaped its creation and are evident in its form and structure of the narrative. This method involves identifying the structure of each text; the similarities and differences between the structures of each text; an explanation of why a particular structure exists; and how this is used to create a form of social reality.

Conversational analysis provides a way of examining the structure that underlies social interactions (Bryman 2001). Jones and his colleagues (Jones et al. 2000; Jones and Candlin 2003) used diaries to explore the ways in which men who have sex with other men accounted for their actions. They recruited 18 gay men who kept diaries in which they recorded their sexual activities and their reflections on sex and AIDS. In these diaries they identified 49 'sexual narratives', which they defined as 'accounts of specific sexual encounters with specific partners in specific settings which contained three or more clauses arranged in chronological order' (Jones and Candlin 2003: 203). They found that most of these narratives had a distinctive form, as they took the form of 'paired actions'. This structure was used to present the reported behaviours, even when these were 'risky' such as having unprotected sex, as reasonable and rational within the specific context.

Narrative analysis provides a further approach that explores the structure of the text. Rather than examining the structures of interactions which underpin the text, it addresses the ways in which the narrator structures and uses the narrative. It examines the role of the author in telling the story in a convincing way. Thus in a narrative analysis the focused interest is in the production of the text; the identity and intention of its author; the extent to which the author appears in the text; and the devices used in the text. In the case of documents such as letters, the identities and relationships of the person writing the letter and the person receiving it may be important in interpreting the narrative. For example, Honkasalo (2006) has contrasted the suicide notes of men and women in Finland noting that women write mostly to family or closest ones and men tend to write for, and justify themselves to, a wider audience.

Crossley (2003) used a narrative approach to analyze John Diamond's account of living with oral cancer which was originally published as a regular column in *The Times* and then reprinted in a posthumous collection of writings (Diamond 2001). Crossley treated Diamond's account as a text in which the author tried to make sense of challenges to his very existence. Crossley suggests that Diamond uses four main devices to structure and communicate his experience of cancer. The first related to the early pre-cancer stage in which Diamond raised the possibility of cancer, but distanced himself from the experience. The second and main device of the narrative involved detailed descriptions of treatment or therapeutic employment when Diamond was engrossed in the treatment process. This alternated with periods of remission when the third device, relative silence about the cancer, was used – before culminating in the final unspoken narrative of dying.

HOW DOCUMENTARY MATERIAL CAN BE USED WHEN PRESENTING FINDINGS

Using numbers

If a researcher uses numbers and statistical analysis, it is important to present these in an interesting way, for example by using visual presentations. Generally, the simpler the analysis, the easier it is to present visually. For example, the products of univariate analyses can be presented as bar charts, pie charts or histograms. Bivariate analyses can be presented as scatter diagrams, though it may be more difficult to present the results of multivariate analyses visually.

Coxon (1996) in his analysis of the Project SIGMA diaries started his analysis and discussions of sexual sessions with the simple description of the number of sexual acts per session that:

> The average (mean) is quite low (1.75 for most data-sets), but there is a very long tail: some sessions are quite long, and a few very long. (1996: 109)

He then moved on to more complex analysis to explore the structure of acts, that is the relationship between different sex acts. He used multidimensional scaling to produce a table of the co-occurrence of sex acts and a map in which each act was positioned to indicate its association with other acts. Using this analysis, Coxon was able to explore the relationship between sex acts showing that some acts such as oral sex tended to be reciprocal whereas others such as penetrative sex tended to be asymmetric or 'gendered'.

Developing themes in qualitative data

Content analysis of documents involves taking a number of written texts, breaking them into their constituent parts and reassembling these parts into a new scientific text. The most effective way of presenting such ideas is to describe how they developed out of the analysis of the text and to provide illustrative sections of that text. Griffiths and Jordan (1998) used this approach in their study of the patients' experiences during recovery from lower limb fracture and have identified the ways in which individuals reconstructed their lives. They use quotes from their texts to illustrate key themes such as loss of control:

> The last few months I really lost control over my life, and I feel I am just existing at the minute. That is how I feel. I feel I am on pause, as if someone has turned on a pause button on my life ... I know it is not going to last. (Griffiths and Jordan 1998: 1281)

Identifying structures

Structural analysis relies on identifying the ways in which documents are created and how they achieve their effect. This involves a comparison of key features of different texts and therefore the findings are often presented in the form of broad comparisons. Geertz (1988) showed how ethnographers have created accounts of other cultures that their readers can understand. He compared, *inter alia*, two journal-like ethnographies, the diary of Malinowski (1989) with its account of fieldwork in the Melanesian Islands and the account by Read (1965) of life in Highland New Guinea:

> Instead of the Dostoevskian darkness and Conradian blur [of Malinowski's text], the Readian 'I' is filled with confidence, rectitude, tolerance, patience, good nature, energy, enthusiasm, optimism — with an almost palpable determination to do what is right and think what is proper. If the Diary presents the image of the womanizing café intellectual cast among savages, The High Valley presents one of an indefinite country vicar. (Geertz 1988: 85)

Case study: **Using documents to examine the ways in which nurses learn to manage risk in everyday practice**

This example draws on a project that ran from 1996 to 1998, funded by the English National Board for Nursing, Midwifery and Health Visiting. The project was designed to evaluate whether current nurse education adequately prepared nurses to identify and manage the risks associated with supporting vulnerable people in the community (Alaszewski et al. 1998; Alaszewski et al. 2000). In one part of the project, we examined the types of risk nurses identified in their practice and the ways they addressed these. In the other part, we examined current nurse education and the ways in which it prepared nurses to mange risk. In both parts we used documents alongside other sources of data. To examine risk in nursing practice we invited a number of nurses to record their everyday practice in diaries and to examine current education we accessed course documentation.

For the study of current practice we used an interview/diary approach. We felt that using interviews alone would introduce recollection bias, for example a tendency to remember dramatic events and forget more mundane activities, and was likely to result in generalized and idealized accounts. Observation was an alternative but it would have

CASE STUDY

(Continued)

(Continued)

intruded into the potentially sensitive relationship between the nurses and their clients and might have distorted the very processes that we were seeking to capture. We therefore decided to use a less intrusive approach and invited nurses to act as self-observers and to record their observations in diaries (Alaszewski et al. 2000). We recruited 26 diarists, 10 student nurses, 8 new practitioners and 8 experienced nurses. To examine educational preparation, we sampled 24 current nurse education programmes. We interviewed lecturers, practice teachers and students engaged with each programme and examined course documentation – especially programme validation documents. We found that the latter were especially useful as they were very detailed.

In our analysis of the diaries we started by identifying decisions – the choices which the diarist made between different courses of actions. Some decisions could be identified relatively straightforwardly, for example the diarist wrote: 'Decision 1: to allow client to make her own choice where she slept.' Other decisions were embedded in a general discussion of the interactions and activities and we needed to examine whether the diarist had implicitly identified a choice, but chosen not to make it. For example, 'Next chap regular. Contriving to support wife regarding catheter care although I end up doing work; wife prefers to watch.' Although the diarist was reporting an activity, she had chosen not to confront the issue of handing over responsibility to the carer and she noted: 'I am allowing the wife to accept her responsibilities slowly'. Having identified the decisions, we then examined them to consider their nature, especially the ways in which nurses identified and managed the risk and uncertainty intrinsic to each decision. From each diary we selected two contrasting decisions to discuss with the diarist in more detail in a follow-up interview.

Our research team also analyzed the content of all the documentation from the 24 selected courses. Each set of documents was read by at least one member of the team and a sample read by two to check for the accuracy of coding. In some documents risk was explicitly identified within the documentation. But usually risk-related teaching was identified using other categories such as 'safety', 'empowerment', 'advocacy' or 'challenging behaviour'. Using these categories we were able to identify how, and in what ways, risk was identified and treated within each teaching programme. We could then compare this with lecturers', practice teachers' and students' discussions of risk in a teaching situation.

(Continued)

The documentary material in our study made an important contribution to our published findings. It added both interest and authenticity. For example, entries in the diaries help to establish the seriousness and urgency of some decisions:

> Message on answer phone from Client M. She needs to talk to me. When I phone back she says she doesn't need me she is going to [famous landmark on English coast] ... My decision is to cancel my first client and go round to M. I find her staring from the window, refusing to let me in. Eventually I persuade her to open the door... She then indicated to me that she is going to drive off [famous landmark on English coast] to join her sister. I arrange for ward to take her ... and she is admitted.

The diary material also enabled us to explore the content, complexity and difficulty of many of the risk assessments and of risk management. In focus group interviews, nurses tended to emphasize the importance of identifying and managing hazards. In the diaries and follow-up interviews a richer and more complex picture emerged. Nurses were often managing dilemmas and conflicts of interest rather than obvious hazards. For example, one set of diary and follow-up interviews allowed us to explore the ways in which a district nurse dealt with the pressure from the family of a terminally ill patient to move beyond pain management, to an acceleration of the dying process.

The material from the course documentation provided an insight into the ways in which nurse education prepared nurses for the risks of everyday practice. Overall coverage of risk management was patchy. In only 13 of the 24 sets of documents could we identify risk-related issues and, in most of these, risk did not form a prominent theme in the curriculum. For example, in one registration course on adult nursing, risk was only identified as a theme within a health promotion unit. However, we did identify courses that highlighted risk. In one learning disability course, risk formed one of the 12 units of competence that successful students were expected to develop. Furthermore, a clear and coherent rationale was given for risk teaching within the documentation that included a well-developed statement of the importance of risk management within professional practice.

CONCLUSION

This case study of nursing illustrates the practical use of documentary analysis in health research, the relevance and applicability of which have been clarified in this chapter – as well as the resources that it requires, its strengths and weaknesses, and the way that data so derived can be coded, analyzed and presented. As this chapter shows, the value of this comparatively neglected qualitative method in health research cannot be understated, particularly given the insights it provides into areas that are otherwise often difficult or impossible to access directly through the use of other research techniques. While further qualitative and quantitative methods are examined in detail in subsequent chapters of this book, its distinctive value is further underlined by the exercise set out for the reader below on the experience of stroke over the past three centuries in the United Kingdom.

Exercise: The use of documents in research into the experience of stroke

The following exercise is designed to make you think about the ways in which documents can be used in health research. While the material contained in this chapter may help you consider many of the issues, you may wish to access additional material from a library or the Internet. If you would like to prepare a formal answer, then write a research proposal or protocol.

   You want to apply to a charity for funding to undertake a study of the ways in which the experience of stroke has changed over the last 300 years in the United Kingdom.

1   What sort of documents could you use?

   • Consider the range of possible documents including personal documents such as diaries and letters, literature, newspapers and pamphlets, medical textbooks, records of care and treatment.
   • Consider where such documents might be held for different time periods.
   • How could you access appropriate documents?

(Continued)

2   How will you select the documents for your study?

- Consider what sort of design you want to use.
- Consider whether you wish to concentrate on one type of document or compare and contrast.
- How will you judge how 'typical' documents are?

3   How will you analyze documents?

- Will you need to transcribe them?
- Will the analysis be primarily qualitative, quantitative or both; do you have access to appropriate support such as statistical advice or support for qualitative software packages?
- Will you want to use a software package to help with the analysis?

4   What sort of resources will you need?

- Can you calculate an approximate time budget and identify travel and equipment costs?

5   How will you present your findings?

- Who do you see as the main users of your findings and what are their needs?
- How will you structure the publications, such as reports, articles and presentations?
- How will you present the evidence supporting your findings?

RECOMMENDED FURTHER READING

Alaszewski, A. (2006) *Using Diaries for Social Research*. London: Sage.
This book provides a comprehensive overview of the different ways in which diaries can be used for social and health research, describing their development and examining how the method can be most effectively used in all the stages of the research process.

Plummer, K. (2001) *Documents of Life 2: An Invitation to Critical Humanism*. London: Sage.
This is a key text that explores the ways in which personal or documents of life can and should be used in social health research, arguing that they can restore the humanism to research.

Prior, L. F. (2003) *Using Documents in Social Research*. London: Sage.
This is an overview of the strategies and debates surrounding the diverse range of documents that can be employed in research, giving examples of their use.

REFERENCES

Alaszewski, A. (2006) *Using Diaries for Social Research*. London: Sage.

Alaszewski, A., Alaszewski, H., Manthorpe, J. and Ayer, S. (1998) *Assessing and Managing Risk in Nursing Education and Practice: Supporting Vulnerable People in the Community*. London: ENB.

Alaszewski, A., Alaszewski, H., Ayer, S. and Manthorpe, J. (2000) *Managing Risk in Community Practice: Nursing, Risk and Decision Making*. Edinburgh: Ballière Tindall.

Bolger, N., Davis, A. and Rafaeli, E. (2003) 'Diary methods: capturing life as it is lived', *Annual Review of Psychology*, 54: 579–616.

Brewer, J. (2003) 'Content analysis', in R.L. Miller and J.D. Brewer (eds), *The A–Z of Social Research*. London: Sage.

Bryman, A. (2001) *Social Research Methods*. Oxford: Oxford University Press.

Charmaz, K. (2003) 'Grounded theory: objectivist and constructivist methods', in N.K. Denzin and Y.S. Lincoln (eds), *Strategies of Qualitative Inquiry*. Thousand Oaks, CA: Sage.

Clarkson, L. (2003) 'Documentary sources', in R.L. Miller and J.D. Brewer (eds), *The A–Z of Social Research*. London: Sage.

Corti, L. (2003) 'Documentary sources', in R.L. Miller and J.D. Brewer (eds), *The A–Z of Social Research*. London: Sage.

Coxon, A.P.M. (1996) *Between the Sheets: Sexual Diaries and Gay Men's Sex in the Era of AIDS*. London: Cassell.

Crossley, M.L. (2003) '"Let me explain": narrative employment and one patient's experience of oral cancer', *Social Science and Medicine*, 56: 439–48.

Diamond, J. (2001) *Snake Oil and Other Preoccupations*. London: Vintage.

Elliott, H. (1997) 'The use of diaries in sociological research on health experience', *Sociological Research Online*, 2(2). Available at: http://www.socresonline.org.uk/socres online/2/2/7.html

Geertz, C. (1988) *Works and Lives: The Anthropologist as Author*. Cambridge: Polity Press.

Griffiths, H. and Jordan, S. (1998) 'Thinking of the future and walking back to normal: an exploratory study of patients' experiences during recovery from lower limb fracture', *Journal of Advanced Nursing*, 28: 1276–88.

Honkasalo, M.-J. (2006) 'Fragilities in life and death', *Health, Risk and Society*, 8(1): 27–41.

Jones, R.H. and Candlin, C.N. (2003) 'Constructing risk across timescales and trajectories: gay men's stories of sexual encounters', *Health, Risk and Society*, 5: 199–213.

Jones, R.H., Kwan, Y.K. and Candlin, C.N. (2000) *A Preliminary Investigation of HIV Vulnerability and Risk Behavior among Men who have Sex with Men in Hong Kong*. Hong Kong: City University of Hong Kong.

Jordanova, L. (2000) *History in Practice*. London: Arnold.

MacFarlane, A. (1970) *The Family Life of Ralph Josselin: A Seventeenth-Century Clergyman: An Essay in Historical Anthropology*. Cambridge: Cambridge University Press.

Malinowski, B. (1989) *A Diary in the Strict Sense of the Word*. London: Athlone.

Miller, K.A. (1985) *Emigrants and Exiles: Ireland and the Irish Exodus to North America*. New York: Oxford University Press.

Moser. C.A. and Kalton, C. (1971) *Survey Methods in Social Investigation*. London: Heinemann.

Parkin, D., Rice, N., Jacoby, A. and Doughty, J. (2004) 'Use of a visual analogue scale in a daily patient diary: modelling cross-sectional time-series data on health-related quality of life', *Social Science and Medicine*, 59: 351–60.

Penn Library (2004) *Finding Diaries – Research Guide*. Available at: http://gethelp.library. upenn.edu/guides/general/diaries.html

Plummer, K. (2001) *Documents of Life 2: An Invitation to Critical Humanism*. London: Sage.

Pollock, L.A. (1983) *Forgotten Children: Parent–child Relations from 1500 to 1900*. Cambridge: Cambridge University Press.

Read, K.E. (1965) *The High Valley*. New York: Scribner.

Robinson, D. (1971) *The Process of Becoming Ill*. London: Routledge and Kegan Paul.

Sahlins, M. (1995) *How 'Natives' Think: About Captain Cook, For Example*. Chicago: University of Chicago Press.

Sheridan, D. (ed.) (1991) *The Mass-Observation Diaries: An Introduction*. The Mass-Observation Archive (University of Sussex Library) and the Centre for Continuing Education, Falmer: University of Sussex. Available at: http://www.sussex.ac.uk/ library/massobs/diaries_1939-65.html and http://www.sussex.ac.uk/library/massobs/ diary_booklet.html

Stone, A.A., Shiffman, S., Schwartz, J.E., Broderick, J.E. and Hufford, M.R. (2003) 'Patient compliance with paper and electronic diaries', *Controlled Clinical Trials*, 24: 182–99.

Thomas, W.I. and Znaniecki, F. (1958) *The Polish Peasant in Europe and America*, Volume 1. New York: Dover.

WW2 People's War Team (2004) *About WW2 People's War*. Available at: http:// www.bbc.co.uk/dna/ww2/About

Zimmerman, D.H. and Wieder, D.L. (1977) 'The diary-interview method', *Urban Life*, 5: 479–98.

5

Unstructured Interviews and Health Research

JACQUELINE LOW

INTRODUCTION

The unstructured interview, also referred to as the in-depth, the open-ended, the narrative or the long interview, has become a favoured method in research into health and health care (Miczo 2003; Silverman 1998). This is the case not only in the social sciences but also, to the extent that 'lay knowledge' has been deemed essential to the development of health policy and practice, in the field of nursing (Sorrell and Redmond 1995) and evidence-based medical and other clinical research (Boulton et al. 1996). The methodological techniques employed in the unstructured interview are standard irrespective of context (Booth and Booth 1996). However, in health research, especially where there are sensitive issues or vulnerable informants, the researcher faces particular challenges (Corbin and Morse 2003).

In this chapter, the advantages of the unstructured interview as a technique are explored, followed by an account of the stages of a project using this method. Issues of data collection and techniques for data analysis are considered. The validity and reliability of this form of research are discussed and a checklist provided for ways of demonstrating its rigour. A final section indicates how to present research findings in such a way that enhances their credibility, followed by a case study.

THE ADVANTAGES OF USING THE UNSTRUCTURED INTERVIEW

The unstructured interview has certain advantages over survey research and the structured interview. As discussed in Chapter 2, while these methods set out with particular questions in mind to test a particular hypothesis, interpretivist or constructivist theoretical perspectives using qualitative methods provide access to the subjective perceptions of individuals, as well as the means by which they give meaning to their experiences. For example, a survey can furnish data concerning the number and demographic characteristics of people with a chronic illness, but can tell us little about the experience of living with chronic illness or the kinds of service that people think would be most appropriate to meet their needs as they perceive them.

One such interpretivist or constructivist method is the unstructured interview that many argue is the best way to gain access to the experience of health and illness where people already feel disempowered by their illness. It is an essential tool too in gathering data from people who, due to illness and/or disability, may be physically unable to participate in other types of research. For instance, Higgins and Daly (1999) used unstructured interviews successfully with people on mechanical ventilation.

Corbin and Morse (2003) have discussed with clarity the advantages of the unstructured interview and these can be summarized as follows:

- It is a cost-effective way of collecting a great deal of data in a relatively short time frame.
- It is useful when exploring research areas where little is known or which are complex.
- It can address how and why questions from the perspective of subjective experience: that is, it allows researchers to explore the perceptions of individuals and how they give meaning to, or interpret, their experiences.
- It is flexible. It allows the researcher to follow the lead of the interviewee into how they construct particular phenomena, pursue emergent themes and thus gain new insights.
- The pace of the interview can be adjusted throughout. This is particularly useful in dealing with people on matters of health and illness. For example, people may be ill, beginning to feel tired or may be in pain.
- It allows the researcher the opportunity to seek ongoing informed consent – this is important when dealing with sensitive issues in research in health and illness (Miczo 2003).
- It can give voice to the lay perspective (Low 2003), an important consideration in health and illness both from the perspective of the health professional and the research perspective.
- It gives informants more power and control over what gets discussed in the interview, and how it gets discussed.

THE STAGES OF RESEARCH USING AN UNSTRUCTURED INTERVIEW TECHNIQUE

Having decided on the questions you wish to address in your research as well as having carried out a literature review resulting in the decision that an unstructured interview is the best method to use, there are a number of steps in planning the research. The first step is to recruit informants.

Recruiting research participants

Most commonly, 'purposeful' sampling is used where informants are selected who have specific knowledge about the research question (Glaser and Strauss 1967). This is made easier if informants are members of a pre-existing group or if they congregate at one locale (Johnson 2002). Alternatively, physicians' organizations, and particularly a health consumer group such as the Multiple Sclerosis Society, might be approached in order to make contact with potential informants. Hospital administrators could also be asked for help in recruiting health personnel to participate in health service research. In a situation where the contact is not being made directly by a researcher, a two-stage process should be followed. The third party has privileged access to people's names and addresses. In the first instance, they should approach the individuals concerned with an outline of the project and what it would involve, to ask if they would be prepared to take part. Only when permission has been received should details be given to a researcher. Chapter 15 discusses this and other ethical issues in research further.

However, in many cases, there simply is no setting in which to recruit people to take part in interviews, unstructured or otherwise. For example, when I first began researching the lay use of alternative therapies in Canada, there were few holistic health centres and, as I did not want to limit my analysis to the clients of any one alternative practitioner, there was no one setting in which to recruit informants (Low 2004a). I therefore had to use a combination of snowball sampling (that is, asking one informant to suggest another) and convenience sampling (that is, contacting known, rather than randomly selected, informants) in making contact. The technique of sampling is discussed further in Chapter 9. Using 'insider awareness', where the researcher has personal experience of the substantive topic or social world under study, I began convenience sampling by approaching an acquaintance who had used alternative health care (Douglas 1976). Snowball sampling occurred at the end of each interview when I asked informants if they knew of anyone else who would be interested in taking part in the study. Researchers should keep track in field notes of how they have made contact with informants as well as noting the nature of any relationships between informants. They can then differentiate in their analysis between patterns that reflect friendship or other related networks from more general patterns in the data (Low 2004a).

Decisions must also be made about how many informants to recruit as well as how many interviews to conduct. For instance, in grounded theory research it is the concept or the basic item being counted or studied, not the informant, which is the unit of analysis. Theoretically, therefore, one interview is sufficient provided it is adequate in terms of conceptual richness. In reality, however, one interview is seldom enough. A commonly used guideline is that at least 20 to 30 informants should be interviewed and reinterviewed. In narrative analysis, and some types of linguistic or discourse analyses, the number of interviews is typically very small. Nonetheless, enough data must be collected to enable the researcher to reach 'theoretic saturation'. Theoretic saturation is satisfied when no new information is generated by subsequent interviews, and when the data reflect a conceptual richness that both accounts for 'variations' in the data and allows for detailed description of the 'processes' informants experience – as well as enabling the researcher exhaustively to analyze the relationships between concepts and the categories identified (Glaser and Strauss 1967; Strauss and Corbin 1990).

Structuring the unstructured interview

As the name suggests, unstructured interviews do not follow a set path, but may vary in length and/or richness. However, in practice there is no interview that is totally devoid of structure. At the very least it must be informed by a research question or questions and researchers should have some idea of how they will begin the interview. The questions employed in the unstructured interview should be open ended and as non-directive as possible. McCracken (1988) likens this type of interview to a conversation where the researcher says as little as possible, allowing informants to tell their stories in their own fashion. The unstructured interview is a dynamic event that 'often takes unexpected turns or digressions that follow the informant's interest or knowledge' (Johnson 2002: 111). Both the informant and the researcher are deeply involved in the emergent narrative.

The unstructured interview typically opens with a 'grand tour' question (McCracken 1988). These are questions that encourage informants to begin speaking without directing the content or substance of their discourse. For instance, a researcher might begin by saying something like: 'tell me about your experiences with ...'. Subsequent questions are based on what the informant says and prompts are used to support informants in telling their stories, and to solicit further information, clarification or explanation. According to McCracken (1988), 'floating prompts' like features of everyday speech – such as eyebrow raises or repetition of a keyword – are used to maintain the flow of responses without undue interruption of their narrative. In contrast, planned prompts, or probes, are used when further explanation is required, or when the researcher wishes to delve deeper (Crabtree and Miller 1991). Recapitulation probes are also used where informants are asked to 'retell parts of stories'. In so doing, they may add new details (Sorrell and Redmond 1995). When to prompt is a matter of researcher judgement. Some researchers choose to wait until the interview is complete before probing, as they believe that any type of interruption of the informant's speech will affect the meaning of the findings (Corbin and Morse 2003). Demographic characteristics such as age, sex, class and ethnic background should be listed after informal conversation as this aids the development of trust and rapport between the researcher and informant.

The researcher must also be aware of the implications of silences in the unstructured interview (Sorrell and Redmond 1995). As Charmaz (2002: 303) points out:

> Not all experiences are storied, nor are all experiences stored for ready recall. Silences have meaning too. Silences signify an absence — of words and/or perceivable emotions ... [and] may ... reflect active signals — of meaning, boundaries, and rules.

Silences may also indicate that the informant is becoming tired, that illness and/or disability is compromising their ability to speak, or that they are in pain. Silence may also indicate a breach of communication norms. For example, something the researcher says may literally 'silence' the informant. Finally, informants may silence the researcher as well when they decline to answer a question (Charmaz 2002). The researcher therefore must listen carefully and prompt judiciously in response to what informants say, or do not say. Silences should be noted and accounted for in the analysis.

Resourcing the interview

For unstructured interviews both technical and interpersonal skills are required, as well as access to resources. One such resource is willing and informed research participants. Not all potential informants have sufficient motive or interest to participate in an unstructured interview given the greater commitment in terms of time and emotional energy required (Johnson 2002). Furthermore, not all informants are articulate and not all interviews result in an equally high degree of conceptual richness (Charmaz 2002). However, it would be a mistake for the researcher to equate succinct responses with a lack of richness of the data, especially in cases where illness or disability constrain the informant's speech. As Booth and Booth (1996: 66) argue, 'it is possible for people to communicate a story in one word answers. Even single words can leave a big wash.'

If the unstructured interview requires more of informants, it also requires more from the researcher. Glaser and Strauss (1967) argue that researchers must develop 'theoretic sensitivity' so that they can judge when theoretic saturation and conceptual richness have been reached. Furthermore, locating and contacting informants, especially in medical settings, can be difficult as it requires reserves of energy and ingenuity. Unstructured interviews also mean that researchers need to invest more of themselves, including their emotions (Charmaz 2002). Corbin and Morse (2003: 344) argue that unstructured interviewers 'become involved in the story and reach out with empathy to participants'. Consequently, this method is always demanding and can often be exhausting for the researcher.

COLLECTING AND ANALYZING UNSTRUCTURED INTERVIEW DATA

Recording data

It is important to audio-tape the unstructured interview as an informant's words must be presented verbatim in the analysis to preserve meaning (Johnson 2002). However, there are situations where audio taping is difficult. An informant may refuse to give permission for a tape recorder to be used or the interview might take place in a location not conducive to audio taping. In these cases, researchers must use their note-taking skills during and after the interview to preserve as much of the informant's actual words as possible. Field notes should also be taken that include non-verbal aspects of the interview such as facial expressions, body language, the setting and informant/researcher interaction, as these may affect the interpretation (Miczo 2003). Silverman (1998) advocates the use of video taping to record better the interactive aspects of the unstructured interview. However, this may be felt to be too intrusive and to jeopardize confidentiality.

Allowing time

A fundamental resource required using the unstructured interview technique is time. Setting up and conducting interviews, and particularly transcribing and analyzing data, are time-greedy activities.

Time is required to recruit informants, schedule interviews and allow for reinterviews. In health research more time may be required as, for example, informants with chronic illnesses may tire easily and several short interviews may be necessary. Analysis of the vast amount of data which results from unstructured interviews is also time consuming. Unstructured interviews are long, and transcription of one audio-taped interview can take 'several hours … generat[ing] 20–40 pages of single-spaced text' (Pope et al. 2000: 114). Crabtree and Miller (1991: 148–9) report that it took them up to six hours 'to highlight and make notations on a twenty-four page transcript' when using a fairly simple coding scheme. More complex methods of coding, such as comparative coding, where transcripts are read and reread several times throughout the analysis, can take much longer.

Methods for data analysis

Discussions about how to analyze, like making decisions about how to collect, unstructured interview data are informed by the theoretical assumptions held by the researcher (Kvale 1996). For instance, if the researcher is aiming to develop a grounded theory, analytic induction is a technique for deriving theory from empirical research, in contrast to a deductive approach, where data are collected to support or refute an existing theory. In this case, theoretic sampling from the data collected and comparative coding are the forms of analysis modes employed. According to Glaser and Strauss (1967: 45), theoretic sampling is a method by which 'the analyst jointly collects, codes, and analyzes … data and decides what data to collect next and where to find them, in order to develop … theory as it emerges'. Open coding is 'the process of breaking down, examining, comparing, conceptualizing, and categorizing data' (Corbin and Strauss 1990: 61; also see Chapter 6). For example, in research that I conducted with people who use alternative therapies, an alternative model of health emerged through the process of comparative coding. This model is made up of the interconnected categories of holism, balance and control. Through the process of comparative coding the category of balance was broken down into the concepts of balance in the body and balance in the self (Low 2004a).

  Other theoretical approaches dictate other types of coding. For instance, Baker (2002: 778) asserts that within ethnomethodology, informants' stories are understood 'as accounts rather than reports'. Such analysis therefore involves coding individuals' explanations for their beliefs and behaviour. Depending on the mode of analysis followed, the style of transcription will also vary. Thus, in the case of narrative analysis transcription, this will include the recording of pauses, hesitations, timing of responses and other linguistic devices, in addition to the words spoken by the informant. This is so the analyst is able to discern how a text is structured and organized in order to bring out its meaning (Kvale 1996).

Data coding

Regardless of the particular mode of analysis chosen, coding of unstructured interviews takes the form of a thematic content analysis. More specifically, it is the rigorous and systematic analysis of data that results in the development of concepts and categories that emerge from the words of informants, culminating in the development of explanatory models – what Glaser and Strauss (1967) would call 'formal theory' (Silverman 1998). This kind of content analysis means more than merely counting occurrences of key terms. Rather, the researcher analyzing unstructured interviews more often codes for similarity of meaning as the words informants use in expressing themselves are hardly ever exactly the same. That they are rarely the same, however, does not mean that they are not consistent in terms of their conceptual meaning. For example, in my analysis of the lay model of alternative health and healing, one informant used the words 'inner self' while another spoke about her 'higher self', but what they were both talking about was the importance of drawing on their own spiritual power to heal themselves (Low 2004a).

How the researcher goes about the practical task of coding and categorizing is a matter of preference. Some highlight transcripts; others use word processing search, copy and paste functions; still others photocopy and physically cut up the transcripts to categorize data. Qualitative computer software can also be of use in the coding and categorizing phase of analysis. However, it is important to be aware that qualitative analysis software such as *Ethnograph* or *NUD*IST* does not do the conceptual or analytic work. The researcher must still develop concepts and categories by reading and rereading the transcripts and making analytic notes. Software merely helps in storing, moving and collating large amounts of text-based data – to paraphrase Silverman (1998): 'garbage in, garbage out'.

Regardless of the type of analysis or the practical method of coding employed, attention must be paid in the analysis to divergent themes: what some researchers call 'deviant cases' (Silverman 1998). This is essential for capturing the conceptual richness and validity of unstructured interview findings (Corbin and Strauss 1990). For instance, only one participant in my research on the users of alternative health care said that a desire for control over her healing process motivated her use of these therapies. This was significant as it allowed me critically to address assumptions in the literature about what motivates people to seek out alternative health care (Low 2004a). It is also important to pay attention to discordant elements or seeming contradictions within the discourse of informants as they can give insight into its deeper meaning (Corbin and Morse 2003). Divergent cases can also illuminate the way in which an informant's story has been influenced by the researcher (Miczo 2003).

ENHANCING RIGOUR: VALIDITY, RELIABILITY AND GENERALIZABILITY

Silverman (1998) argues that attention to the historical, cultural, political and contextual grounding of informant discourse is necessary to enhance the reliability, validity and generalizability of the findings from unstructured interview research. Analyses must be situated in the historical context and the political factors behind informants' experiences must be addressed. Attention must also be paid to how cultural constructs and discourses are both reflected in, and shape, informants' beliefs and action. For example, Lupton and Chapman (1995) ground their analysis of media coverage of the role played by cholesterol in heart disease in the socio-cultural context of contemporary discourses about food as being healthy or unhealthy. Contextual grounding refers to the fact that social phenomena take on a variety of meanings in different contexts and that individuals construct contexts for their actions. Thus analyses of unstructured interview data must also take account of how salient aspects of informants' personal biographies shape their experience and behaviour (Lupton 1997). For instance, health status, such as living with chronic illness, may be one such biographical factor that shapes experiences, perceptions and actions (Low 2004b).

Validity

The validity of unstructured interview findings centres on the richness of the data that are generated by this method. The information disclosed by informants is so detailed that it guards against:

> bias by making it difficult for [informants] to produce data that uniformly support a mistaken conclusion, just as [it makes] it difficult for observers to restrict [their] observations so that [they] see only what supports [their] prejudices and expectations. (Becker 1970a: 52)

This richness derives, in part, from the fact that the researcher allows the informant to direct the flow of conversation, saying as little as possible. This bolsters the validity of the finding as statements volunteered by informants are 'likely to reflect the observer's preoccupations and possible biases less than [those] made in response to questions posed by the researcher' (Becker 1970b: 193). Furthermore, the non-directive nature of open-ended questions enhances validity as informants are able to articulate their experiences, rather than having to conform to predetermined answer categories imposed by the researcher (Cicourel 1982). It has been said by advocates of this method that unstructured interview data are not valid or invalid in relation to 'objective' truth. Instead, the unstructured interview is seen as a 'social occasion' (Johnson 2002) governed by power relations and rules of communication (Miczo 2003). The narrative or story which emerges from the unstructured interview is one which is jointly constructed between the researcher and the informant, making it both 'process and product' of that interaction (Charmaz 2002).

Reliability

The quantitative notion of reliability, that research instruments 'continually yield an unvarying measurement', is not only inappropriate to research employing the unstructured interview, but also impossible to achieve using this method (Kirk and Miller 1986: 42). This is because the social world is dynamic, not static. Consequently, two researchers who interview the same informant at different times using the same questions will invariably collect different data (Becker 1970a). However, this should not be taken as an indication that the unstructured interview method is unreliable. Rather, it is that the social context and the informant's perspective have changed over time. The unstructured interview, though, must satisfy the standards of synchronic reliability – 'the similarity of observations within the same time period' – as well as the consistency of observations with regard to the researcher's conceptual concerns (Kirk and Miller 1986: 42). More simply, the words that informants use will rarely be the same, yet they can still be conceptually consistent.

Techniques to enhance validity and reliability so that the reader can assess the overall credibility of the findings are:

- Audio taping interviews and taking comprehensive field notes.
- Systematic transcription and analysis allowing others to assess how researchers have analyzed their data and developed theoretic constructs.
- Triangulation, or using a combination of methods, with other sources of information, such as observation or documentary analysis (see Chapter 6 and Chapter 16 for discussions of triangulation).
- Using inter-judge or inter-rater techniques. Here more than one researcher codes the transcripts. Comparing coding can increase consistency, reliability and validity in coding and subsequent analysis.
- Using a 'member test' or informant validation. Here analysis and early findings are assessed through the informant's confirmation that these reflect accurately their perspectives and experiences.

Generalizability

However valid and reliable the findings from unstructured interview research are, the analyst must also pay attention to the nature of the generalizations that can be made from the findings. For instance, what Williams (2000) refers to as 'moderatum generalization' or 'generalizations about every-day life' are appropriate to research where the intention is theoretic or conceptual, rather than statistical generalization. This is where an informant's individual perceptions, beliefs and experiences can be seen as indicators of larger socio-cultural features or generic social processes (Blumer 1969). Williams (2000: 215) illustrates what he means by moderatum generalization by invoking Geertz's classic ethnographic analysis of the cockfight, in writing:

> Geertz's claim … 'that every people loves its own form of violence' is an example of such a general feature, which is then reworked and enriched through the specific inferences about the [particular] 'cockfight'.

PRESENTING UNSTRUCTURED INTERVIEW FINDINGS

Techniques to ensure credibility

How the findings from unstructured interview analysis are presented impacts directly on the credibility of the research. For example, informants' speech should be used verbatim in presentation of the findings as rewording or summarizing inevitably reduces validity by changing the meaning of words. It also detracts from the reliability of the findings as readers cannot assess the validity of the data for themselves. Research questions in addition to informant responses should also ideally be presented as answers that are inextricably linked to the questions to which they are a response. Furthermore, in order to allow the reader to assess their validity, an indication should be given of whether or not the concepts and categories presented in the findings emerged from the actual words of the informants or are researcher constructs.

Sufficient informant quotations must also be included such that readers are able to evaluate the findings (Boulton et al. 1996). Here, it is important that researchers indicate if the quotations selected are representative of some, many or all of the participants in the research. Researchers must also make plain how contradictory cases have been accounted for. To this end Silverman (1998) argues that counts of 'events-quasi statistics' should be included in presentations. However, others caution that presenting findings in the form of percentages or relative frequencies may be misleading when the findings are derived from a small number of interviews (Pope et al. 2000). In contrast, presenting precise counts can sometimes be important. The finding, for instance, that only 1 out of 21 informants in my study of the lay use of alternative therapies said that they had a desire for control over health and healing was essential to the credibility of my conclusion that the generic social process of problem solving, not individual motivating factors, better explained informants' health-seeking behaviour.

Demonstrating credibility in presentations

Demonstrating credibility in presentations can be achieved through the following:

- Setting out the theoretical perspective taken in the study.
- Giving detailed descriptions in research reports or publications of how reliability and validity have been ensured.
- Including excerpts from field notes that describe how the data were collected, transcribed and analyzed to provide a paper trail.

Including all of the aspects of the unstructured interview method described above can fill several pages of the article or report in which researchers write up their findings. Consequently, researchers should be aware that many journals, especially medical and nursing journals, typically publish very short articles. Editors of such journals may object to lengthy methodology sections or to the inclusion of the large amount of data necessary adequately to present the findings. This may inhibit the publication of qualitative studies (Boulton et al. 1996). It may therefore be wise for health researchers using this method to include, in the covering letter accompanying their submission for publication, the argument that such information is essential to the assessment by both referees and readers of the reliability and validity of the study. The publication process is discussed more generally in Chapter 21.

THE WEAKNESSES OF THE UNSTRUCTURED INTERVIEW METHOD

While conducting unstructured interviewing can be more cost effective than survey research, a corresponding weakness of the method is the greater amount of time invested in the analysis of unstructured interview data compared with statistical analysis. In addition, Silverman (1998) concludes that the unstructured interview should never be used as a substitute for observation, calling into question its usefulness as a stand-alone method. He asserts that while unstructured interviews are an effective method of gathering data about what people say, they are less useful as a means of capturing what they do. However, what people say about what they do provides valid and useful information, as an account of their experience of what they do. As Trow (1970) convincingly argues, observation and interviewing are different methods that measure different things. One is not inherently better than the other.

Silverman (1998) also asserts that a weakness of the unstructured interview method is that the data collected are retrospective. It is an informant's description of event(s) that happened in the past and therefore cannot be an accurate account of their experience at the actual time the event(s) occurred. However, the moment we experience something it becomes part of our past, thus we always make sense of our lives retrospectively. In the end, all methods have strengths and weaknesses. Good researchers are aware of them and use their informed judgement in selecting the method appropriate to the research question at hand. This applies no less to the use of unstructured interviews in health research.

Case study: **The use of unstructured interviews in alternative and complementary health care**

The research I conducted on how people assess the efficacy of the alternative and complementary therapies is illustrative of many of the methodological issues already discussed in this chapter. In this study I used the unstructured interview method to collect data from people with Parkinson's disease who used alternative and complementary health care. In addition to the symptoms of Parkinson's disease and the adverse reactions caused by Parkinson's medication, some of the people I spoke with also experienced difficulty with verbal and non-verbal communication (Lesser and Whitworth 1999). Thus, having Parkinson's disease is a salient aspect of these informants' personal biographies that needed to be taken account of in recruitment, data collection and analysis.

Contacting informants

I was able to make contact with informants through the pre-existing groups of the Parkinson's Disease Society (1999) and Young, Alert, Parkinson's Partners and Relatives. In the end, 14 people were eligible to participate in the interviews, a relatively small number of informants. However, this did not present a problem concerning the generalizability of my findings as the data collected were conceptually rich and my intent was to develop a theoretical explanation of how these people determined efficacy, not to make statistical generalizations about how people assess efficacy.

(Continued)

Conducting interviews

This research demonstrated the flexibility of the unstructured interview approach to data collection which allowed me to start and stop the interviews in responding to informants when they became tired, were experiencing pain, and when the effectiveness of their medication began to wear off. Moreover, the method also proved invaluable in coping with the communication difficulties that occurred during some of these interviews. This flexibility meant that there was more scope for probing for clarification; repeating questions or keywords; and checking and rechecking that we had understood each other.

Some communication difficulties resulted in several virtually unintelligible portions of the taped interviews, reinforcing the need to take systematic field notes in addition to audio taping. Transcription and analysis of the interviews took much longer than anticipated as it was necessary to verify with informants that I had interpreted their voices correctly. This also meant noting the length of informant pauses, the types of questions that generated problems in communication, and informant requests for repetition. The symptoms of Parkinson's disease also impacted on the nature of the data collected. Some interviews were quite short and, due to speech difficulties, some informant responses were very brief. However, it was possible to probe in order to expand upon brief responses (Low 2006).

Selecting deviant cases

Finally, the importance of accounting for contradictory cases, and attention to contextual grounding, in the analysis of unstructured interview data was highlighted by this research. Through the process of comparative coding, for instance, I noted that some informants believed that a therapy is effective if it works for one person — arguing that, even if it did not work for them, it might for someone else. In seeming contradiction, they also believed that therapies need to work for most people to be considered efficacious. However, what appeared to be a contradiction was actually a reflection of these informants' internalization of both an alternative healing ideology, which posits an individual notion of efficacy, and the view that the state-subsidized health service lacks the funds to provide services that do not work for all (Low 2003).

CONCLUSION

The strengths and weaknesses of unstructured interviews in health research have been covered in this chapter – along with the issues that they raise in practice in the various stages of research, from recruiting research partici- pants and resourcing the interviews to analyzing the data and presenting the research findings. These highlight that unstructured interviews can be extremely helpful as a qualitative research method, but are not as straightfor- ward to carry out as first meets the eye. The contrast with more structured interview approaches can be made by referring to Chapter 10 in this volume which covers quantitative survey methods in health research. It is hoped, though, that this chapter will help the reader to negotiate some of the poten- tial challenges of unstructured interviews – not least with reference to the brief case study on their use in alternative and complementary health care. Questions now follow in a practical exercise which should further highlight the benefits and limitations of the method and the issues that it poses, specif- ically in the context of research into the experience of burns.

Exercise: The use of unstructured interviews to conduct research into the experience of burns

Using the unstructured interview, you intend to conduct research focused on how individuals who have suffered serious burns experience and cope with pain. The burns have left those concerned with severe scaring over large portions of their bodies. Address the following questions:

1 How would you go about purposeful sampling in this research?
2 What problems would you anticipate in recruiting informants for your study?
3 How many informants would you need to participate in the interviews?
4 What kind of probing questions do you anticipate would be useful in interviews with these informants?
5 What aspects of informant biographies would you have to be aware of?
6 What particular socio-cultural, historical and political contexts would you have to ground your analysis in?

(Continued)

7 How might class, gender, stigma and cultural notions of beauty, among other contextual factors, shape the experiences of your informants?
8 In addition to unstructured interviews, are there other sources of data you could draw on in increasing the validity, reliability and generalizability of your analysis?

RECOMMENDED FURTHER READING

Corbin, J. and Morse, J.M. (2003) 'The unstructured interactive interview: issues of reciprocity and risks when dealing with sensitive topics', *Qualitative Inquiry*, 9 (3): 335–54.
This is a very focused article that highlights the issues that make aspects of unstructured interviewing unique in the context of health research.

Gubrium, J.F. and Holstein, J.A. (eds) (2002) *Handbook of Interview Research: Context and Method*. Thousand Oaks, CA: Sage.
This is an accessible and comprehensive text covering the unstructured interview method in general.

McCracken, G. (1988) *The Long Interview*. Newbury Park, CA: Sage.
This is a classic book on the unstructured interview, in which unstructured interview techniques such as probing are very nicely described and explained.

REFERENCES

Baker, C.D. (2002) 'Ethnomethodological analyses of interviews', in J.F. Gubrium and J.A. Holstein (eds), *Handbook of Interview Research: Context and Method*. Thousand Oaks, CA: Sage.
Becker, H.S. (1970a) *Sociological Work: Method and Substance*. Chicago: Aldine.
Becker, H.S. (1970b) 'Problems of inference and proof in participant observation', in W.J. Filstead (ed.), *Qualitative Methodology: Firsthand Involvement with the Social World*. Chicago: Markham.
Blumer, H. (1969) *Symbolic Interactionism: Perspective and Method*. Englewood Cliffs, NJ: Prentice Hall.
Booth, T. and Booth, W. (1996) 'Sounds of silence: narrative research with inarticulate subjects', *Disability and Society*, 11: 55–69.

Boulton, M., Fitzpatrick, R. and Swinburn, C. (1996) 'Qualitative research in health care: II. A structured review and evaluation of studies', *Journal of Evaluation in Clinical Practice*, 2(3): 171–79.

Charmaz, K. (2002) 'Stories and silences: disclosures and self in chronic illness', *Qualitative Inquiry*, 8(3): 302–28.

Cicourel, A.V. (1982) 'Interviews, surveys, and the problem of ecological validity', *American Sociologist*, 17: 11–20.

Corbin, J. and Morse, J.M. (2003) 'The unstructured interactive interview: issues of reciprocity and risks when dealing with sensitive topics', *Qualitative Inquiry*, 9(3): 335–54.

Corbin, J.M. and Strauss, A.L. (1990) 'Grounded theory research: procedures, canons, and evaluative criteria', *Qualitative Sociology*, 13(1): 3–21.

Crabtree, B. and Miller, W.L. (1991) 'A qualitative approach to primary care research: the long interview', *Family Medicine*, 23(2): 145–51.

Douglas, J.D. (1976) *Investigative Social Research: Individual and Team Research*. Beverley Hills, CA: Sage.

Glaser, B.G. and Strauss, A.L. (1967) *The Discovery of Grounded Theory: Strategies for Qualitative Research*. Chicago: Aldine.

Higgins, P.A. and Daly, B.J. (1999) 'Research methodology issues related to interviewing the mechanically ventilated patient', *Western Journal of Nursing Research*, 21: 773–84.

Johnson, J.M. (2002) 'In-depth interviewing', in J.F. Gubrium and J.A. Holstein (eds), *Handbook of Interview Research: Context and Method*. Thousand Oaks, CA: Sage.

Kirk, J. and Miller, M.L. (1986) *Reliability and Validity in Qualitative Research*. Newbury Park, CA: Sage.

Kvale, S. (1996) *Interviewing: An Introduction to Qualitative Research Interviewing*. Thousand Oaks, CA: Sage.

Lesser, R. and Whitworth, A. (1999) 'Communication in Parkinson's with cognitive impairment: a diagnostic and therapeutic medium?', in R. Percival and P. Hobson (eds), *Parkinson's Disease: Studies in Psychological and Social Care*. Leicester: British Psychological Society Books.

Low, J. (2003) 'Lay assessments of the efficacy of alternative/complementary therapies: a challenge to medical and expert dominance?', *Journal of Evidence-based Integrative Medicine*, 1(1): 65–76.

Low, J. (2004a) *Using Alternative Therapies: A Qualitative Analysis*. Toronto: Canadian Scholar's Press.

Low, J. (2004b) 'Managing safety and risk: the experiences of people with Parkinson's disease who use alternative and complementary therapies', *Health: An Interdisciplinary Journal for the Study of Health, Illness and Medicine*, 8(4): 445–63.

Low, J. (2006) 'Communication problems between researchers and informants with speech difficulties: methodological and analytical issues', *Field Methods*, 18(2): 153–71.

Lupton, D. (1997) 'Consumerism, reflexivity and the medical encounter', *Social Science and Medicine*, 45(3): 373–81.

Lupton, D. and Chapman, S. (1995) '"A healthy lifestyle might be the death of you": discourses on diet, cholesterol control and heart disease in press and among the lay public', *Sociology of Health and Illness*, 17(4): 477–94.

McCracken, G. (1988) *The Long Interview*. Newbury Park, CA: Sage.

Miczo, N. (2003) 'Beyond the fetishism of words: considerations on the use of the interview to gather chronic illness narratives', *Qualitative Health Research*, 13 (4): 469–90.

Parkinson's Disease Society (1999) *The Drug Treatment of Parkinson's Disease: For People with Parkinson's and their Families*. London: Parkinson's Disease Society.

Pope, C., Ziebland, S. and Mays, N. (2000) 'Qualitative research in health care: analysing qualitative data', *British Medical Journal*, 320: 114–16.

Silverman, D. (1998) 'The quality of qualitative health research: the open-ended interview and its alternative', *Social Sciences in Health*, 4(2): 104–18.

Sorrell, M.J. and Redmond, G.M. (1995) 'Interview in qualitative nursing research: differing approaches for ethnographic and phenomenological studies', *Journal of Advanced Nursing*, 21: 1117–22.

Strauss, A.L. and Corbin, J. (1990) *Basics of Qualitative Research: Grounded Theory Procedures and Techniques*. Newbury Park, CA: Sage.

Trow, M. (1970) 'Comment on participant observation and interviewing: a comparison', in W.J. Filstead (ed.), *Qualitative methodology: Firsthand Involvement with the Social World*. Chicago: Markham.

Williams, M. (2000) 'Interpretivism and generalisation', *Sociology*, 34(2): 209–24.

6

Participant Observation in Health Research

DAVID HUGHES

INTRODUCTION

This chapter considers the method of participant observation (PO) in health care settings. The term PO is sometimes used interchangeably with 'sociological ethnography', although ethnography is a broader category that includes methods such as the ethnographic interview and the analysis of cultural artefacts, as well as observation. PO is one of the oldest and least 'high-tech' research methods, emphasizing as it does the importance of gathering data through observing, interacting with, and listening to, the human subjects under study. The participant observer typically spends an extended period of time in a natural setting, such as a hospital ward or an intensive care unit, following the activities of staff members, observing particular classes of activities, or generally 'hanging out' with a view to understanding what is going on. It is this requirement for the researcher to participate in social interaction as part of the research process that separates PO from the systematic observational methods used in psychology and organizational studies where the observer simply looks on and records (Emerson 1981; McCall 1984). In consequence, there is an extensive literature on field relations and the participant observer role. Although naturalistic observation takes many forms and involves varying degrees of participation, all PO methods share the need to manage social interaction with subjects in the field (Gold 1958).

This chapter examines the characteristics of PO and the types of study that have been carried out in health care settings. It looks at the strengths and weaknesses of the approach, the methods and techniques for collecting, coding and analyzing data, and identifying and writing up findings, and presents a case study to illustrate how the method was used in practice.

THE CHARACTERISTICS OF PARTICIPANT OBSERVATION

Almost all recent PO research takes the form of a case study where there is intense observation in a specific setting. PO would not, for example, undertake an investigation of the ecology of a city nor would it be the method of choice to examine the characteristics of a geographically dispersed social group. In the health field, most PO studies examine a patient or staff group or particular social processes associated with selected settings, such as the emergency ambulance service, the accident and emergency department, the outpatient clinic, hospital ward, hospice or the nursing home. A typical study might last between six months and two years, with the researcher spending several observation periods each week in the setting. Usually a period of relatively unfocused fieldwork, where the researcher 'feels out' the setting and attempts to develop an appropriate field role, will be followed by a strategy to spread observations between different categories of subjects and aspects of activity that need to be covered.

Typically, access will be negotiated first with senior staff who act as formal gatekeepers to the setting, and then with the various levels of actors who will be the subjects of the study. Usually access will need to be maintained or renewed on an ongoing basis, so that it will remain a preoccupation throughout the period of fieldwork. A handful of studies in settings such as mental hospitals or acute wards (Caudill et al. 1952; Porter 1995) have been carried out covertly, without the knowledge of people in the setting, but most studies now for ethical reasons depend on explicit access agreements, with researchers operating in an open researcher role.

The origins of PO are often traced back to anthropology and the Chicago School of Sociology but the method as we know it today derives more directly from the work of later 'neo-Chicagoan' sociologists, particularly in the sociology of deviance and medical sociology (Fine 1995). The initial classic health studies focused on the process aspects of health care, such as:

- Professional socialization in medical school (Becker et al. 1961)
- The temporal experience of polio (Davis 1963) and TB care (Roth 1963)
- The management of death in hospital (Sudnow 1968) and organization of terminal care (Glaser and Strauss 1965).

All involved long periods of fieldwork spent observing and talking with research subjects in naturally occurring settings, charting the various stages, transitions or attitudinal shifts associated with professional education, patient 'careers' or illness trajectories.

There is some evidence that changes in the nature of health care systems have resulted in a change in the focus of research. Zussman (1993) has pointed out that the once flourishing tradition of studies of hospitalized patients' social worlds has all but disappeared as patient throughput speeds up and special-ized units replace traditional wards. He contends that the focus of research has shifted from ward culture and felt experience to detailed studies of specialized locales. More exacting ethical requirements for informed consent by patient research subjects may have accentuated this trend (Edgerton et al. 1984; see also Chapter 15). Most recent American studies focus on staff rather than patient perspectives in settings, such as:

- The intensive care unit (Zussman 1992)
- The neonatal unit (Anspa ch 1993)
- The surgical training programme (Bosk 1979)
- Paramedic ambulances and emergency rooms (Timmermans 1999)
- The construction of post-traumatic stress disorder in psychiatric facilities (Young 1995).

A similar trend is discernable in British work, for example:

- The study by Atkinson (1995) of haematologists
- Research by Fox (1992) on surgeons
- The study by Allen (2001) of the division of labour in acute wards
- Research on the health service as an organization by Strong and Robinson (1990), Bennett and Ferlie (1994) and Flynn et al. (1996).

THE RATIONALE FOR EMPLOYING PARTICIPANT OBSERVATION AS A RESEARCH METHOD

The rationale for using the PO method is bound up with its instrumental effec-tiveness in answering particular kinds of research question. Qualitative meth-ods have traditionally been concerned with questions of explanation and understanding, rather than questions about frequency or quantity. Such meth-ods may be used at the exploratory stage of research to map out variables in a field and generate hypotheses for testing in later quantitative studies. They can also have a role in making sense of observed correlations or patterns in quanti-tative data by elucidating the social processes that produce these patterns.

Qualitative studies can provide a snapshot of the behaviour or perspectives of a hard-to-reach or stigmatized group inaccessible via other methods (Lambert et al. 1995). They have shed light on seemingly illogical aspects of illness behaviour, poor compliance with drug prescribing, unsafe sex practices, teenage smoking behaviour, and have demonstrated some of the reasons for the limited effectiveness of programmes such as the controversial World Health Organization 'Directly Observed Therapy, Short Course' (DOTS) strategy for TB control. In any situation where the context of a health care intervention or programme or policy is likely to affect outcomes, qualitative studies can help identify real-world factors that may slip below the gaze of experimental or survey research.

In an early and influential paper, Becker and Geer (1957) suggested that PO has clear advantages over interview studies where special in-group languages (such as medical argot) are used; in situations where informants are unwilling to talk or find it difficult to describe an unfolding or complex social process; or where group myths and stereotypes feature centrally in accounts. Other writers have emphasized the importance of obtaining accounts that give an authentic representation of the social world by 'being there' and 'telling it as it is' with respect to the group being studied (Melia 1982). However, while PO undoubtedly provides data that could not be obtained via other methods (Mays and Pope 1996), it is important to avoid a naive realism that overlooks the role of the observer in 'interpreting' or making sense of observational data. It is tempting to assume that direct experience of a setting provides greater validity for research findings (Hammersley 1992). However, as discussed further below, PO raises issues of differential focus and selective perceptions on the part of the researcher that rules out any simple equation between direct observation and the one true account of events.

THE RESOURCES REQUIRED FOR PARTICIPANT OBSERVATION

PO is resource intensive in terms of human resources rather than technology. It makes heavy time demands, but usually involves individuals or small teams rather than the large teams characteristic of survey research. The need to build up field relationships over time militates against the kind of 'hired-hand' research common in quantitative projects (Roth 1999). In recent times, many researchers have supplemented the classic tool of the research notebook with the tape recorder to collect and record data and the computer to analyze data using various kinds of qualitative data based on the software discussed below.

Tape recording permits more rigorous recording of organizational discourse and is particularly useful when focused interactions, such as patient consultations, case conferences, ward rounds or management meetings occur at key junctures of organizational processes. Several contemporary ethnographies combine elements of field-note-based data collection with recording conversation or discourse so that a general description of organizational processes may be illustrated through a series of detailed exemplars. However, the decision to tape-record has significant implications for costs and the nature of data analysis.

Transcribing and analyzing recordings is an expensive and time-consuming process – a much slower process than the reading of conventional field notes – and will probably be beyond the capabilities of a lone researcher who cannot afford secretarial support. Making sense of data collected typically involves forms of sequential or discourse analysis which are very different from traditional forms of content analysis of documents that were described in Chapter 4, and will represent a steep learning curve for many qualitative researchers.

A number of packages such as *Ethnograph*, *NUD*IST* and *ATLAS*™ have been produced to assist with the management of field note and interview data (Kelle 1995). Most of these applications are essentially 'chunkers and coders', which attach electronic labels to passages of text and allow the retrieval of extracts coded under a chosen index term. Although most packages permit more complex operations such as Boolean searches using the three logical operators 'or', 'and' and 'not' for search terms (see Chapter 3), searches for co-occurring categories, the merging of codes and so on, they are no substitute for the sophisticated processes of interpretation, synthesis and theory generation that researchers have traditionally performed on field data (see below). Such programmes are useful as a support tool for conventional thematic content, but can create problems with forms of process analysis where change over a series of data entries or the narrative structure of a text are important.

More recent packages such as *Hypertext* use embedded links to preserve the overall structure of field notes, and may reduce the risk of fragmentation or de-contextualization of data but, in this researcher's view, the technology remains an imperfect one. My informal questioning of a small number of well-known qualitative health researchers revealed very mixed views on this subject, with many preferring to stick to the traditional manual approach to data analysis.

THE STRENGTHS OF PARTICIPANT OBSERVATION

The strengths of PO studies lie in their ability to shed light on issues that other methods are less effective in investigating. Becker and Geer (1957) spell out the advantages of PO as a tool for exploring local cultures and the unfolding of social processes over time. However, in practice there are different sets of arguments about the strength of PO in illuminating culture and subjective experience and its strength in examining social organization and organizational practices.

The argument that PO is a naturalistic method concerned with immersion in the culture and the authentic representation of what the famous anthropologist Malinowski (1922: 25) termed 'the native's point of view … his vision of his world', still holds sway but has become increasingly controversial. It is clear that observation does not in itself provide the researcher with access to the inner mental states of research subjects, and research which claims to provide a window into the social worlds of staff or patient groups must back this up with supporting evidence that goes beyond inferences about what outward appearances indicate about subjective perceptions. Some naturalistic studies have made a convincing case about the value of examining previously neglected user perspectives, and strongly support this with data (for instance, Daly et al. 1992). However, several influential commentators argue that observational research should be about documenting *practices* rather than ascribing *meanings* to participants' action or talk, and advocate a refocusing of analysis to centre on propositions that can be plausibly derived from observational data (see, for instance, Dingwall and Strong 1985; Silverman 1998).

Indeed, for observational researchers of a more policy-oriented nature, organizational processes and practices have been of greater interest than meanings, and they have seen PO as a promising alternative to interviews for seeing inside the 'black box' of health care organizations and understanding service delivery and change. PO can be viewed as a pragmatic way of 'reaching the parts other methods cannot reach' (Pope and Mays 1995). It can reveal routines of which participants are unaware; probe the micro-level behaviours that lie between known differences in outcomes; and shed light on how policies or programmes may be subtly reshaped in the course of implementation. For instance, the following studies in the United Kingdom have documented:

- Hospital reception work (Hughes 1989)
- Waiting list management (Pope 1991)
- Bed management (Green and Armstrong 1995)
- Patient's Charter targets (Sbaih 2002).

These studies have shown a gap between official policy and actual practices that is highly relevant to the organizational evaluation of health services.

THE CHALLENGES OF PARTICIPANT OBSERVATION

In the fieldwork phase

Some major disadvantages of PO, particularly in a contemporary British context preoccupied with outputs and the Research Assessment Exercise, are the time-consuming nature of fieldwork and the strain of sustained contact with subjects. While some accounts of the research experience may have overdramatized the emotional traumas of fieldwork (see Punch 1986), researchers undoubtedly face taxing challenges in terms of managing their identity in the research setting; mediating between different actors and interest groups; presenting the research in different situations; deciding just how much participation is appropriate; and determining when, and how, to put information into the public domain. There are also well-documented ethical dilemmas concerning trust and disclosure which arise when researchers build up social relationships for research purposes.

Furthermore, given that research funding bodies are often seeking a review of a whole service or population, there is often a temptation to tack a limited observational component on to an interview study covering multiple settings, and to come away with very limited data that are hard to contextualize. Malinowski (1922: 7) emphasized the importance of 'close contact', and cautioned that: 'There is all the difference between a sporadic plunging into the company of natives, and being really in contact with them.' One of the risks associated with contemporary mixed-method studies is that the PO element is so episodic and dispersed across settings that it cannot examine the process aspects of social organization that the method has traditionally coped with so well.

Methodological problems and solutions

The fact that some studies trade wider coverage against some loss of depth often reflects a quest for increased representativeness and generalizability. PO has traditionally been seen to be weak in these areas, but this is a topic about which more than a few misconceptions exist. There are undoubtedly situations where PO studies can illuminate general social patterns affecting a wide range of settings and where sampling may be appropriate (Bryman 1988). Yet the model of statistical inference from sample to population seems unsustainable in real-world situations where the 'population' of organizations from which a researcher might select the sample is itself small and diverse.

For example, some years ago, I was involved in planning a project which required the research team to select three or four study hospitals from all hospitals in Scotland that accommodated teenagers with learning disabilities. Yet the then 10 or so candidate hospitals differed on a range of dimensions: some admitted both children and adults while a few were children's facilities; most were specialist learning disabilities hospitals while at least one also contained psychiatric wards; some provided special education on site while others used outside schools; some allowed extensive mixed-sex activities, while others did not. Then, there were issues of urban versus rural locations and significant size differences. It took only a little reflection to conclude that any idea of selecting a case to represent a larger group of similar institutions would be flawed.

As a consequence of problems of this kind, examples of conventional sampling in PO studies are thin on the ground. Instead, some PO researchers have opted for purposive samples, intended to facilitate observations and comparisons that will help to build theory. Case studies may permit theoretical generalization rather than statistical generalization (Mitchell 1983), so the issue is not whether the events observed in the case study site precisely represent events elsewhere, but whether the analysis of social processes produced by the research has more general applicability. For Yin (1984) and other exponents of case analysis, the path towards generalizability is not about filling in the gaps by progressively achieving more complete population coverage, but about replication studies which will disconfirm, or leave in place, the theoretical propositions generated by earlier case studies.

The problem of researcher influence

A problem that features prominently in many textbook accounts of PO is 'reactivity' – the possibility that the researcher's presence influences the behaviour observed. This phenomenon, also known as the *Hawthorne effect*, featured centrally in the classic study by Roethlisberger and Dickson (1939) of human relations in the Hawthorne plant of the Western Electric Company in Chicago. Here a series of 'experiments' carried out by production engineers on a small group of telephone relay assembly workers appeared to show that almost any change in the factory environment led to improved productivity, including both increasing and reducing the lighting (although the data have subsequently been questioned). Clearly research subjects may very well modify aspects of their behaviour under observation, but arguably this is usually more of a problem in the early stages of a research project than when field relations are well established. Certainly it is not unknown for a study to be prematurely terminated because of non-cooperation or resistance from subjects (for example, Clarke 1996).

However, even where attempts are made to conceal things from the researcher, many features of social organization are difficult to change without disrupting the work of the setting. In my own experience, the kinds of data that subjects do not want recorded are more likely to involve individual mistakes or indiscretions, like negative comments about colleagues, than routine work practices. Once the researcher has become familiar to them, subjects may be surprisingly open in discussing sensitive and potentially problematic issues.

DATA CODING, ANALYSIS AND INTERPRETATION IN PARTICIPANT OBSERVATION

Most PO studies rely on some form of thematic content analysis. In line with PO's neo-Chicagoan influences, many observational researchers base their approach to analysis on analytic induction (Becker 1958) or grounded theory (Glaser and Strauss 1967). Both approaches typically start with a general orientation to an issue rather than definitive hypotheses for testing, and move through a process where problems and concepts relevant to an organization are identified, and theoretical propositions for further investigation formulated. Analysis goes on as data are collected and further data collection takes its direction from the provisional analysis. At this stage the analysis must necessarily remain provisional because of the exigencies of fieldwork, and final comprehensive analysis will only take place when fieldwork is completed.

Analytic induction and grounded theory

Analytical induction, as originally conceived by early Chicago researchers, was an approach concerned with the systematic search for falsifying evidence and the progressive refinement of theory until no disconfirming evidence could be found. In the work by Lindesmith (1947), this involved the progressive modification of a hypothesis, set out as a formal proposition at the start of the study. For Znaniecki (1952), analytical induction offered the prospect of producing universal propositions which could then be used to predict future patterns of behaviour. Later writers built on the core notions of inductive inference of theory from data and deviant case analysis, but abandoned the quest for empirical prediction and often avoided any initial hypothesis.

The approach by Glaser and Strauss (1967) to grounded theory emerged out of this period of reappraisal, and represented an extension and elaboration of analytic induction. Grounded theory studies start with a general area of concern rather than a hypothesis, and move to identify the concepts and theoretical connections emerging from the data. Where some contemporaneous qualitative studies (as well as almost all quantitative studies) were concerned mainly with verifying theories, Glaser and Strauss placed primary emphasis on generating theory by discovering relevant concepts and hypotheses through fieldwork. The core ideas of the constant comparative method and theoretical sampling have over time been supplemented by guidelines for a complex system of coding (Strauss and Corbin 1990).

However, the increasing formalization of grounded theory has led to considerable controversy among its exponents (Melia 1996), and may have made the approach less attractive to pragmatically inclined health service researchers. Many contemporary health researchers utilize modified versions of analytic induction or grounded theory. These make use of techniques like thematic coding, constant comparison and deviant case analysis, but do not adhere strictly to the original models (Murphy et al. 1998).

The growth of interest in the use of language has led to the emergence of more sophisticated approaches to the analysis of spoken interaction, such as the ethnography of communication, conversation analysis and discourse analysis. This has led many PO researchers to question whether their field notes represent adequately the interactions they have observed. *The Social Organization of Juvenile Justice* by Cicourel (1968) marked an important step because it encouraged researchers to pay greater attention to language and to produce field notes that were as near verbatim as possible. The emergence of linguistically sensitive forms of PO has changed the way many PO researchers present data (Dingwall and Strong 1985). It has led some to supplement observations recorded in field notes with tape recordings of key events or meetings, and to combine thematic content analysis with sequential analysis of transcribed talk based on conversation analysis or discourse analysis techniques.

Data selection

The process by which a researcher observes and records events, and then analyzes them to build descriptions and theories in published form, has led to a good deal of soul searching for several generations of participant observers. There are difficult issues concerning the selection and representation of observations that are not easy to resolve, even when data are presented in considerable detail. There are questions of trust, and also about just how ethnographic accounts might be said to represent reality. This quickly leads into the deep waters of epistemology and ontology which are beyond the scope of this chapter.

Many pragmatically inclined researchers have opted for a position of 'subtle realism' (Murphy et al. 1998; Mays and Pope 2000), which accepts that research reports can never encapsulate a single 'truth' but rejects the relativism of postmodern ethnography. They argue that a researcher's aim is to produce a credible account of social processes, which are acknowledged to be representations rather than reproductions of social reality. This may be used to build theories that can be developed in the light of findings from later studies.

WRITING UP AND PRESENTING THE FINDINGS

Different PO studies address different aspects of social organization and rest on different theoretical foundations, and this is reflected in striking differences in how findings are written up and presented. A classic interactionist ethnography like *Boys in White* (Becker et al. 1961) takes a very different form from an anthropology-influenced study like *The Cloak of Competence* by Edgerton (1967), just as the linguistically sensitive study *Medical Talk and Medical Work* by Atkinson (1995) is presented in a different style from the policy ethnography of Flynn and associates (1996). In recent years, styles of writing have come under increasing scrutiny (Hammersley 1993). For example, there is extensive debate about issues such as the viability of realist ethnography (and representational devices such as the invisibility of the author), and the use of alternative forms of textual organization such as chronology, narrative and analytic themes. From a practical perspective, researchers are often required to produce outputs for multiple readerships, which need to meet the stylistic requirements of different journals. In my own work, straddling sociology, socio-legal studies and health policy, it has been necessary to vary the mode of presentation to suit the particular audience targeted (see Chapter 21 for further discussion).

Case study: **Participant observation and contracting in the NHS internal market**

My research on the NHS internal market with Lesley Griffiths illustrates some of the dilemmas and trade-offs discussed above (see, for instance, Griffiths and Hughes 2000; Hughes and Griffiths 2003). The main component of the research was an observational case study of contracting between a health authority and its main providers, but this was supplemented by an interview study of all Welsh health authorities and NHS Trusts, which provided a context for the case study. We were also aware that the observational data could be utilized to examine both general socio-legal and economic aspects of contracting behaviour, and micro-level issues concerning language and social interaction in contracting meetings, and that we would need to produce different kinds of outputs to cover our full range of interests.

The study was conceived as a 'policy ethnography' (Strong and Robinson 1990) and takes a broadly naturalistic stance to data collection, influenced by interpretive sociology, while also seeking to influence policy. Compared with earlier work, we incorporated a larger observational component and paid more attention to the specifics of discourse by making extensive use of verbatim transcriptions of meetings. Over 80 contracting meetings were observed over two annual cycles, and supplemented with in-depth interviews with key participants. Most meetings and interviews were tape recorded and transcribed, resulting in a corpus of data amounting to about 2,800 sheets of typescript. Analysis took a broadly inductive form. We sought to identify themes emerging from the transcripts, which were then used to code and index relevant textual segments.

The qualitative data package NUD*IST allowed us to automate this process to some extent. However, chronology was an important consideration, and was less amenable to analysis via this 'chunking and coding' approach. It was necessary to read transcripts in context and track issues through a series of meetings.

(Continued)

As fieldwork began, two researchers shared the task of observing weekly meetings of the health authority's core contracting team, and also its negotiation and monitoring meetings with providers. Later we were also able to negotiate access to the corresponding weekly contracting team meetings in a local trust. This regular round of observations was supplemented by attendance at public health authority meetings, a small number of one-off events and visits to carry out informal interviews with key staff and review documents. Although a policy ethnography of this type centres mainly on a series of timetabled events and appointments, and thus falls short of the full 'immersion' in the field described in classic observational studies, we visited research sites three or four times in an average week.

In retrospect the key finding emerging from the observational data was the discrepancy that existed between official policy and the actual implementation of the internal market. In several areas informal social organization was crucial to the operation of the reforms, something that was missed in most interview studies. Although health authorities complied with some high-profile government directives, such as the instruction for purchasers to use contracts to require trusts to reduce surgical waiting times, other 'rules' of the internal market were not enforced to the same extent (Hughes et al. 1997). For example, the Department of Health's 'pricing rules' required that NHS Trusts should calculate the price of treatments on a full-cost basis, with no cross-subsidization of services, and publish standard prices (tariffs) which all purchasers would pay. But our observations revealed that prices were usually not specified in advance, and were often derived during contract negotiations by mechanically dividing the sum available by the agreed number of treatments. Tariffs might be the starting point for negotiations, but were frequently not published at all. This meant that different health authorities frequently ended up paying different prices for the same treatments, depending on historic funding levels and the available monies.

Attempts by health authorities to get trusts to reduce surgical waiting times usually took the form of penalty clauses in contracts, which would lead to a loss of income for the hospital if waiting times targets were not achieved. The official policy in most health authorities was that monetary penalties would be imposed when trusts missed their targets, and that the sanction would apply equally to all providers. However, the informal reality was that penalty clauses were often not

(Continued)

CASE STUDY

(Continued)

invoked when problems arose (Hughes and Griffiths 1999a). Some trusts had confidential 'side letters' containing a promise from the health authority not to impose the penalty specified in the contract. In a few other cases, trusts were able to get the penalty level reduced so that the figures specified in their contract were lower than those in the standard contract.

This led some health authorities and trusts to bend another official rule — the one that said that NHS contracts were public documents, available on request once signed. Health authorities had an incentive to keep secret the concessions forced by individual trusts. Trusts had an incentive not to reveal price differentials and unequal loading of costs between purchasers. In practice, it could be very difficult to obtain complete contracts at the beginning of the financial year. It was common for signing to be delayed for many months, or for certain schedules or price information not to be supplied with the main contractual document (Hughes and Griffiths 1999b; Hughes et al. 2000).

One of the most revealing indications of the nature of a market comes when disputes between buyers and sellers occur. Official policy required that NHS contract disputes should be settled through special conciliation arrangements, or if these failed, by arbitration by the Secretary of State (a government minister) or an appointee. At that time this involved 'pendulum arbitration', which meant that the decision would favour one side or the other, rather than proposing a compromise. Actually the official system was rarely used, largely because purchasers and providers were unwilling to take the risk of losing everything under a pendulum judgement (Hughes et al. 1997). In practice, senior NHS officials devised a variety of informal 'arbitration' arrangements which allowed compromises, and also made frequent use of direct management intervention. One high-profile contract dispute in Wales led to the sacking of the chief executives in the health authority and trust involved, and the preparation of a 'recovery plan' devised by senior NHS managers seconded from other areas to solve this problem.

Our work influenced the then Department of Health and Welsh Office to rewrite their guidance on resolution of NHS contract disputes. However, the major impact came from a raft of contemporaneous studies that delivered similar messages. Programmes of research with observational components, such as work at Warwick University funded by the Department of Health and the Economic and Social Research Council's *Contracts and Competition Programme*, provided ammunition for policy makers critical of the internal market reforms. Policy on the internal

(Continued)

market had been heavily influenced by the discipline of economics, and particularly by principal/agent theory and transactions cost theory.

The observational studies showed that many of the predictions about the likely impact of contracting in the NHS had not taken sufficient account of real-world constraints. The findings highlighted some of the negative features of adversarial contracting and the limited development of health care markets in the NHS. They showed that the early emphasis on complete and binding contracts, close monitoring, and clear incentives and sanctions had not delivered the expected benefits. These findings influenced the decision of the new Labour government after 1997 to end annual contracts and move towards longer term agreements. A number of research teams which had been involved in the ESRC *Contracts and Competition Programme*, including our own, were approached for advice by Department of Health officials tasked with developing guidelines on the new contracting framework.

CONCLUSION

The argument put forward in this chapter is that PO has a number of strengths in addressing particular kinds of research questions. In health research, PO can help researchers penetrate the social processes and, handled with care, the understandings of social actors, in particular settings. Most recently, it has been used to penetrate the 'black box' of health care organizations, and probe gaps between public accounts and informal behaviour. Moreover, most PO studies incorporate flexible research designs, which are not derailed by rapid and unpredictable organizational change.

The underlying argument in the chapter has supported the case for a pragmatic selection of methods according to the research question. This runs somewhat counter to the recent enthusiasm in health service research circles for enumerating the 'hierarchy of evidence' (see Chapter 3) that favours experiments and particularly randomized controlled trials and the other quantitative methods discussed in the next part of the book. These are the preferred methods of many British funding bodies and tend to marginalize qualitative studies, and to expand the application of experimental methods in programme and policy evaluation (Russell 1996). However, experimental methods do not work well when organizational structures and boundaries are subject to constant rejigging. Indeed, there are no published large-scale studies of this type dealing with the recent health service reforms. This is a less persuasive vision than the one set out some years ago by Illsley (1980) when he called for a multifaceted research programme that includes both randomized controlled trials and observational studies. Illsley (1980: 135) notes that there are many real-world situations where:

> The data are not cut and dried in the tradition of the natural sciences, instead they trace and reflect what is and what must be a fragmented, complex process. The data have to be put together and the process reconstructed with various forms of logical analysis but also with judgements about the relative weight and influence of actors and items.

This is what Illsley termed 'illuminative evaluation'. The case study presented above shows that observational research can influence policy, albeit in rather unpredictable ways, and as part of a larger body of research findings. To shed further light on PO as a health research method, a practical exercise based on the use of the method in a health contracting meeting follows.

Exercise: Participant observation and a health contracting meeting

The following exchange occurred in a health authority contracting team meeting. The first speaker, the finance director (FD), is the team leader. The other speaker, the contracts manager (CM), is the team member with hands-on responsibility for managing provider contracts. Caerbrook is a regional specialist hospital providing children's cancer services – indeed the only hospital offering some treatments in this geographical area. Metro is a regional hospital providing a wider range of tertiary services. The tape recording was made openly with the team's permission. No special assurances were requested after this meeting. Like many Welsh NHS purchasers, this health authority sought to impose a cash penalty on hospitals which 'breached' the guarantees offered by the Patient's Charter – a high-profile government initiative offering a commitment about the maximum surgical waiting times for different categories of patients – and to insert a clause to this effect in service contracts with providers.

(Continued)

FD: You'll have to be careful how you minute this. What we've agreed with Caerbrook ... is that the penalties for Patient's Charter will only be a thousand pounds this year, not five thousand or ten thousand. The reason for that is that they weren't prepared to sign a contract if we insisted on the other penalties. Their contract is a quarter of a million and they have never incurred a penalty with us.

CM: We need to be careful George.

FD: I got a personal assurance from their chief executive, Neil Hayward, that the deal is strictly confidential and not to be leaked to any other East county provider, and that they will not incur any penalties. If they do, we will review. But given that they were only a quarter of a million; given that, well, my figures say, and certainly his were, that they haven't incurred any penalties – that seemed to be confirmed by the budget reports – that we wouldn't ... it's not in our interest not to sign a contract. But we wouldn't want the same to apply to Metro, because Metro is a completely different provider. They have incurred fifty penalties in the last year, and ...

CM: It's vital that information doesn't get out. Once that gets out we haven't got much of a contract there.

FD: We've got to hold the line here. Nobody has heard that.

We were already aware from other observed meetings that three local providers had been arguing hard against the inclusion of penalty clauses but had been told that they would be applied in all contracts, and that another regional specialist hospital was also said to be unhappy with penalties.

Answer the following questions:

1   What does this extract show about the use of penalty clauses in the NHS quasi-market?
2   What, if anything, does the extract show about the problem of 'reactivity'?
3   What weight can be attached to a single observation, without corroborating information? How could such corroboration be obtained?

(Continued)

(Continued)

4 What questions does this data extract suggest should be explored in later interviews?

5 What practical problems does knowledge of this arrangement pose if any for the research team in managing field relations?

6 The researchers decided to use this extract but not until after this health authority was reorganized and the people concerned had moved to new jobs. What ethical problems does this raise, if any?

RECOMMENDED FURTHER READING

Allen, D., Griffiths, L. and Lyne, P. (2004) 'Accommodating health and social care needs: routine resource allocation in stroke rehabilitation', *Sociology of Health and Illness*, 26 (4): 411–32.
This is an example of the use of PO in a policy-oriented study of resource allocation at the boundaries of health and social care.

Griffiths, L. and Hughes, D. (2000) 'Talking contracts and taking care: managers and professionals in the NHS internal market', *Social Science & Medicine*, 51: 209–22.
This is an article from the case study discussed in this chapter, which illustrates the use of PO and its application to the topical issue of management/professional relations.

Timmermans, S. (1999) *Sudden Death and the Myth of CPR*. Philadelphia: Temple University Press.
This is a modern PO study in mainstream treatment settings, which uses the classic approach.

REFERENCES

Allen, D. (2001) *The Changing Shape of Nursing Practice*. London: Routledge.
Anspach, R. (1993) *Deciding Who Lives: Fateful Choices in the Intensive-Care Nursery*. Berkeley, CA: University of California Press.
Atkinson, P. (1995) *Medical Talk and Medical Work: The Liturgy of the Clinic*. London: Sage.
Becker, H.S. (1958) 'Problems of inference and proof in participant observation', *American Sociological Review*, 28: 652–60.
Becker, H.S. and Geer, B. (1957) 'Participant observation and interviewing: a comparison', *Human Organization*, 16: 28–32.

Becker, H.S., Geer, B., Hughes, E.C. and Strauss, A.L. (1961) *Boys in White: Student Culture in Medical School*. Chicago: University of Chicago Press.

Bennett, C. and Ferlie, E. (1994) *Managing Crisis and Change in Health Care: The Organisational Response to HIV/AIDS*. Buckingham: Open University Press.

Bosk, C.L. (1979) *Forgive and Remember: Managing Medical Failure*. Chicago: University of Chicago Press.

Bryman, A. (1988) *Quantity and Quality in Social Research*. London: Unwin Hyman.

Caudill, W., Redlich, F.C., Gilmore, H.R. and Brody, E.B. (1952) 'Social structure and interaction processes on a psychiatric ward', *American Journal of Orthopsychiatry*, 22: 314–34.

Cicourel, A. (1968) *The Social Organization of Juvenile Justice*. New York: Wiley.

Clarke, L. (1996) 'Participant observation in a secure unit: care, conflict and control', *Nursing Times Research*, 1: 431–40.

Daly, J., McDonald, I. and Willis, E. (1992) *Researching Health Care: Designs, Dilemmas, Disciplines*. London: Routledge.

Davis, F. (1963) *Passage Through Crisis: Polio Victims and Their Families*. Indianapolis: Bobbs Merrill.

Dingwall, R. and Strong, P.M. (1985) 'The interactional study of organisations', *Urban Life*, 14: 205–31.

Edgerton, R. (1967) *The Cloak of Competence*. Berkeley and Los Angeles: University of California Press.

Edgerton, R.B., Bollinger, M. and Herr, B. (1984) 'The cloak of competence: after two decades', *American Journal of Mental Deficiency*, 88: 345–51.

Emerson, R. (1981) 'Observational fieldwork', *Annual Review of Sociology*, 7: 351–78.

Fine, G.A. (ed.) (1995) *A Second Chicago School? The Development of Postwar American Sociology*. Chicago: University of Chicago Press.

Flynn, R., Williams, G. and Pickard, S. (1996) *Markets and Networks: Contracting in Community Health Services*. Buckingham: Open University Press.

Fox, N. (1992) *The Social Meaning of Surgery*. Buckingham: Open University Press.

Glaser, B.G. and Strauss, A.L. (1965) *Awareness of Dying*. Chicago: Aldine.

Glaser, B.G. and Strauss, A.L. (1967) *The Discovery of Grounded Theory: Strategies for Qualitative Research*. New York: Aldine.

Gold, R.L. (1958) 'Roles in sociological field observations', *Social Forces*, 36: 217–23.

Green, J. and Armstrong, D. (1995) 'Achieving rational management: bed managers and the crisis in emergency admissions', *Sociological Review*, 43: 743–64.

Griffiths, L. and Hughes, D. (2000) 'Talking contracts and taking care: managers and professionals in the NHS internal market', *Social Science and Medicine*, 51: 209–22.

Hammersley, M. (1992) *What's Wrong with Ethnography*. London: Routledge.

Hammersley, M. (1993) 'Ethnographic writing', *Social Research Update* 5. Available at: http://www.soc.surrey.ac.uk/sru/SRU5.html

Hughes, D. (1989) 'Paper and people: the work of the casualty reception clerk', *Sociology of Health and Illness*, 11: 382–408.

Hughes, D. and Griffiths, L. (1999a) 'On penalties and the Patient's Charter: centralism v decentralised governance in the NHS', *Sociology of Health and Illness*, 21 (1): 71–94.

Hughes, D. and Griffiths, L. (1999b) 'Access to public documents in a study of the NHS internal market: openness vs. secrecy in contracting for clinical services', *International Journal of Social Research Methodology: Theory and Practice*, 2 (1): 1–16.

Hughes, D. and Griffiths, L. (2003) 'Going public: references to the news media in NHS contract negotiations', *Sociology of Health and Illness*, 25 (5): 571–88.

Hughes, D., McHale, J. and Griffiths, L. (1997) 'Settling NHS contract disputes: formal and informal pathways', in R. Flynn and G. Williams (eds), *Contracting for Health: Quasi-Markets in the NHS*. Oxford: Oxford University Press.

Hughes, D., Griffiths, L. and Lambert, S. (2000) 'Opening Pandora's box? Freedom of information and health services research', *Journal of Health Services Research and Policy*, 5 (1): 59–61.

Illsley, R. (1980) *Professional or Public Health? Sociology in Health and Medicine*. London: Nuffield Provincial Hospitals Trust.

Kelle, U. (ed.) (1995) *Computer-aided Qualitative Data Analysis: Theory, Methods and Practice*. London: Sage.

Lambert, E.Y., Ashery, R.S. and Needle, R.H. (1995) *Qualitative Methods in Drug Abuse and HIV Research*, NIDA Research Monograph 157. Washington, DC: US Department of Health and Human Services, National Institutes of Health.

Lindesmith, A. (1947) *Opiate Addiction*. Bloomington, IN: Principia Press.

Malinowski, B. (1922) *Argonauts of the Western Pacific*. London: Routledge & Kegan Paul.

Mays, N. and Pope, C. (1996) 'Observational methods in health care settings', in N. Mays and C. Pope (eds), *Qualitative Research in Health Care*. London: BMJ Books.

Mays, N. and Pope, C. (2000) 'Qualitative research in health care: assessing quality in qualitative research', *British Medical Journal*, 320: 50–2.

McCall, G.J. (1984) 'Systematic field observation', *Annual Review of Sociology*, 10: 263–310.

Melia, K.M. (1982) 'Tell it as it is – qualitative methodology and nursing research – understanding the student nurses world', *Journal of Advanced Nursing*, 7 (4): 327–35.

Melia, K.M. (1996) 'Re-discovering Glaser', *Qualitative Health Research*, 6: 368–78.

Mitchell, J.C. (1983) 'Case and situation analysis', *Sociological Review*, 31: 187–211.

Murphy, E., Dingwall, R., Greatbatch, D., Parker, S. and Watson, P. (1998) 'Qualitative methods in health technology assessment: a review of the literature', *Health Technology Assessment*, 2: 16.

Pope, C. (1991) 'Trouble in store: some thoughts on the management of waiting lists', *Sociology of Health and Illness*, 13: 193–212.

Pope, C. and Mays, N. (1995) 'Qualitative research: reaching the parts other methods cannot reach: an introduction to qualitative methods in health and health services research', *British Medical Journal*, 311: 42–45.

Porter, S. (1995) *Nursing's Relationship with Medicine: A Critical Realist Ethnography*. Aldershot: Avebury.

Punch, M. (1986) *The Politics and Ethics of Fieldwork*. London: Sage.

Roethlisberger, F.J. and Dickson, W.J. (1939) *Management and the Worker: An Account of a Research Program Conducted by the Western Electric Company, Hawthorne Works, Chicago*. Cambridge, MA: Harvard University Press.

Roth, J.A. (1963) *Timetables*. New York: Bobbs Merrill.

Roth, J.A. (1999) 'Hired-hand research', in A. Bryman and R.G. Burgess (eds), *Qualitative Research, Volume One: Fundamental Issues in Qualitative Research*. London: Sage.

Russell, I. (1996) 'Methods of health service evaluation: the gospel of Archie Cochrane after 25 years', *Journal of Health Services Research and Policy*, 1: 114–15.

Sbaih, L.C. (2002) 'Meanings of immediate: the practical use of the Patient's Charter in the accident and emergency department', *Social Science and Medicine*, 54: 1345–55.

Silverman, D. (1998) 'Qualitative research: meanings or practices?', *Information Systems*, 8: 3–20.

Strauss, A.L. and Corbin, J. (1990) *Basics of Qualitative Research: Grounded Theory Procedures and Techniques*. Newbury Park, CA: Sage.

Strong, P. and Robinson, J. (1990) *The NHS: Under New Management*. Milton Keynes: Open University Press.

Sudnow, D. (1968) *Passing On: The Social Organization of Dying*. New York: Prentice Hall.

Timmermans, S. (1999) *Sudden Death and the Myth of CPR*. Philadelphia: Temple University Press.

Yin, R. (1984) *Case Study Research: Design and Methods*. Beverly Hills, CA: Sage.

Young, A. (1995) *The Harmony of Illusion: Post-Traumatic Stress Disorder*. Princeton, NJ: Princeton University Press.

Znaniecki, F. (1952) *Cultural Sciences*. Urbana, IL: University of Illinois Press.

Zussman, R. (1992) *Intensive Care: Medical Ethics and the Medical Profession*. Chicago: University of Chicago Press.

Zussman, R. (1993) 'Life in the hospital – a review', *Milbank Quarterly*, 71 (1): 167–85.

7

The Use of Focus Groups in Research into Health

JUDITH GREEN

INTRODUCTION

Focus groups are an important qualitative research method in researching health. Some authors use the term 'focus group' to describe one specific research technique, in which a number of strangers are brought together by the researcher to discuss a topic in a 'focused' way. The roots of this kind of focus group lie in market research, where the aim is to gather consumers' views of new products and services as an aid to marketing. However, it can be used as another term for a group interview, which has a long history in social research. Since the 1980s, focus groups have become increasingly popular as a data generation technique for a range of purposes, with health researchers being some of the most enthusiastic proponents. Focus groups have been used in projects with aims as broad ranging as needs assessment, users' perceptions of services and sociological studies of the understanding of health by the public.

This chapter examines the typical structure of a focus group and the kinds of questions that can be explored in a focus group setting. It then examines the different types of resource required for running a focus group and the strengths and weaknesses of the method covering methodological and ethical considerations. Questions of data management, analysis and presentation are a particularly challenging issue when using the focus group method and the chapter argues that the researcher must keep in mind that it is the group, rather than individuals within it, that is the focus of the analysis. A case study example demonstrates the various stages of a project using a focus group method in practice.

FOCUS GROUP SIZE AND STRUCTURE

Although there are many variations, a focus group typically consists of between 6 and 12 people brought together to discuss a topic, with one or more facilitators (sometimes called 'moderators') who introduce and guide the discussion and record it in some way. Sometimes the group is also asked to carry out exercises together, such as sorting a set of cards with statements on them, or ranking a list of priorities. A typical focus group might include the following stages as set out in Box 7.1.

Box 7.1   *The stages of a focus group*

- *Welcome*: The facilitator(s) welcome the participants, ask for consent forms to be completed, and perhaps provide refreshments
- *Icebreaking exercise*: Once the group is together and seated, and the aims of the group outlined, an introductory exercise is used to introduce the participants to each other and establish a relaxed, informal atmosphere. This might be an invitation for each participant to say their name and one thing about themselves (such as their favourite food, or something related to the topic in question)
- *Introductory exercise*: This is designed to introduce the topic, and get participants discussing it. Examples would be inviting participants to sort or rank pictures or phrases
- *Group discussion*: A series of questions (the topic guide) is used to 'focus' the discussion. These usually move from the general to the more specific. For instance, in a study to explore patient satisfaction with nursing care among inpatients, Lois Thomas and colleagues included the following questions in their topic guide:

  – What's it like being in here?
  – What have the nurses done for you today?
  – Can you think of a time when a nurse did something for you that you thought was an example of good nursing?
  – Can you think of a time when something struck you as an example of not very good nursing care, something that was not quite up to par?
  – *Summing up*: The facilitator summarizes the key issues raised, and asks for any additional comments people have

---

Source: Thomas et al. (1995)

WHY FOCUS GROUPS FOR HEALTH RESEARCH?

Focus groups provide an opportunity to research not only people's experiences and attitudes, but how these are communicated in a relatively 'naturalistic' setting. As health topics are often readily discussed in everyday contexts such as workplaces and social environments, a group setting often works well for generating talk about health and health services. One rationale for using focus groups follows the market research tradition, in which focus groups are used to ask users about their views of health services. Where there are policies to develop health services that are more user centred, focus groups are a useful tool for proactively seeking the views of communities. Unlike user surveys, focus group discussions allow participants to frame their concerns in their own terms rather than that of the researcher, and to bring issues to the agenda that researchers might not have considered. Analyzing discussion, rather than single opinions, allows the complexity of views to be studied. Bringing together people with something in common (such as using the same hospital services, or having similar religious views) can be a direct way for service providers and commissioners to find out how satisfied users are with services.

The potential for discussion also means that focus groups have advantages for studies of broader views about health and illness, such as investigating what people know, how they know it, and how this knowledge is communicated in social interaction. Health researchers have therefore made extensive use of focus groups (either on their own, or in combination with individual interviews or other methods) to explore the public understanding of health and how accounts of health and illness are used in everyday talk. One example is from Evans et al. (2001) who explored parents' decisions about accepting the combined measles, mumps and rubella (MMR) immunizations for their children. In the wake of considerable media coverage of controversy about the safety of the MMR vaccine in the United Kingdom, there was concern that rates of immunizations were falling to dangerously low levels. The study is an example of the role of focus groups in exploring beliefs about these kinds of controversial issues. The researchers used group interviews to explore in detail how parents made decisions, and asked about the sources of knowledge they drew on. They found that most parents found the decision of whether to immunize their children or not very stressful, and that they were dissatisfied with the information available to help them make the decision. Parents wanted more open and informed discussion with health professionals about the risks and benefits. By bringing together groups which included only parents who had immunized, or only those who had not, Evans and her colleagues provided a safe environment in which parents could discuss their views.

One advantage of focus group methods cited by some researchers is their potential for redressing some of the traditional power imbalances between researchers and research participants. A group may be able to exert more control over the research agenda than a single interviewee, and the process of being a focus group participant may encourage individuals to become involved in the research, if focus groups are used as part of a participatory approach. At the end of a project, focus groups can be a very useful way of getting feedback from participants on draft reports. However, focus groups in themselves are not inevitably more, or less, likely to lead to participation. Such factors as how far participants are involved in early stages of setting the research agenda and how committed the research commissioners are to implementing recommendations will obviously shape the extent to which the research is participatory. If commissioners are committed to a participatory approach, deliberative methods such as citizen's juries may be more appropriate than one-off focus groups. These involve a greater time commitment from participants, who have the task of developing a consensus view in the light of expert witness presentations and structured discussions.

Finally, focus group discussions are widely used in preparatory work within larger health research projects, for instance to generate data to help in survey design or in the development of patient-based outcome measures. Thomas et al. (1995) used focus groups, as well as individual interviews, in this way as part of their development work on measure of patient satisfaction with nursing care. Focus groups were held with groups of patients in medical and surgical wards and with one group of post-discharge patients in a family doctor's surgery. The aim was to use the data from these groups and interviews to develop a multidimensional concept of satisfaction with nursing care, which could then be used in a scale of satisfaction that was patient based. The researchers identified key elements of satisfaction from these focus groups and interviews, such as availability, attentiveness and information.

RESOURCES REQUIRED FOR FOCUS GROUPS IN PRACTICE

Focus groups are often selected in health research because they appear to be a relatively cost-effective data generation method, compared with alternatives such as individual interviews or ethnography. A small number of groups can certainly generate a large data set, without the labour-intensive commitment of long-term ethnographic fieldwork. However, it is perhaps a mistake to assume that focus groups are necessarily a cheap option. Identifying participants and organizing the groups is resource intensive, and there are a number of hidden costs. Some of the key issues to consider when thinking about the resources needed for a focus group study are: how participants will be recruited; identifying a suitable location; whether professional facilitators will be needed; payments to participants; and costs of data preparation.

Recruitment

Depending on the aims of the study, participants can be recruited through advertising for volunteers; working with personal contacts or established gate-keepers (such as community leaders, school heads or trade unions) to recruit from particular groups in the population; or paying for professional recruit-ment (for instance, through a market research company). The advantages and disadvantages of these recruitment methods depend on the aim of the study, but all incur some costs. Advertising is relatively cheap, but rarely effective; few people respond to calls for volunteers unless there are financial or other incentives. Moreover, developing relationships with gatekeepers in the com-munity takes up considerable researcher time. Professional recruitment agen-cies are often very effective (especially if the participants you need come from very specific sub-populations), but expensive, with additional direct payments to participants.

Location

The location needs careful consideration, in that a relatively neutral location with good facilities for refreshments, seating and transport access is needed to maxi-mize attendance and goodwill. The specific location also shapes the kind of data collected (Green and Hart 1999), and a range of locations may be required. People's accounts are context dependent and if you talk to them in the workplace, for example, they are more likely to be in work roles, and their accounts will reflect this. In their study of children's views of risks for accidental injury, Green and Hart found that children gave very different accounts depending on whether the group was held in school premises or in youth club premises, with those in the school-based groups more likely to stress their 'sensible' views, and the youth club groups more likely to tell stories in which they had taken risks.

Facilitators and other assistants

Facilitating a focus group discussion is a skill, and not one all researchers have developed, so a professional facilitator may be needed. For most groups, two people will be needed to run the discussion. One leads the discussion, making sure the topic guide is covered. The other has responsibility for practical issues such as meeting and greeting participants, organizing refreshments, checking that tape recorders are working and perhaps taking notes or summarizing at key points. In addition, professional help may be needed for translation, child-care or other special needs.

Payments to participants

Participants recruited by a market research company will usually expect payment for their time, in addition to travel expenses. Professionals will expect payment for their participation, if the research is conducted outside their working hours. This can be expensive if a study has to include large numbers of health care workers. There is some debate about both the ethical and methodological implications of paying participants. Offering incentives may make it difficult for low-income people to decline to participate, and paying people may make them more likely to say what they think the researcher wants to hear. It is difficult to judge these concerns empirically, but there are some justifications for perhaps paying focus group participants, who (unlike those in one-to-one interviews) usually turn up at a time and place of the researcher's choosing, devoting several hours to a study. There are ways of minimizing any potential impact of payment on the quality of data, such as not advertising the payment, but offering store vouchers at the end of the group as a 'thank you'.

Costs of data preparation

Most social research in health adopting this research method uses transcripts of focus group discussions as the basis of the analysis. The costs of producing transcripts vary considerably, but a skilled audio-typist can take four to six hours to transcribe each hour of focus group discussion. If a more detailed transcript is required, or the discussion is difficult to hear, this obviously takes longer.

Other resources

Other costs incurred will include refreshments; travel for participants; tape recorders and tapes; and pens, paper and flip charts for exercises and summing up. Some groups will have special needs that have to be considered, such as crèche facilities or interpreters. If the topic is a sensitive one, it may be appropriate to provide facilities for debriefing.

Focus group research is, then, rarely a cheap option, but it is cost effective if the data generated address the research question. Costing obviously also depends on how many groups are to be included, and there may be trade-offs between a perfect research design (such as one which continues sampling groups until theoretical saturation has been reached) and that which is available within the resources allocated.

FOCUS GROUPS IN HEALTH RESEARCH: METHODOLOGY

The first issue to be considered here is the strengths and weaknesses of focus groups as a method in health research. In this respect, the decision to use focus groups should be based primarily on methodological considerations. Are the data that they generate likely to address the research question posed? Like other qualitative data generation techniques, focus groups are appropriate when there is a need to identify participants' perspectives, and to understand their frames of meaning. The key methodological advantage of using group rather than individual interviews is that they provide access to interaction between participants. Focus groups are therefore the method of choice when an ability to explore interaction is needed to address the research question. In this vein, Bloor et al. (2001) suggest that focus groups are the method of choice when:

> *researching topics relating to group norms, the group meanings that underpin those norms and the group processes whereby those meanings are constructed* ... Focus groups are a particularly advantageous method where these group norms, meanings and processes are hidden or counter-cultural. (Bloor et al. 2001: 90, italics in original)

However, other issues will also influence the decision to use focus groups, including the resources available and the topic – is it one, for example, which is easier for participants to talk about in a group setting? Like all methods, the strengths and weakness of focus groups relate to the specific research question, topic and setting; what is a strength for one study may be a weakness for another. Three particular issues illustrate how strengths and weaknesses need to be considered in the light of a specific research project. These are access to interaction, naturalism and talking about sensitive issues.

Access to interaction

The main methodological advantage of using group interviews compared with individual interviews is that the researcher has access to interaction between participants, rather than just to talk between the researcher and one participant. This potentially allows access to rather more 'naturalistic' talk about the topic of interest, which (it is assumed) might reflect the ways in which people discuss issues in everyday life. This advantage is maximized when the focus group consists of people who might ordinarily interact in work, domestic or other settings. Khan and Manderson (1992) note how useful it is to tap into social networks such as kin groups or neighbours when doing research on health:

Such natural clusterings of people represent, in a loose fashion, the resources upon which any member of the group might draw, both in material terms and with respect to information and advice … It is precisely this natural social network which provides the scripting for the management of an illness event — what to do with a child with bloody diarrhoea, for example, or how to nurse a high fever; or who to call in the case of a threatened miscarriage … As a result, discussions with such groups provide fairly accurate data regarding the diagnosis and treatment of illness, choices of health services and so on. (Khan and Manderson 1992: 60)

Although Khan and Manderson are discussing informal interviews in rural settings, this captures neatly the advantage of utilizing 'natural' groups in more formal focus group research. To some extent, the researcher has access to the kinds of discussions that might happen in non-research settings about treatment decisions, or health services, rather than the supposedly more artificial 'opinions' that are more readily offered in one-to-one interviews. Kitzinger used natural groups in a study of how media messages about HIV/AIDS were understood by various audiences in a UK context. She notes that in the study:

We chose to work with pre-existing groups — clusters of people who already knew each other through living, working or socialising together. We did this is order to explore how people might talk about AIDS within the various and overlapping groupings within which they actually operate. Flatmates, colleagues and friends — these are precisely the people with whom one might 'naturally' discuss such topics … The fact that research participants already knew each other had the additional advantage that [they] could relate each other's comments to actual incidents in their daily shared lives. They often challenged each other on contradictions between what they were professing to believe and how they actually behaved. (Kitzinger 1994: 105)

Focus groups allow exploration of interaction and this has great advantages for many of the kinds of questions health researchers wish to address. We are often interested not just in the content of knowledge, but in how decisions come to be made, or how information about health is transferred between people within social networks. Individual interviews are often criticized for providing information on what people say, but not on what people do. As Kitzinger (1994) suggests in the quote above, in focus group discussions between people who know each other, stories about how people say they behave are challenged, corroborated or undercut, giving some information on the relationship between behaviour and how people talk about it.

 A good example of how focus groups can generate data on the gaps between professed beliefs and behaviour comes from a European study on attitudes to food risks discussed further later in the chapter (Green et al. 2003). In the focus groups held with adolescents, some of the young people in both the United

Kingdom and Italy talked during the discussions about how they avoided 'fast food' as 'unsafe'. However, as the group discussion progressed, friends challenged each other, with reminders of how they had eaten burgers from street stalls, especially when they were returning late from clubs or concerts. In analyzing focus group data, the researcher can contrast what might be called the 'public' accounts (such as 'we don't eat fast food') with stories of examples of everyday experience. This can provide data on normative ideas about health (what people think they should do), as well as information on the situations in which these normative accounts do not, in practice, shape behaviour.

Naturalism

However, the 'naturalism' that generates such useful interaction for analysis presents some practical, and more methodological, problems. There is perhaps a trade-off between facilitating the kind of natural discussions that happen in everyday life, with people interrupting and talking over each other, and generating a discussion in which people's talk can be heard, transcribed and analyzed. The researcher has to make a decision about the main aim of the study: is it to reproduce 'natural' talk, in order to analyze how ideas are transmitted and knowledge about health discussed? If so, the facilitator will allow discussion to continue in a more natural way. If the main aim is to access a range of views, and ensure that the group's views on every topic are heard, then the discussion may have to be more tightly controlled.

A more methodological limitation is perhaps the seductiveness of a natural focus group discussion: it appears like 'everyday talk' and it is tempting to treat it as such. Nonetheless, even if relatively informal, a specially constituted focus group is still an artificial setting. Given that people's talk is contextual (that is, it is shaped by, and for, specific contexts) we cannot assume that what is said in a research setting reflects what might be said in the home, workplace or other environment. The stories recounted in focus groups may be different from those recounted in one-to-one interviews, but we cannot assume that they are any more valid as representations of 'what really happened'. It cannot be assumed that the accounts provided in a focus group setting reflect in any simplistic way 'real life'. For this reason, focus groups are not a substitute for detailed ethnography. If the aim of the study is to research social behaviour in context, a design that uses long-term observational methods would be a more appropriate choice.

Talking about sensitive issues

A practical strength of a group setting is that it can offer a more supportive environment for participants to discuss sensitive issues. One example is dissatisfaction with health services. In a one-to-one interview, it may be difficult to express dissatisfaction, especially if the interviewer is known to be a health professional, or associated with the provider service. In a group, other participants can legitimate negative views, and one participant's story about their experiences can trigger off other participants' recollections.

Again, though, this strength is a potential weakness, depending on the research aims and the topic. First, the supportive environment of a group can lead people to 'over-disclose' and perhaps talk about issues in a way that they regret later, especially if they are part of a natural group that exists outside the research setting. Vissandjée et al. (2002), in their report of how they used focus groups in a study of women's health behaviour in rural Gujarat in India, discuss this as a particular problem in doing research in small communities. People have to interact with each other long after the research team have gone home. There is an ethical obligation therefore to make sure that participants did not reveal information they had not intended to, which might make them vulnerable in their everyday lives.

Second, there are some topics for which a focus group might not be an appropriate setting, unless the participants all share a particular experience. Using focus groups to explore deviant behaviour, or socially stigmatizing experiences, may be inappropriate if some participants are likely to feel uncomfortable.

SAMPLING GROUPS AND PARTICIPANTS

A second issue relating to the use of focus groups in researching health concerns sampling. When sampling, both the selection of groups and the selection of individual participants have to be considered. As in most qualitative research, the sampling strategy is usually dictated by identifying what Patton (1990) describes as 'information-rich' cases. These are the groups that are most likely to furnish the data needed to address the research question. However, other concerns are likely to influence both the sample size and who is included. Often, focus group research is done with an aim of influencing policy, whether at the immediate local level (such as improving service provision) or at a more national level. To provide convincing data for policy makers, the sample also has to be credible, in that it should include representatives of all the constituencies that policy makers are likely to be interested in.

The number of groups needed depends largely on how many constituencies there are within the population of interest. In a local study of health care users, it may be enough to convene two groups of patients, perhaps segregated by gender, as men and women tend to talk very differently in mixed- and single-gender groups. In a study with a broader research question, such as the one reported in the case study at the end of this chapter on how consumers in four

European countries choose safe food, there might be a large number of population segments in terms of characteristics such as gender and age, especially if the researcher also wants to include some homogeneous and some more heterogeneous groups. Rather than including groups that reflect every possible combination of factors, it is worth designing a sampling grid and selecting groups across the grid. The sampling grid for the study of European consumers is shown in Table 7.1 which appears later in this chapter.

Within each group, one decision is whether to sample participants for homogeneity (so that they share some characteristics) or heterogeneity. Traditionally, market researchers sampled for heterogeneity, with an aim of generating a range of views within each group. The advantages of homogeneity are that shared experiences can provide a more supportive environment for discussing a difficult or sensitive issue. Including a range of participants can also be a useful way to trigger participants' accounts of issues that they may consider too 'common sense' to mention unless prompted by someone who does not share their perspective. In practice, of course, researchers may have little control over the individuals who participate, especially if recruitment is done by inviting volunteers or through gatekeepers.

ETHICAL CONSIDERATIONS

A third area for exploration in relation to focus groups and health research is ethical issues. In a focus group, participants outnumber researchers and this can be an important element in shifting the balance of power towards participants. In projects that aim to listen to communities, or access the voices of groups that are traditionally marginalized in the public arena, this can be an important ethical advantage. In work with young people, for instance, using group interviews as opposed to individual ones can be a very useful way of redressing the power imbalance between interviewer and interviewee (Green and Hart 1999). However, as Michell (1999) warns, in the context of her study of young people's peer groups, the focus group reproduced the hierarchical relations of the friendship group, meaning that the voice of those low down in the pecking order was not heard. Experiences of bullying and victimization were only accessible through individual interviews. So the group setting may facilitate access to marginalized communities, but at the same time it may reproduce local hierarchies and limit access to marginalized individuals within those communities (see also Chapter 18).

This also applies to opportunities for participation. Discussions of ethics tend to focus on informed consent, and ensuring that participants have not been cajoled or bullied into taking part. However, there are also ethical concerns about those who do not get the opportunity to take part. For young people, the need to secure parents' consent may mean that some children are disenfranchised (Green and Hart 1999). Similarly, if using community leaders to aid recruitment, it is worth considering who is not being asked to participate, as well as ensuring that those who do have provided their genuine consent.

Taking part in focus groups can provide some personal advantages for participants, especially if they are relatively isolated. In a study of patients with glaucoma (Green et al. 2002) participants in the focus group reported that they valued the chance to meet with other people coping with similar problems, and some participants exchanged contact details at the end of the research to keep in touch. Ethical issues such as those involving confidentiality constantly need to be considered in health research, though, and they are discussed more generally in Chapter 15 for interested readers.

THE MANAGEMENT, ANALYSIS AND PRESENTATION OF FOCUS GROUP DATA

A fourth issue related to the use of focus groups in researching health is centred on the handling of the data that they generate. A first decision is whether to work with full transcripts. In social research, it is usual to transcribe fully all the group discussions and use these as a basis for analysis. However, in many projects it may be enough to use notes of the discussion, transcribing only those sections of the tape that are most relevant. This would be justifiable if only a summary of key concerns was needed, or if the aim was to access the groups' consensus views on a particular topic, rather than research how they came to the decision. If it is not possible to tape and transcribe the discussion (for instance, if working in a setting where this would be either practically or politically impossible), the facilitators should ensure that detailed notes are taken, and perhaps the group's opinions summarized at key points throughout the process.

If there are complete transcripts of all, or most, of the groups, there are a number of strategies for analysis. Essentially, these are no different from techniques for analyzing any other qualitative data set, and there are now a range of textbooks that advise on a range of approaches to analysis (see, for example, Miles and Huberman 1994; Silverman 1993; Strauss and Corbin 1990). As in any other type of study, choosing a strategy for analysis depends on the aim of the study (in terms of the research question and the commissioner's expectations) and the methodological orientation of the researcher. If the focus groups were convened to provide a broad-brush overview of community views, or to identify some common issues to feed into later studies, then a fairly simple content analysis of transcripts of the discussion, or notes taken, will suffice.

Thematic content analysis

This involves identifying the recurring themes within the data, exploring typologies of these themes and looking at variations and relationships between, and within, themes. Analysis is an iterative process that begins with the first data collected, and continues into the writing up of the project. It involves moving between the data, empirical and theoretical literature that helps make sense of the data and discussion between the research team about 'what is going on here'. This is clearly not just a technical exercise in coding extracts of talk, but one that involves some analytical imagination. However, there are some steps that can help with a simple thematic analysis. They are:

- *Familiarization with the transcripts*: Reading and rereading the transcripts, and listening to the tapes, to get an overall sense of key issues for participants. What made participants angry, enthusiastic, nervous? A summary can be written of each group discussion.
- *Developing a coding frame*: It is worth doing this in a group, with either a team of researchers or colleagues. Read early transcripts in detail, identifying in each segment the key concept: what the participant is 'talking about'. Try to label these concepts in as abstract a way as possible. These can then be built up into a coding frame, which is essentially a list of the concepts and their labels (the 'codes').
- *Coding*: When you have a coding framework, the entire set of transcripts can be 'coded' by identifying each segment as an instance of a code. This will be modified as more data are analyzed.
- *'Cut and paste'*: All the instances of the same code can now be gathered together, either manually by literally cutting up the transcripts, or using a word processor or specialized software. Now look at the list of extracts under each code to identify the range of talk about each topic.

This kind of thematic content analysis is fine for mapping out the range and strength of views and comparing the kinds of issues that arise across the group. To exploit the strengths of focus group data and maximize the chance of producing useful policy-relevant findings, a more detailed and sociologically informed analysis will probably be needed, which takes interaction into account.

Social interaction: Analysis and presentation

A common criticism of much focus group research is that researchers often stress the advantage of interaction, but rarely show in published papers how this has been used in the analysis. One exception is from Wilkinson and Kitzinger (2000) who, in their study of women's talk about 'thinking positive' in the context of cancer, provide a very nice illustration of how analyzing interaction in focus groups can generate a much more sophisticated understanding of health knowledge than merely identifying some common themes. They note that their data on women's talk could have furnished a number of quotes such as 'You just have to think positive.' In a superficial content analysis, these could be identified as 'evidence' of the importance of 'thinking positive' in cancer patients' lives.

However, a more subtle analysis of this talk as discourse enabled Wilkinson and Kitzinger to reflect on how and why such comments are used in talk. First, such comments as 'thinking positive' are, they argue, a common idiom in English: a taken-for-granted summary of common-sense knowledge that is utilized as a general purpose statement within everyday talk to move the conversation along, and move it specifically from a personal to a general frame. Participants invoke such idioms when they want to cite a shared norm, something the audience can agree with, and turn a conversation from a potentially difficult one about personal difference to an inclusive one about affiliation. Thus, through paying attention in the analysis not just to the content of what is said (through stripping out phrases or paragraphs without any sense of context), but to how interaction works discursively, Wilkinson and Kitzinger are able to specify much more precisely what participants are doing when they invoke such phrases as 'thinking positive', and to uncover the social contexts in which such statements might be made. In this case, it was reflected in a broad cultural norm expressed in a setting where 'thinking positive' was the expected and morally required response.

The group should be the unit of analysis

Given that focus group studies often include a large number of individual participants, it can be tempting to treat any data derived from individuals quantitatively. This is a mistake: individuals are not selected as representatives of a broader population, but as part of a group, and the group should properly be the unit of analysis. When writing up, it is inappropriate to report on the characteristics or beliefs of individuals as if they were a population sample. The focus should be on the groups, and sufficient context given about their compositions to enable the reader to judge how the data were generated. This might include details of how the groups were recruited, what social characteristics they share, and what they were asked to discuss. It will also ideally involve providing discursive context, rather than merely using individuals' statements as indicators of their beliefs, to indicate how particular utterances were used within the discussion. This might include details of the issues over which participants agreed or disagreed; which topics were difficult to discuss; and how persuasive particular kinds of accounts were in interaction.

Case study: Exploring accounts of food risks using focus groups

As part of a large European study of the public perceptions of the risks associated with bovine spongiform encephalopathy (BSE), we wanted to explore public concerns about food risks in general, and to identify what kinds of information on food safety were trusted (Green et al. 2003; Green et al. 2005). The aim was to include people from four European countries, which had been chosen to represent a range of 'food cultures' (Germany, Italy, the United Kingdom and Finland), and to include people from different stages in the life cycle theoretically associated with different approaches to food choice (adolescents, young single people, those responsible for shopping for young children and older citizens). In addition to providing detailed data on how these population groups talked about their food choices, we also aimed to compare findings across the four countries and the four life cycle stage groups. An international study presents particular challenges (see Chapter 20), but many are typical of the kinds of decisions researchers in any focus group study have to take. The first is selecting an appropriate sample of groups.

Given our comparative aim, we wanted a similar range of groups in each of the four countries. However, within each country, of course, the meaning of the life cycle groups and other population groups is rather different. As an example, young single men in Italy had rather less experience of choosing their own food than those of similar age in other countries. In some countries, regional or rural/urban differences were more pronounced than in others. Second, focus group methodologies have to resonate with local cultural norms about interaction. In some countries, it became clear it would not be productive to run single-gender groups, as there are few situations in which men would interact normally in this way and the focus group setting simply would not reproduce 'natural' talk in the way that it might for other groups. We therefore created a sampling grid, which aimed to select a range of life cycle groups in each country, but to also select within each country a range representing other factors theoretically linked to food cultures, such as geographical location or social class. A total of 36 groups were sampled to generate a data set that would enable us to compare countries and life cycle groups, and within each country to take account of differences in location or social class, as illustrated in Table 7.1.

The aim was to recruit natural groups wherever possible, to maximize the methodological advantages discussed above. Research teams used a mixture of methods to do this, including contacting community groups such as church-based or local associations, and working with schools to recruit friendship groups of adolescents. However, for the 'young single' groups, which may consist of relatively mobile individuals with few

(Continued)

Table 7.1 *Sampling grid for the food risks study – including the location and life cycle stage of the focus groups*

Country and location	Adolescents	20–25s	Family food purchasers	55+
Finland:				
Kuopio	X	XX	XX	XX
Germany:				
Kiel	X	X	XX	X
Eckernförde	X	X	X	X
Italy:				
Bologna	X	X		X
Naples		X	X	
Trento	XX		X	X
UK:				
London and environs	X	X	XX	X
Midlands	XXX	X	X	X

X = one focus group.
Source: Green et al. (2005)

obvious community allegiances, we relied on market research companies to recruit.

The protocols for running the groups also had to balance comparability with flexibility. We used icebreaking exercises, asking participants to rank pictures of foodstuffs in terms of their 'riskiness' to generate discussion in all groups, but the pictures reflected the kinds of foods eaten locally. The list of topics to cover in each group was the same, but facilitators worded prompts appropriately for local participants.

Typically, health research is done by teams of people rather than individual researchers. In this project we had research teams in each of the four countries, and had to coordinate the analysis of data collected in four languages. First, pilot data from each country were transcribed and translated into English so all the project teams could carry out an initial thematic analysis. At a project meeting, these transcripts and the initial thematic analyses were discussed, and we then generated a combined coding scheme to aid a comparative analysis across all countries. This was used within each country to generate a country report and more detailed analysis. These reports were then subject to a 'meta-analysis' to produce integrated results across the study.

Access to interaction in the groups provided useful data on not just accounts of choosing safe food, but how these were used in everyday life. In

(Continued)

(Continued)

the transcripts we could see what sources of knowledge people referred to, and also how effective these sources were in persuading others. Personal anecdotes about food risk were seen to be much more effective, in interaction, for convincing others. Analyzing interaction, rather than just individual accounts, also enabled us to look at the social consequences of talk about risk. As one example, we were interested in how 'risk' has become a relatively neutral discourse for discussing social difference. Looking at how talk about 'differences' such as ethnicity and religion was reframed in many group discussions into talk about how aspects of risk illustrated some of the social uses of the rhetoric of risk in a multicultural society. This example is from a group of women in the United Kingdom, who quickly reframed one participant's religious rationale for avoiding pork into a frame of 'hygiene':

A: We don't eat pork in any case ... for religious reasons.
B: A lot of the religious things to do with meat come from the hygiene aspect anyway, like Jewish people, they won't store meat in the same fridge as dairy produce ... a lot of that is down to hygiene.
C: They are dirty, pigs.
D: Absolutely, it has been proved apparently, many years ago.
B: So it all comes down to hygiene.

(Green et al. 2003: 42)

However, as suggested above, we cannot assume that the interaction we record is in any unproblematic way 'natural'. First, recruiting people within particular life cycle segments (or indeed any other homogeneous characteristic) raises some methodological problems. In a group consisting only of those responsible for household shopping, for instance, participants arrive already attuned to one particular social role (usually that of 'mother'), and we are to some extent generating the kinds of discourse we analyze as an artefact of our sampling strategy. The same individuals, if recruited as part of a group with some other characteristic in common (such as profession, or political affiliation), may focus on rather different aspects of food choice and risk. Second, the process of taking part in a focus group on 'food risks' is in itself one way in which participants learn about the topic. Indeed, many of the participants in the groups said they had enjoyed themselves because they had learnt a lot, or commented that the discussion itself had changed their opinions. Whilst this is very useful data, in that we can explore what kinds of talk are likely to lead to people saying they will change behaviour, it does suggest that the setting (an hour and a half devoted to one topic) is not one that really reflects the kinds of everyday talk people are likely to have.

CONCLUSION

It has been argued that the focus group method has a number of advantages in gaining access to the way in which people discuss issues and deal with problems related to health in everyday life. Particularly if people in a focus group already share a common background and know each other, this can enable the researcher to understand frameworks of meaning, what resources people use and how they draw on social networks to deal with matters that arise on a day-to-day basis. Focus groups based on population samples that deliberately seek to bring together a group of people from different backgrounds to discuss a particular topic can also serve to demonstrate the range of views about a specific issue. However, using the focus group method can be challenging in terms of management, resources, process, data recording and analysis, particularly for the lone researcher. It is also important for researchers using the method and analyzing the data to concentrate their attention on aspects of social interaction within the group in terms of understandings, views and attitudes and the lines of agreement and divergence.

The case study demonstrates how focus groups can be used in relation to exploring people's understandings of food risks. The exercise below provides the opportunity for readers to consider employing the method in finding out about people's experience of maternity services and their priorities in any reorganization. As an additional background to this, there is also discussion of focus group research in Chapter 16 where focus groups were used as one method in a study of user involvement in cancer services and in Chapter 18 where the method has been used in a range of studies on service development for ethnic minority communities.

Exercise: Planning a focus group study of maternity services

There are plans to reorganize maternity services in a health district, and a research programme has been commissioned to find out the views of staff and users on what could be improved in the new system. You have been asked to carry out some focus groups, with professionals and users, to explore their views of current service provision and their priorities for change.

(Continued)

(Continued)

Write a brief (500-word) proposal for a focus group study. This should cover the following issues:

1   Sampling:

- Which groups of users and professionals should be included?
- How many will be needed to cover the main constituencies of interest?
- Are there particular sub-groups of the population that should be included?
- Will the groups be homogeneous or heterogeneous, and what is the rationale for your decision?

2   A protocol for running the groups:

- Think of an introductory exercise that would be appropriate for the groups of professionals and users.
- List 5–6 prompts for a topic guide.

3   Resources:

- What resources are needed to conduct your study?

4   Ethical issues:

- What particular ethical issues are raised by your proposed study?
- How will these ethical issues be addressed?
- Consider ethical issues in conducting the study and disseminating the findings.

5   Assessment:

- What are the main advantages and disadvantages of using focus groups for this study?

RECOMMENDED FURTHER READING

Barbour, R. and Kitzinger, J. (eds) (1998) *Developing Focus Group Research: Politics, Theory and Practice*. London: Sage.
This collection of papers stimulates more thoughtful use of focus groups by addressing methodological and practical issues, including researching sensitive topics, ethical considerations and different styles of analysis.

Bloor, M., Frankland, J., Thomas, M. and Robson, K. (2001) *Focus Groups in Social Research.* London: Sage.
This book usefully discusses the more methodological issues raised by employing focus groups in social research in health, and is particularly strong on issues of analysis and interpretation.

Kreuger, R. and Casey, M.A. (2000) *Focus Groups: A Practical Guide for Applied Research.* London: Sage.
The authors of this text use their experience of a range of studies/participants to provide excellent practical advice on all stages of an applied focus group study – planning and recruiting, moderating, coping with problems and managing and reporting data.

REFERENCES

Bloor, M., Frankland, J., Thomas, M. and Robson, K. (2001) *Focus Groups in Social Research.* London: Sage.
Evans, M., Stoddart, H., Condon, L., Freeman, E., Grizzell, M. and Mullen, R. (2001) 'Parents' perspectives on the MMR immunisation: a focus group study', *British Journal of General Practice*, 51: 904–10.
Green, J. and Hart, L. (1999) 'The impact of context on data', in R. Barbour and J. Kitzinger (eds), *Developing Focus Group Research.* London: Sage.
Green, J., Siddall, H. and Murdoch, I. (2002) 'Learning to live with glaucoma: a study of diagnosis and the impact of sight loss', *Social Science and Medicine*, 55: 257–67.
Green, J., Draper, A. and Dowler, E. (2003) 'Short cuts to safety: risk and "rules of thumb" in accounts of food choice', *Health, Risk and Society*, 5: 33–52.
Green, J., Draper, A., Dowler, E., Fele, G., Hagenhoff, V., Rusanen, M. and Rusanen, T. (2005) 'Public understanding of food risks in four European countries: a qualitative study', *European Journal of Public Health*, 15: 523–27.
Khan, M.E. and Manderson, L. (1992) 'Focus groups in tropical diseases research', *Health Policy and Planning*, 7: 56–66.
Kitzinger, J. (1994) 'The methodology of focus groups: the importance of interaction between research participants', *Sociology of Health and Illness*, 16: 103–21.
Michell, L. (1999) 'Combining focus groups and interviews: telling how it is; telling how it feels', in R. Barbour and J. Kitzinger (eds), *Developing Focus Group Research.* London: Sage.
Miles, M. and Huberman, A.M. (1994) *Qualitative Data Analysis: An Expanded Sourcebook*, 2nd edition. Thousand Oaks, CA: Sage.
Patton, M.Q. (1990) *Qualitative Evaluation and Research Methods*, 2nd edition. Newbury Park, CA: Sage.
Silverman, D. (1993) *Interpreting Qualitative Data: Methods for Analysing Talk, Text and Interaction.* London: Sage.

Strauss, A. and Corbin, J. (1990) *Basics of Qualitative Research*. London: Sage.

Thomas, L., MacMillan, J., McColl, E., Hale, C. and Bond, S. (1995) 'Comparison of focus group and individual interview methodology in examining patient satisfaction with nursing care', *Social Sciences in Health*, 1: 206–20.

Vissandjée, B., Abdool, S. and Dupéré, S. (2002) 'Focus groups in rural Gujarat, India: a modified approach', *Qualitative Health Research*, 12: 826–43.

Wilkinson, S. and Kitzinger, C. (2000) 'Thinking differently about thinking positive', *Social Science and Medicine*, 50: 797–811.

8

Action Research and Health

HEATHER WATERMAN

INTRODUCTION

Action research is a participative method of research that both seeks to gain more knowledge and aims to change people's circumstances for the better by engaging them in the research process. The process of action research is therefore complex and requires participants to develop skills in research, practice, education and change management. This chapter outlines some of the challenges of action research and how difficulties can be overcome. Despite the pitfalls, the literature on action research shows that this approach can have a positive impact on people's health and health services.

From a personal perspective as an action researcher, I have shifted from a position of viewing action research as a technical approach to solving problems in health care, to seeing the method as one that aspires towards empowerment and democracy. In this case, empowerment refers to enabling research participants to take action, often in difficult situations, and democracy refers to encouraging people from diverse backgrounds to debate freely and work towards improving their circumstances through research. As a practitioner, a ward manager, I was enthusiastic about the immediacy of action research and by the idea of studying a situation and changing practice at the same time. Later, after participating in several action research projects, I came to appreciate the significance of group critical reflection and deciding on action in empowering participants, both practitioners and patients, in health care settings. The increased knowledge and confidence that occurs enables changes to be made by those who are experiencing a problem, whether they are patients or staff, in areas related to direct patient care, management, administration or education. Action research by its nature is an exercise of democracy as it encourages a group of people who normally may not be heard, or enabled to change their lives, to work together actively and take responsibility for changing their situation.

However, over time, I have become more realistic and critical of the method. In this chapter, I will expand on these issues by:

- Examining the main characteristics and rationale for action research in health care settings, and the resources required to apply it in practice.
- Considering the strengths and weaknesses of action research and the challenges of data analysis, and report writing.
- Providing an example of action research still in progress and an exercise to help the reader understand the interrelationships between theory, method and data.

ACTION RESEARCH: RATIONALE, PRINCIPLES AND RESOURCES

Definition and methods

Action research is defined by Kemmis and McTaggart (1988: 5) as 'simply a form of collective self-reflective enquiry undertaken by participants in social situations in order to improve the rationality and justice of their own situations, their understandings of these practices and the situations in which these practices are carried out'. This definition captures the essence of action research in highlighting its participatory and action-oriented goals. It also underlines that learning is an important part of the process. In practice, action research has been variously interpreted and applied depending on the research paradigm and discipline base of the action researcher. For example, action research in a health education setting will tend to play out differently to that found in commercial organizations (Hart and Bond 1995). The former is likely to focus on a small group of teachers who have chosen to improve the quality of their teaching and the latter will tend to concentrate on institution-wide problems as identified by senior managers.

Research may be undertaken using a range of methods: surveys, interviews with patients and practitioners, focus group interviews, observation of practice, and the secondary analysis of previous research. Qualitative and quantitative research methods are employed depending on the nature of the problem and the scope of the project. The research should aim to provide insight into different perspectives on a problem and may be undertaken throughout the process of action research in order to help assess what needs to be done, and to monitor and evaluate any changes introduced. In the study discussed, patients' perspectives were sought through letters and focus group interviews, staff views were gathered via interviews, clinical nursing care was observed and the effect of different posturing regimes were measured (Waterman et al. 2005a; Waterman et al. 2005b).

The rationale for action research: Improving practice through critical reflection

In discussing the principles of action research, and its strengths and weaknesses, illustrative examples will be drawn mainly from this one study, referred to throughout the chapter as 'the posturing study' (for full details see Waterman et al. 2005a; Waterman et al. 2005b). This action research study was undertaken at a regional eye hospital in the United Kingdom, and the study aimed to encourage patients to maintain a regime of 'face-down posturing' following retinal surgery. This had been recommended as a regime to maintain healing, but there was uncertainty about how best to support patients in following the regime at home. The first phase of the action research project consisted of interviews with nurses and doctors from both inpatient and outpatient settings to learn about current practice and how this could be improved. This led to consensus among staff that the best way forward was to make 'take-home' specialist equipment available for patients to help them to 'posture' for longer and, in consequence, achieve more cost-effective treatment.

This illustrates the first principle of action research: the overriding purpose is to improve practice and the experience and outcome of patient care (Kemmis and Wilkinson 1998). Action research aims to assist both practitioners and patients to understand their problems better and to enlighten and inform them so that they can decide on action. The research moves beyond describing the 'status quo' as in traditional research to speculating on what 'might or ought to be', introducing changes and assessing the results. Thus, the research is about producing knowledge for action (Cornwall and Jewkes 1995).

A second important ingredient in action research is critical reflection. Critical reflection, while presented for the purposes of explanation as separate from research method, has an interdependent relationship with it. It binds together all activities associated with the research process and leads to empowerment and action. In practice, critical reflection in a group setting refers to the process of identifying and examining assumptions that underpin daily activity, and asking whether the ideologies and attitudes that influence practice are those that best serve the interests of patients and staff. It means examining critically professional values and assumptions and assessing whether these are carried into practice. Professionals will have their own views of what actually happens in practice and a further test is to investigate the views of patients. Critical reflection aims to examine the (power) relationships between practitioners and patients, and between, and within, professional groups. Different perspectives on a problem are deliberately sought to help illuminate an issue and to prevent one viewpoint from taking precedence. Some techniques are to enable patients and practitioners to discuss issues together, and for professionals from different disciplines to share their experiences with one another. An example of this process is described by Waterman and colleagues (2005a; 2005b) in the posturing study. Here, the key stakeholders in the project on post retinal surgery – namely, nurses, a specialist registrar and managers – watched a number of videos of patient focus group interviews. These showed that patients were critical of the lack of warning about, and information on, posturing. This provoked discussions critical of the ethos, practicalities and effects of the existing forms of nursing and medical care.

A synthesis of different perspectives occurs over time both in the group and individually. By drawing on experiences and integrating these with other types of evidence, conclusions can be drawn about how, and why, practice could be changed. The main result of the critical reflection in this study led to the setting up of nurse-led, pre-operative clinics so that patients could be provided with detailed information about 'posturing' two weeks in advance of their surgery. The process of critical reflection is challenging. It takes time and, as indicated later, may not always be successful.

Participation

A third important principle in action research is participation. This is linked to ideas of democracy and the belief that people should be able to inform the health care service and participate or be consulted about health care decisions defined in the broadest sense. Compared with traditional approaches to research where research participants play a passive role in that they do not determine the research questions or affect practice, participants in action research are active. Cornwall and Jewkes (1995) argue that action research was borne out of methodological critiques of conventional research that ignored issues of power in the research process, especially with regard to the subjugated position of the research subject. A partnership between researchers and participants is seen as equitable and liberating in action research (Stringer 1996).

The level of participation may vary within a project, and between projects. Cornwall (1996) identifies six types of participation ranging from co-option and token representation with no real input, to collective action where local people set, and carry out, the research agenda without assistance from professional researchers. In many action research projects in health, the participants have been practitioners – that is, mainly nurses and doctors (Waterman et al. 2001). This has parallels in educational action research and the teacher-as-researcher movement (Elliott 1991). In health and social care, clients and carers are consulted and may cooperate with a project but they tend not to be placed in an equal position with health care practitioners to make decisions about the research. As Cornwall and Jewkes (1995) describe, they are 'participants in a process' over which they have no real control. Research by Bradburn and Mackie (2001) is an exception. In their project, clients with cancer jointly led an action research project where the aim was to raise awareness of the needs of cancer service users in cancer service planning meetings of the local health authority. The clients were directly involved in determining the course of the project. Further examples are given in this volume in Chapters 16 and 18. One hazard of research with patients who have a particular illness is that some patients may be, or become, too ill to participate actively. Researchers in these circumstances must take care to respect the wishes of participants.

Introducing change

A fourth fundamental aspect of action research is the inclusion of a change intervention. The process is often described as a 'spiral' (Kemmis and McTaggart 1988) or 'cycle' (Lewin 1947) of different phases that incorporate fact finding (also known as reflection or reconnaissance), planning, action and evaluation, reflection, planning, action and so on. Each phase is the foundation for the next. Readers from a nursing or quality assurance background will find the outline of this process similar to the nursing process and the audit cycle respectively. However, it is fundamentally different to either as there is an iteration between reflection, action and research and because of the ethos of empowerment and democracy that is fundamental to action research.

Action may come in several forms as follows. There may be:

- *Technical advancement*: This was the case referred to above where new equipment was purchased to encourage patients to maintain 'face-down postures' following retinal surgery (Waterman et al. 2005a; Waterman et al. 2005b).
- *The development of educational programmes for staff*: An example is the project to develop a multisensory environment for patients with dementia (Hope and Waterman 2004).

- *Developments in professional roles*: For example, advanced nurse practitioner roles have been developed in caring for patients with dementia (Rolfe and Phillips 1997).
- *Service reorganization*: For example, acute medical care was reorganized in a district general hospital following an action research project (Hanlon et al. 1997).

This does not take into account the more subtle changes in thinking and behaviour that will occur through participating in research and critical reflection.

Action research may be an appropriate choice of research methodology when the problem being addressed is complex, poorly understood, culturally bound, causes conflict, gives rise to ethical issues, or when resolution is required. Complexity typically refers to the different factors which may influence a problem. For example, poor pain management on a ward may be a result of poor assessment, lack of staff knowledge on analgesia, lack of empathy, poor leadership and poor communication. To improve pain management, a holistic strategy including action research may be needed. Action research may also be suitable in situations where there is conflict between groups or one occupational group dominates another. Meetings and forums for critical reflection can allow for the discussion of ethical and cultural issues and help to empower all participants. Again to draw on the posturing study referred to above, the iterative action research process demonstrated differences in perception between staff. Nurses felt they were doing their best to encourage patients to posture. Patients, however, found it difficult to carry out the instructions given by doctors while doctors themselves thought that their post-operative instructions were being ignored. Through meetings and research, the nurses and doctors realized that their discussions with patients on posturing in the outpatients clinic had been too superficial to convey to patients the importance of following a face-down posturing regime. Furthermore, the lack of information given to patients on their responsibilities on discharge prevented them from preparing themselves properly for post-operative face-down posturing at home.

Resources: Human, technical and support staff

Action research is resource intensive. For instance, the action research project described above involved eight members of staff in the core action research team, as well as costs for the author as research director. Costs were also incurred in the development and implementation of changes in practice, although these costs were absorbed later by the hospital. A systematic review on action research projects suggests that the majority of projects do not secure external funding (Waterman et al. 2001). Funding is essential as participants must be released from their day-to-day activities to attend meetings, undertake research, and resources are required to implement changes (McNiff et al. 1996; Stringer 1996). Action researchers often have to seek resources as part of their task and some examples of strategies follow.

Webb and colleagues (1990) were invited to carry out an action research project by nurses on a ward caring for elderly people. Their aim was to move from a drug-round administration of medicines to a system where patients were permitted to take medicines without supervision. Webb managed to secure funding to replace staff who were then able to attend meetings to develop a strategy. In contrast, in the project on posturing following retinal surgery, we had to meet on a side ward so that the nurses were accessible in an emergency. Although there was strong internal support for the project, no external funding was secured. This meant that meetings occurred less frequently and, when they did take place, they were sometimes hurried or interrupted. Generally, funding should be gained prior to the commencement of a project so that planning and implementation can take place within a budget (McNiff et al. 1996).

External funding may be gained from health authorities, charities and research funding agencies, or government agencies. However, action researchers face certain barriers. Proposals for action research may not fit the conventional research template. Ways of overcoming such problems are to ensure that there is a match between what action researchers want to do and the objectives of the organization from which they hope to obtain funding and to work closely with others experienced in developing research applications for a particular funding body.

Table 8.1 outlines the main resources needed to carry out an action research project and what they are likely to be needed for. The budget should be worked out between participants so that all their costs are accounted. Sometimes full economic costing is required, including overheads and costs of supervision. Action researchers should seek advice on what they need to cost from research accountants, business managers and experienced action researchers.

Table 8.1 *Resources typically required for an action research project*

Item	Purpose
Research assistant	To facilitate the research and the process of critical reflection. To work closely with clinical team
Time for all stakeholders	To pay for staff replacements
Travel expenses including accommodation	To pay for travel costs incurred. For example, by clients to attend meetings and to pay for a hotel
Tape recorder and transcribing machines	To record meetings/interviews and to speed up the process of transcribing
Transcribing costs	To pay for a typist for checking by participants
Educational costs for educational qualification	To pay for MSc, MPhil or PhD fees
Miscellaneous costs	To pay for unforeseen costs that may occur in action research including implementation costs

THE STRENGTHS OF ACTION RESEARCH

The main characteristics and rationale for action research indicate three main strengths. First, it can lead to contextually relevant changes or innovations in practice, education or management that will have a positive effect on clients' experiences and the outcome of health care interventions. Second, the knowledge and theory are directly relevant for action. Third, participants are helped to take responsibility for their own circumstances. Each of these strengths will now be explored in turn.

Action research and change/innovation

The rhetoric of action research focuses on how it can improve people's situations. There are many examples of action research where this ultimate goal has been achieved. These include the reorganization of in- and outpatient services; the identification and development of new professional roles for nurses and allied health professionals; new care planning documentation; better assessment and management of clients; and the development of educational packages for students and educational videos for patients. However, not all projects bring about successful changes as defined by the researchers and participants (for positive and negative examples see Waterman et al. 2001). There is no single cause for a lack of success, which is likely to be a combination of the following factors: over-ambition; the imposition of researchers' goals upon participants; a high staff turnover so that group cohesion is lost; power relations where one professional group dominates another; poor or no external supervision; a lack of research skills; poor interpersonal skills on the part of the researcher; a lack of, or withdrawal of, organizational support; and, lastly, deliberate sabotage. Action research is more likely to succeed when realistic expectations are set; where there are good collaborative relationships; when there is supervision of the researcher; when the researcher has been educated in action research and has good people management skills; and where the organization is supportive of the project.

It has been argued that action research can also promote professional development (Koch et al. 2002). As staff can reflect critically on their situation and participate in various activities, this is thought to lead: first, to greater self-confidence as the process is self-validating; second, to enhanced competence as it is a learning exercise; and, third, to a reassessment and consolidation of professional values as these are dissected and reconstructed. However, it is not easy to demonstrate whether and how these changes in practice have taken place, let alone to attribute them to action research. A self-reflective diary and interviews may record personal views of changes in understanding or observations of nursing care in practice may demonstrate that changes have taken place.

Action research, knowledge and theory development

Another of the main advantages of action research is that it produces knowledge and theory that are relevant to a particular context (Coghlan and Casey 2001). Typically, knowledge and theoretical ideas are identified in the first phase of a project and then tried out and evaluated. Findings are reflected upon and action plans amended. In other words, practice is studied in order to change it and then to change it again in light of this assessment (Kemmis and Wilkinson 1998). The interaction between reflection, research and action broadens the developing theory and makes it more applicable to the particular research setting. As Hope and Waterman (2003) argue, the dialectical process of action research prevents premature closure and provides opportunities for further study to enhance the depth and breadth of analysis. Again, the posturing project may be used to illustrate this process of change and reassessment. While initially research participants thought that the purchase and use of specialist equipment would facilitate adherence to the post-operative posturing instructions, as the equipment was utilized it became apparent that there were other issues. An analysis suggested that both better communication with patients and further education were necessary.

The theory that is generated through action research may be informal or formal. Informal theory development takes place within individuals as they expand their understanding and experience of the issue under study. The 'theory' is locally bound, unwritten, practical and experiential, and could be described as helping to develop personal explanatory frameworks for action. For example, in the posturing project, the discussions among nurses of how they could help patients' posture showed they felt competent in what they were doing to help patients and the reasons that underlay their practice. This was tantamount to an informal explanatory theory (Waterman et al. 2005a; Waterman et al. 2005b).

Theory may also be formal, communicable and generalizable beyond the specific setting. An example may be taken from a study (Waterman et al. 2006) of HIV/AIDS home-based care coordinators in an action research project in Kenya that is described more fully below. The care coordinators applied sociological theories on how to reduce stigma in the analysis of qualitative interview data collected as part of the project. As this analysis was presented in a theoretical framework, it could be transferred to assist HIV/AIDS work in other settings in Africa. Findings from quantitative data may also be generalizable beyond a specific action research setting. For example, Waterman (2002) undertook a pilot randomized controlled trial as part of the posturing project described above. The hypothesis stated that a group of patients who held a face-down posture for 45 minutes with a 15 minute break would comply with instructions to a greater extent, and feel less depressed, than a group who postured for 55 minutes and had a 5 minute break. The aim of this research was to generate information on the sample which would be useful in the development of a full randomized controlled trial that could test the hypothesis.

In action research, most theory development is of the informal variety. It is practical and based on experience. This could be perceived as a missed opportunity to make the findings more widely accessible. However, formal theory development requires good supervision as well as education and training in research methods.

In action research, there is undoubtedly a tension between undertaking rigorous research to develop theory that is generalizable and the pragmatic concerns of the staff group or institution to improve practice. In the posturing project, for example, managers wanted changes to practice to be made before we had completed the research into patient experiences of face-down posturing. We carried on with the research knowing that some changes were taking place, so we documented these parallel changes and noted their effect. This meant that the research was used as a basis for change and as a tool for monitoring the changes. However, there was some loss of rigour and the possibilities for generalizability to other settings. This is discussed further below. Both Coghlan and Casey (2001) and Williamson and Prosser (2002) underline the importance of understanding the institutional context in action research to identify potential hazards early on in a project.

Action research and empowering participants

A common justification for action research is the empowerment of those who are oppressed or marginalized in society. As practitioners, Koch et al. (2002) argue that this is a key advantage of this approach. Empowerment is a subtle process that occurs as participants gain in confidence, knowledge and understanding of their situation. However, it takes time to gain sufficient insight to decide on the best action to take in ways that are likely to be sustainable. Again, an example can be drawn from the posturing project. It took a number of phases in the project, and a variety of practical difficulties had to be overcome, before finally introducing nurse-led instruction in outpatient pre-operative clinics.

LIMITATIONS AND DILEMMAS IN ACTION RESEARCH

As well as strengths, there are a number of limitations and dilemmas in action research which include empowerment and management issues; the challenge of data collection and analysis; ethical issues; and writing up and presenting findings. These will now be considered in turn.

Empowerment and management issues

Empowerment is not always achieved in action research. For example, Sturt (1997) attempted to carry out action research in a primary health care trust in a study to improve health promotion practices for smoking cessation. She reports that the practice nurses were effectively disempowered by the doctors when they took a decision to halt the project. This led to frustration and dissatisfaction for all concerned. Ironically, although empowerment is thought to be useful in conflict resolution, when power relations hitherto hidden are revealed, this may lead to surprise, shock or even explicit conflict. Cornwall and Jewkes (1995) suggest that while action researchers may be enthusiastic about empowerment, participants may prefer the status quo of hierarchical relationships. Inevitably, empowerment means going outside one's 'comfort zone' provoking anxiety and uncertainty. It is important also for the researcher not to raise expectations at the beginning of the study by discussing the possibilities of empowerment. The starting point of any project is a careful analysis of the original problem and an assessment of how the project fits into the wider organization (Coghlan and Casey 2001).

Closely connected to the issue of empowerment is the question of whether a project should be managed by an insider or outsider. Action researchers may be insiders holding a formal position of employment in the research institution, or they may be an outsider who is facilitating a project in an organization where they have no formal position. In practice the two positions are often blurred. For example, a researcher may be an employee, that is an insider, but an outsider to the group taking part in the research. Both situations have advantages and disadvantages in terms of empowerment. An insider will have knowledge of the organizational structure and this is useful in getting support and approval for the project. On the other hand, they may be constrained by unwritten organizational rules and may have to live with the consequences of the action research process (Coghlan and Casey 2001). In contrast, an outsider will have to spend time getting to know the formal organizational structures and informal social relationships. However, they may be in a better position to see the opportunities for change.

Titchin and Binnie (1993) suggest ways in which the advantages of the insider and outsider roles are combined in a 'double act'. They argue for shared responsibility between an insider and outsider with the former responsible for the clinical component of the action research and the latter facilitating and leading the research and critical reflection. This was a model adopted in the posturing project already described. Initially, I led the research and the changes in clinical practice, but subsequently the roles were split.

The challenge of data collection and analysis

A further challenge in action research is how to collect and analyze data. Winter and Munn-Giddings (2001) identify three reasons for undertaking data analysis in action research. Data may be analyzed to provide insights into what changes can be made in future; data interpretation helps to make findings generalizable; and, lastly, data can be used to provide a baseline to explore what learning has taken place. If participants discuss and plan their approach to data analysis in advance, then any tensions between these objectives will be reduced.

In a conventional research project, the researcher is 'detached' from the research setting and has sole responsibility for data collection and analysis. In action research, not only are there difficult and possibly conflicting purposes for data collection but priorities may shift over time. Moreover, there may be various sources of data that will be available at different points in the life of a project. How data are to be analyzed, by whom, and for what purpose, will require active management in a participative manner (Christensen and Atweh 1998; Winter and Munn-Giddings 2001). In the posturing study, for example, a staff nurse and I undertook most of the detailed analysis of patient focus group interviews. Then, the team as a whole participated in the process through reflective discussions based on the results. In the subsequent randomized controlled trial, a research student undertook all the statistical analysis so that results could be presented for discussion.

Ethical issues in action research

Some ethical issues arise in the course of health research, while others can be predicted in advance. In either case, these matters require discussion and negotiation. Confidentiality is likely to be an issue. For example, it should not simply be assumed that participants will want the contents of their interviews and observations to be shared by other participants whether colleagues or clients. The matter requires discussion in advance. Maintaining the anonymity of participants is also a matter for discussion. It should not be assumed that identities are hidden by using anonymous quotes (Williamson and Prosser 2002).

Acknowledgements and contact details can give away information that can lead to the identification of participants. On the other hand, it has been my experience of the Kenyan action research study (Waterman et al. 2006) that participants want to be identified in any report, as participation in a research project that is acknowledged may give recognition and status, but they do not want to be individually cited in quotations.

Writing up and presenting findings

Christensen and Atweh (1998) suggest, rightly, that writing a report is an essential stage in action research. This represents the final and formal end of the reflective activities in which all strands of the study should be pulled together. The submission of a report to a funding agency is a significant act of closure. The public distribution of a report and papers is also important in the external validation of the work and usually involves external peer review (McNiff et al. 1996). Yet, there may be different interests in what kind of report should be written and for what audience.

In preparing to write the report, McNiff et al. (1996: 134) identify four different groups of audience for a research project: 'your boss, your colleagues, your tutor, and your academic peers'. These may require different kinds of report. Managers will want a report that emphasizes organizational and change issues; colleagues may find a report that focuses on practical issues that relate to health outcomes of more value; if some participants are drawing on action research for a higher degree, tutors will want a dissertation that discusses the learning that has taken place; finally, academic peers will be interested in the original contribution to knowledge by the research. Most reports are presented chronologically to tell a 'story' of the different cycles of the project (Henderson 1997). Academic papers may report on the whole project or focus on one part of it (Harker et al. 2002) or discuss methodological issues (Meyer 1993).

In keeping with the rest of the process of action research, writing up should be participative. However, as Christensen and Atweh (1998) identify, the process is not straightforward and can create problems. If a number of researchers undertake different parts of the research, deadlines will have to be coordinated. Some participants may not have the experience or confidence to write, but nevertheless may feel excluded from writing up. To maintain the integrity of the project and to prevent conflict, writing up and authorship should be discussed openly in the early stages of the project and revisited often. Christensen and Atweh (1998) present three strategies for participative writing. First, progressive writing when one person takes responsibility to write the full first draft which is then passed around other participants for comment. Second, accounts may be written by different groups and placed together in a final report. Third, there is 'shared writing' in which a small group of people plan and write together.

In all of these situations, agreement must be reached on whose 'voice' is given priority. This is tied into issues of power and the importance of retaining a sense of shared ownership. Such matters are linked to empowerment. Sharing and learning skills requires time and patience but can be rewarding (McLauchlan et al. 2002). These matters are discussed in more detail in Chapter 21 which explores writing up research and getting published. This brings us to the presentation of a practical case study in action research in countries with limited resources.

Case study: Action research and HIV/AIDS in resource-limited countries

CASE STUDY

The following provides an example undertaken by the author of how action research can be applied in resource-limited countries. Sub-Saharan Africa has been affected by the AIDS epidemic disproportionately compared with Western and Central Europe. There have been 2.4 million deaths from AIDS in Sub-Saharan Africa, whereas there have been only 12,000 in Western and Central Europe (UNAIDS 2005). In Nyanza Province, Kenya, the prevalence rate of HIV/AIDS is 20.2 per cent (Nyanza Provincial Medical Office 2005). The main strategy to deal with HIV/AIDS in Sub-Saharan countries is home-based care. Home-based care is a form of comprehensive community-based care that includes social, economic and health services. In practice, it encompasses hands-on nursing care in people's homes, which helps to reduce stigma; setting up and sustaining health care clinics; finding refuge and adoptive parents for orphans; facilitating income-generating activities for widows and people living with HIV/AIDS; establishing referral mechanisms for clients needing counselling and testing for HIV/AIDS; and treating clients with anti-retroviral therapy.

Little information is available to practitioners and policy makers on how to implement these forms of care. The objectives of our research, therefore, were to clarify the concept of home-based care; to articulate its key constituents; to identify a framework for the introduction of home-based care; and to examine contextual factors that facilitate or hinder its development.

Action research was selected as the preferred method by the key HIV/AIDS health care personnel of a non-governmental organization,

(Continued)

Mildmay International, based in Kisumu, Nyanza. This was because it fulfilled the need to document, reflect and research on practice whilst at the same time endeavouring to deliver the best possible home-based care. The research team consisted of three researchers from the University of Manchester, who worked closely with personnel from Mildmay and the HIV/AIDS home-based care coordinators in Nyanza. The relationship had parallels with the 'double act' as described earlier. The study took place across the 12 districts of Nyanza Province and the main participants were the coordinators and members of the District Health Management Team who became known as co-researchers.

Data were collected from 27 focus group interviews and notes were made on 16 field visits to the community. The topics of focus group interviews varied over the course of the project but included discussions on the significance of stigma, poverty, nutrition and gender on people with HIV/AIDS and the importance of volunteers and the linkages between organizations in delivering care. To date, the action research has consisted of two interrelated cycles: the implementation of a plan to integrate HIV/AIDS home-based care into the existing health system based on a prior needs assessment; and the embedding of policies to provide home-based care.

The focus group interviews encouraged critical reflection and empowerment amongst the co-researchers as they provided the opportunity for the exchange of information between participants and the identification of different perspectives. Among other issues, the reasons why some implementation strategies worked and others did not was explored. The co-researchers reported that the discussions helped to provide some answers to their difficulties so that they could agree on ways forward with their work.

So far, the findings suggest that there is a process through which home-based care may be implemented through preparation, needs assessment, establishing services, mobilizing the community, and embedding and sustaining home-based care. There are several barriers to implementation including poverty, stigma, lack of food, gender issues and a lack of resources. Nevertheless, the action-based approach has enabled a critical approach to the introduction of home-based care in Nyanza and led to findings that will be of interest and use to settings beyond this particular context.

CONCLUSION

The argument underlying this chapter is that the action research method is an appropriate tool where the aim is to change practice or behaviour. And a key aspect of achieving this change is to include the range of professionals who provide a service; those who are the clients or patients using a service; people in groups or communities who stand to benefit from improved practice; and researchers with relevant skills. Depending on the nature of the project, all members of such groups or their representative should be included. The role of the lead researcher in an action research project is a challenging one. Not only are research skills required, but also the ability to play a number of roles as an educator, facilitator and mediator. Furthermore, unlike other forms of research where the researcher tends to act as a detached observer, in action research they should be committed to achieve the outcomes of the research while not allowing this commitment to cloud their judgement in evaluating data and findings.

The case study on action research and HIV/AIDS in resource-limited countries shows that action research is a flexible method that may be used in a variety of settings. It is followed by a brief practical exercise for readers that focuses on applying action research to a health-related work setting with which they are familiar.

Exercise: The use of action research in a health-related work setting

This exercise is intended to help readers critically explore the issues raised in this chapter, and particularly to explore the interrelationship between theory, method and data in action research. On the basis of the practical advice provided in this chapter, draw up a proposal for an action research project based on your own experience in a work setting in which you either work or of which you have some knowledge. First, identify an area of practice that you think causes problems. This may, for example, give rise to conflict amongst professional groups or relate to an aspect of practice that is not up to standard. You should then answer the following questions:

(Continued)

1 Where would you obtain funding to carry out the project?
2 What methods could be used to understand the problem better?
3 Who will be the key participants in the action research team and what is the rationale for inclusion?
4 How will you promote and maintain participation in the project?
5 How will you apply the action research process to your issue and context?
6 What process of critical reflection might be implemented and what part will it play in moving forward the research project?
7 Will you be an insider or outsider to the research setting and what effect will your position have on the project?
8 What ethical issues will be encountered in the course of the project and how will they be addressed?
9 What knowledge and theory will be generated for participants and service users planning to improve the care of patients in your area of interest?
10 What will be the limitations of your project?

RECOMMENDED FURTHER READING

Hart, E. and Bond, M. (1995) *Action Research for Health and Social Care: A Guide for Practice.* Milton Keynes: Open University Press.
This book offers a good introduction to action research, containing a useful typology and history of the methodology involved.

Kemmis, S. and McTaggart, R. (1988) *The Action Research Planner*, 3rd edition. Geelong, Victoria: Deakin University.
This classic book provides a detailed framework for the first phase of action research, providing much helpful advice.

Winter, R. and Munn-Giddings, C. (2001) *A Handbook for Action Research in Health and Social Care*. London: Routledge.
This text is a handbook for action researchers, describing and exploring the theoretical issues underpinning action research.

REFERENCES

Bradburn, J. and Mackie, C. (2001) 'A foot in the door: a collaborative action research project with cancer service users', in R. Winter and C. Munn-Giddings (eds), *A Handbook for Action Research in Health and Social Care*. London: Routledge.

Christensen, C. and Atweh, B. (1998) 'Collaborative writing in participatory action research', in B. Atweh, S. Kemmis and P. Weeks (eds), *Action Research in Practice: Partnerships for Social Justice in Education*. London: Routledge.

Coghlan, D. and Casey, M. (2001) 'Action research from the inside: issues and challenges in doing action research in your own organization', *Journal of Advanced Nursing*, 35 (5): 674–82.

Cornwall, A. (1996) 'Towards participatory practice: participatory rural appraisal and the participatory process', in K. De Koning and M. Martin (eds), *Participatory Research in Health: Issues and Experiences*. London: Zed Books.

Cornwall, A. and Jewkes, R. (1995) 'What is participatory action research?', *Social Science and Medicine*, 41: 1667–76.

Elliott, J. (1991) *Action Research for Educational Change*. Milton Keynes: Open University Press.

Hanlon, P., Beck, S., Robertson, G., Henderson, M., McQuillan, R. and Capewell, S. (1997) 'Coping with the inexorable rise in medical admissions: evaluating a radical reorganization of acute medical services in a Scottish district general hospital', *Health Bulletin*, 55 (3): 176–84.

Harker, R., McLauchlan, R., MacDonald, H., Waterman, C. and Waterman, H. (2002) 'Endless nights: patients' experiences of posturing face down following vitreo-retinal surgery', *International Journal of Ophthalmic Nursing*, 6 (2): 11–15.

Hart, E. and Bond, M. (1995) *Action Research for Health and Social Care: A Guide for Practice*. Milton Keynes: Open University Press.

Henderson, C. (1997) *Changing 'Childbirth' and the West Midlands Region 1995–1996*. London: Royal College of Midwives.

Hope, K.W. and Waterman, H. (2003) 'Praiseworthy pragmatism? Validity and action research: methodological issues in nursing research', *Journal of Advanced Nursing*, 44 (2): 120–7.

Hope, K.W. and Waterman, H. (2004) 'Multi-sensory environments (MSEs) in clinical practice – factors impeding their use as perceived by clinical staff', *International Journal of Social Care and Practice*, 3 (1): 45–68.

Kemmis, S. and McTaggart, R. (1988) *The Action Research Planner*, 3rd edition. Geelong, Victoria: Deakin University.

Kemmis, S. and Wilkinson, M. (1998) 'Participatory action research and the study of practice', in B. Atweh, S. Kemmis and P. Weeks (eds), *Action Research in Practice: Partnerships for Social Justice in Education*. London: Routledge.

Koch, T., Selim, P. and Kralik, D. (2002) 'Enhancing lives through the development of a community-based participatory action research programme', *Journal of Clinical Nursing*, 11: 109–17.

Lewin, K. (1947) 'Frontiers in group dynamics: social planning and action research', *Human Relations*, 1: 143–53.

McLauchlan, R., Harker, R., MacDonald, H., Waterman, C. and Waterman, H. (2002) 'Using research to improve ophthalmic nursing care', *Nursing Times*, 98 (27): 39–40.

McNiff, J., Lomax, P. and Whitehead, J. (1996) *You and Your Action Research Practice*. London: Routledge.

Meyer, J. (1993) 'New paradigm research in practice: trials and tribulations of action research', *Journal of Advanced Nursing*, 18: 1066–72.

Nyanza Provincial Medical Office (2005) Unpublished report. Nyanza Provincial Medical Office, Kisumu.

Rolfe, G. and Phillips, L.M. (1997) 'Development and evaluation of the role of an advanced nurse practitioner in dementia – an action research project', *International Journal of Nursing Studies*, 34 (2): 119–27.

Stringer, E. (1996) *Action Research: A Handbook for Practitioners.* Thousand Oaks, CA: Sage.

Sturt, J. (1997) 'Placing empowerment research within an action research typology', *Journal of Advanced Nursing*, 30 (5): 1057–63.

Titchin, A. and Binnie, A. (1993) 'Research partnerships: collaborative action research in nursing', *Journal of Advanced Nursing*, 18: 858–65.

UNAIDS (2005) 'HIV/AIDS statistics and features in 2003 and 2005', *UNAIDS Epidemic Update: Sub-Saharan Africa*, UNAIDS/WHO AIDS, December.

Waterman, C. (2002) 'A randomised controlled trial to evaluate the effects of two face-down posturing regimes following vitreo-retinal surgery with internal gas tamponade', MSc dissertation, University of Manchester.

Waterman, H., Tillen, D., Dickson, R. and De Koning, K. (2001) 'Action research: a systematic review and assessment for guidance', *Health Technology Assessment*, 5 (23): iii–157.

Waterman, H., Harker, R., MacDonald, H., McLaughlan, R. and Waterman, C. (2005a) 'Advancing ophthalmic nursing practice through action research', *Journal of Advanced Nursing*, 52 (3): 281–90.

Waterman, H., Harker, R., MacDonald, H., McLaughlan, R. and Waterman, C. (2005b) 'Evaluation of an action research project in ophthalmic nursing practice', *Journal of Advanced Nursing*, 52 (4): 389–98.

Waterman, H., Griffiths, J., Gellard, L., O'Keeffe, C., Olang, G., Obwanda, E., Ayuyo, J., Ogwethe, V. and Ondiege, J. (2006) 'Intervening in the process of stigmatization: challenging social inequalities in the context of HIV/AIDS home-based care in Kenya', Unpublished paper.

Webb, C., Addison, C., Holman, H., Saklaki, B. and Wager, A. (1990) 'Self-medication for elderly patients', *Nursing Times*, 86: 46–49.

Williamson, G.R. and Prosser, S. (2002) 'Action research: politics, ethics and participation', *Journal of Advanced Nursing*, 40 (5): 587–93.

Winter, R. and Munn-Giddings, C. (2001). *A Handbook for Action Research in Health and Social Care*. London: Routledge.

PART III
Quantitative Methods and Health

9

Health Research Sampling Methods[1]

PETER DAVIS AND ALASTAIR SCOTT

INTRODUCTION

Sampling a smaller number of respondents so that generalizations can be made about a larger population is an important tool to master for the researcher carrying out a quantitative investigation. In a properly constructed sample, the costs of the research in time and money are kept to a minimum without loss of generalizability. This chapter outlines the basic features of sampling in health research. The emphasis is on probability sampling, both because this is the most widely used approach and because there is a well-established body of theory and practice on sample design and inference. In the chapter we discuss the rationale of sampling and introduce key terms. Different forms of non-probability sampling and the techniques employed in probability sampling are discussed together with issues that arise in sampling and ways of reducing error. The chapter draws examples from four studies undertaken in New Zealand by the authors and others and there is a case study that illustrates the use of sampling in practice.

The studies shown in Table 9.1 are all based on national sample surveys undertaken in New Zealand: a socio-dental survey based on an area sample; an investigation of partner relationships, using telephone interviewing; a

Table 9.1 *Examples of surveys to illustrate sampling techniques*

Survey topic	Dental health	Partner relations	Hospital safety	Primary care
Target population	Adult population, 1975	18—54 year age group, 1991	Hospital in-patients, 1998	All GP patients, 2001—02
Sampling frame	Household enumeration of areas	Random digit dialling	Central admissions register	Telephone page listing of GPs
Sample stages	68 Primary Sampling Units (PSU), 136 Secondary Sampling Units (SSUs), 28 adults	~1,750 clusters of 3, 1 eligible each	13 hospitals, 575 patient admissions	350 GPs, 1 in 4 patients
Size and response rate	3,231 (84%)	2,361 (63%)	6,731 (91.5%)	8,258 (68.5%)
Number of strata	Two (rural and urban)	14 dialling zones	Three (hospital size)	Seven (type of practice, practitioner)
Weighting criteria	Self-weighting	Number of eligibles per household	By hospital size	By practice type
Sources	Cutress et al. (1979) Davis and Scott (1996)	Davis et al. (1993)	Davis et al. (2001)	Raymont et al. (2004)

patient safety study drawing on a sample of medical records held by public hospitals; and a survey of patients attending general practitioners (GPs), which required us first to select a sample of medical practitioners. Throughout the chapter we will draw on these studies selectively for illustration. The details of the studies are found in Table 9.1, and the sources cited accordingly. The terminology and concepts used are standard in the literature and are drawn mainly from Aday and Cornelius (2006) and Korn and Graubard (1999).

SAMPLING AND ITS RATIONALE

Why sample?

The topic of 'sampling' goes to the methodological heart of drawing inferences about human populations. In the cases outlined in Table 9.1, the populations were national in scope and the topics diverse. Typically investigators, whether they are health practitioners, social scientists, managers, clinicians or interested citizens, want to gain information about the features of a particular population group. Yet, information gathering has to be selective, and the process of selection raises issues of the representativeness and accuracy of the knowledge and insights gained from the sample. Thus sampling is the science and practice of selecting information from populations in a manner that allows defensible inferences to be drawn from those data.

The focus of this chapter is on sampling that takes place in a well-defined setting where the probabilities of selection can be attributed to elements in the population. However, it is worth noting that systematic empirical work of any kind requires the analysis of samples of information drawn from a larger universe or population. In the case of qualitative research, the selection of information is based on informed human judgement rather than by technical procedure, and one of the judgement criteria may well be based on a claim to representativeness or typicality (Murphy and Dingwall 2003). In principle, it should be equally possible for qualitative investigators to justify inferences based on samples selected on judgement criteria as for quantitative researchers who draw on probability sample designs.

Basic terminology

The starting point for a sampling scheme is the definition of a 'target population'; this is the population 'of interest' to the proposed investigation. In the case of the four studies outlined in Table 9.1, in the first two the target populations were all adult New Zealanders with an age restriction for the partner relations survey. In the second and third, the focus was on hospital patients and GP patients respectively. In identifying these four populations 'of interest', the aim was to ensure that the results of our sample selection and the subsequent analyses of the data were reflective of, and could be applied to, the four defined sets of the adult and patient populations.[2]

A member of the target population is known as a sampling unit or element. In probability sampling, each one of these units or elements has a specifiable chance of being selected. It is on account of this characteristic that we are able to apply statistical techniques of estimation and inference to the data collected. In many research designs this chance of selection is equal across all units, or self-weighting. However, in others it is not. In the dental health study, for example, people living in larger territorial local authorities had a higher chance of being in a selected territorial local authority because, at the first stage, these units were selected on the basis of probability proportionate to size, as were two second-stage units in each selected territorial local authority. This likelihood of selection then equalized out because of the constant sample size at the third stage (28 respondents in each of the two units in each selected authority).

Conversely, in the case of the primary care study, GPs had different chances of selection depending on what kind of practice they were in, but the final number of patients chosen, one in four, in each case was not uniform but proportionate to workload. This meant the data had to be reweighted in the analysis. This process is illustrated in the example below.

SAMPLE SELECTION USING NON-PROBABILITY DESIGNS

Quota sampling is a non-probability technique commonly used in market research. It involves selecting sample elements according to a predetermined distribution across certain defined categories. For example, respondents may be recruited in such a way as to ensure that there is a roughly equal distribution between males and females, or to cover certain age bands, socio-economic positions or to obtain an area spread such as rural and urban. This is a form of stratified sampling as the predetermined categories are the strata that ensure a predicted sample distribution. However, it is not possible to estimate the probability of selection within those strata because the actual selection process is not a random one. It usually involves working in selected streets or suburbs and trying to accost cooperative respondents (Goupille et al. 2003).

The distinctive characteristic of quota sampling is its non-random basis for selecting sample elements using judgement criteria. This is also a distinctive feature of sampling in qualitative research. The main types are as follows:

- *Convenience sampling*: This is the most rudimentary selection technique. Selection may be based on the ease of recruitment, for example those attending an outpatient clinic, or decision makers who can be easily accessed.
- *Calling for volunteers*: This is a version of the convenience method and is widely used in experimental research.
- *Snowball sampling*: This is a further refinement of the convenience method that requires explicit judgements. With this technique, the investigator starts with an initial group, for example those known to have a particular health condition, and then increases the size of this initial sample by referrals from this group (Momartin et al. 2003).
- *Purposive sampling*: This increases the deliberative or judgemental element by selecting all sample elements according to certain criteria. For example, extreme or unusual cases may be selected to pre-test a questionnaire. In certain study designs, explicit inclusion criteria may be used (Vijayapushpam et al. 2003).
- *Theoretical sampling*: This is a method of selection that is informed by a particular philosophy of qualitative research involving the generating and testing of empirical hypotheses.

PROBABILITY SAMPLE DESIGNS

There is a wide range of probability sample designs that vary along two dimensions – the number of sampling stages and the extent of departure from a simple random selection strategy. The most rudimentary design combines these two features: a single sampling stage with a simple selection strategy. The simplest random sample can be picking names out of a hat, or using a table of random numbers. Where the elements are not returned to the pool after selection, this is called sampling without replacement. According to a strict interpretation of sample theory, this requires a correction factor in estimating standard errors. The impact of this factor reduces as the proportion of the population sampled decreases.

Two departures from the simple random strategy are systematic, or list, sampling and stratification. In the case of the former, a sample is drawn from an existing list that has a degree of organization or ordering of the target population. Approached in the right way, this can be a helpful feature since it ensures a better spread of the sample across implicit strata within the population. For example, an alphabetical ordering by names can ensure a good spread across ethnic groups. We used this method to identify patients by date of admission in the hospital safety study. The New Zealand Health Information Service was able to order patients by date of admission throughout the year for each selected hospital, and then set an interval that would generate the required 575 cases with a random start point, and working from January to December. In this way we ensured a spread of cases that was representative of the mix and volume of workload through the year.

Stratification is a more explicit method for ensuring a desired distribution of a sample across important groups in the population (Pyper et al. 2004). It requires a certain amount of prior knowledge of the population since subsections of the sample will be allocated to predefined strata, usually on a proportionate, that is a representative, basis. There are, however, cases where disproportionate sampling might be used, such as to ensure larger numbers in the sample for a particular ethnic minority group or for more variable strata. In the partner relations survey, we knew from census information how many people in our target age groups there were in the different dialling zones, and we allocated our sample to reflect that distribution. In the case of the primary care study, however, we wanted to ensure a minimum number of practitioners, and their patients, within different practice types. We therefore undersampled doctors in heavily populated strata, such as private GPs, and oversampled in sparsely populated strata, such as GPs in community-governed practices.

Stages in sample design

Looking at the number of stages in sample design, for any but the most concentrated and easily accessible population, cost and logistics dictate more than one stage of sampling (Botman et al. 2000). This helps to localize the requirements of data collection into what are called clusters (usually geographically defined). Another advantage of this approach is that the frame or list of individual population units is required only for the selected clusters, which may be a consideration where there is no simple master frame for the entire population. Both these considerations were important in the dental health study. First, we wished to interview 3,000 adult New Zealanders throughout the country. For reasons of both cost and logistics, therefore, it was essential to concentrate our interviewing efforts. Second, there was no master list of the adult population. We needed to compile such a list, which we did door to door, but only for the 136 geographical areas selected at the second stage.

The trick with constructing an efficient multistage sample design is to strike the right balance between the number and size of clusters (Agarwal et al. 2005). The larger, and fewer, the clusters, the easier the logistics and the lower the costs tend to be. There is also a slightly greater chance that such clusters will be internally more heterogeneous. With smaller clusters, although they will be internally more homogeneous, there will be more of them. This should assist representativeness but the management task and costs will increase with the degree of dispersal.

Frame and coverage

The sampling frame is the list of units or elements assumed to define best the target population (or survey population, if there is a discrepancy or incompleteness in this list), and it is from this list that the sample is drawn. A good frame is one that is up to date and includes all units in a way that ensures they are distinguishable from one another, and are only counted once. Physical lists are commonly used, like the electoral roll or telephone book. Area frames, the enumeration of an area to compile a list, may also be used, or, for example, a conceptual list such as people booking an airline ticket. In the primary care survey there was no complete list of GPs, so we used the electronic White Pages to compile a list, on the assumption that every practice would have to be listed for business purposes. In the dental health survey, we listed household members by going door to door and used an agreed selection procedure for those adults identified.

More complex lists can be constructed by dual or multiple frames and screening surveys (Hosler and Melnik 2005). A dual or multiple frame is one in which more than one list is used in order to achieve adequate coverage of the target population by incorporating a frame that includes a higher concentration of a hard-to-reach group. For example, in order, say, to oversample some identifiable group, a combination of the electoral roll and an area sample in which the particular group lives may be used. Another approach for identifying a hard-to-reach population is to use, either by design or opportunistically, an initial survey to screen a larger population. For example, a survey of people with disabilities could be mounted on a much larger survey of the population, as long as the relevant screening questions for disability were embedded in the first study. The New Zealand official statistical agency conducted two such special post-census surveys following the 2001 Census, to identify two hard-to-reach populations: Maori and disabled people (Statistics New Zealand 2001).

Under-coverage

A complete list is one in which every individual in the target population appears and can be assigned a calculable non-zero probability of selection. This is rarely achieved because usually there are at least some members of the population not entered on the list. This is often due to some systematic bias in the list rather than random error. Such a shortcoming in a list is called incomplete coverage or under-coverage.

Non-response, the failure to collect data on sampled units, is another source of incomplete coverage. Although this source of incomplete coverage occurs at a later stage of the survey process and requires a quite different response, such as through improving contact rates, technically this is a coverage issue. For example, in our partner relations survey those members of the population without phones could not be contacted using our methodology, which was telephone interviewing. This was an example of incomplete coverage in the list, and nothing could be done about it. At the same time, there were a good number of phone numbers for which there was no reply or a refusal. This contributed to our non-response rate. Here, modifications to the approach might have reduced under-coverage.

The impact of under-coverage depends on the proportion of the population that is missing due, for example, either to failures of the list or to non-response and on the difference in the values of key study variables for these missing units compared with those that are adequately covered. This is the degree of systematic bias (Partin et al. 2003). There are a number of methods for trying to correct for the impact of under-coverage. These include weighting, post-stratification, ratio estimation and imputation (Liu et al. 2005). However, none of these methods are as effective as getting the right sample in the first place, and therefore strenuous efforts need to be made to ensure both a complete frame and low non-response rate, concentrating particularly on eliminating bias. Indeed, it may be worth settling for a lower initial sample size if this achieves cost savings that can then be allocated to gaining a higher response rate.

SAMPLE SIZE AND DISTRIBUTION

Sample size is a central consideration when it comes to minimizing the error of sample estimates and maximizing the study value for a given cost. There are two components to the error term associated with a sample-based estimate of a population parameter: accuracy (how close is it to the 'true' value?) and precision (how tightly bunched are the estimates?). Sample size affects precision, but not accuracy. Generally speaking, the larger the size of the sample, the more precise the estimates derived from that sample are likely to be. Indeed, it is possible to work out the size of sample required to achieve a given level of precision (Diehr et al. 2005). For example, in the dental health survey we were able to estimate from other studies the size of sample we needed to get reasonably precise estimates of what we considered a key parameter, namely the average number of teeth that were affected by dental disease, that is decayed, missing or filled.

However, achieving a high level of precision is unlikely to be the only consideration, because the larger the sample, the higher the cost of the study. Usually an investigator is faced with a relatively fixed envelope of field costs, and therefore the objective is to try and maximize sample size to a point where precision is good, while at the same time minimizing costs through sample design. This can be done by clustering and choosing a low-cost method of data collection such as telephone contact as opposed to face-to-face interviews. Again, in the dental health study, precision could be attained by a certain sample size, but that in turn had to be distributed nationally in such a way as to meet a budget. This allowed for three teams working across a prescribed number of geographical clusters in three broad regions: the South Island, the lower and central North Island, and Auckland and the north. For the partner relations survey, a similar sample size calculation around a target measure of precision was made to include the proportion of units with multiple partners in the last year. In this case, moving from face-to-face to telephone interviews halved the cost of data collection, and allowed a doubling of sample size.[3]

For more complex sample surveys an important consideration is the design decisions that need to be made about the way in which the sample is distributed. Again, it is important to balance the minimization of error and the maximization of study value for a given cost. At this point the issue is not so much the sample size as the sample distribution across, say, clusters or strata.

In the case of strata, from the point of view of precision there should be a disproportionate allocation of sample numbers to strata containing units with high diversity or variability (Cardozo et al. 2004). For example, in both the dental health survey and the hospital safety study, sample numbers were allocated proportionately to the size of these units. The reasoning was that large territorial local authorities, such as cities and their associated hospitals, were likely to be the most diverse. On the other hand, there may be other considerations that dictate a strategy that points away from size. Thus, a stratum that is cheap to sample may, other things being equal, justify a higher sampling fraction. There may also be analytical considerations. A stratum of particular interest may justify greater attention. In the primary care survey, we had a higher sampling fraction in the stratum of practices that were community governed.

For sample allocation across clusters, in order to optimize error reduction and cost control, the key questions are the number of clusters and the number of units in each cluster. The optimal cluster sample size increases both with 'within-cluster' heterogeneity or variability and with the cost of adding an extra cluster relative to the cost of obtaining an extra element within a cluster. For a fixed cluster sample size, the ideal is to maximize the number of clusters for a given fieldwork budget (Agarwal et al. 2005).

SAMPLING AND NON-SAMPLING ERROR

The central concern of theory and practice in sampling is reducing overall survey error as far as possible. There are two types of error, random and systematic, and two sources of error, sampling and non-sampling. Usually, effort is focused on sampling error, particularly the random element. This is easy to estimate and to control for. Systematic error, or bias, is harder to identify. Also, the theory and practice for non-sampling error are much less developed than in the case of sampling.

The primary criteria to be assessed in probability sample designs are:

- *Precision*: The minimal random or variable sampling error.
- *Accuracy*: The lack of bias in estimates.
- *Complexity*: The amount of advance information required and the number of stages.
- *Efficiency*: The minimization of cost for given precision and accuracy.

Generally speaking, stratified designs increase precision, and clustering erodes it but also reduces cost. List sampling should have higher precision, although this could be severely eroded if there is a periodic or recurrent pattern in the ordering of the units. Simple random sampling is less complex, but may have lower precision and efficiency.

The main components of non-sampling error are coverage, the frame and non-response rate, and measurement error. Coverage error or bias is hard to estimate and control. In the case of measurement error, there are well-established models for assessing the properties of scales and similar instruments (Diehr et al. 2005), but theory and practice have been less fully developed for questionnaire, respondent and interviewer sources.

Controlling for non-sampling error

Some techniques for controlling for non-sampling error, such as the pilot-test questionnaires, concern approaching respondents in a uniform way with realistic expectations on information recall, and it is better to have more interviewers with smaller workloads than the reverse. Interviewers are able to attend better to a smaller load, and any bias affects fewer respondents. For example, in the dental survey all these points were illustrated (Davis and Scott 1996). First, one item in particular elicited a very large variation in response across interviewers. This was mainly because it asked about an unusual activity, use of disclosing solution, and interviewers had not been provided with a standardized coding response to reflect the lack of knowledge of interviewees. Second, the component of interviewer error was higher for items that aimed to elicit attitudes and required recall. Third, although the errors of interviewers were small, as reflected in the small intra-cluster correlation of their respondents, their workload was high and this small interviewer-specific error therefore translated into quite a major impact across the entire sample.

Stratification and weighting

As already discussed, stratification is a technique whereby information about the structure of the population of interest is used in advance in the design of the sample. Stratification can also be used after the event – that is, after sample selection. This is called post-stratification, and is applied in association with the weighting of sample outcomes. In a typical case, key sample outcomes are compared with known population distributions and weights are then applied to sample units in order to achieve a closer correspondence between sample and population.[4] This approach was used in the partner relations survey to correct for the fact that women were heavily over-represented in the sample.

Although such discrepancies between sample and population could be due to the normal workings of random or variable error, it is far more likely that they are due to bias or systematic error in coverage (such as frame and non-response), and therefore such a practice can be controversial. While weighting in this case may be controversial, its use to correct for features of sample design is completely acceptable; indeed it is desirable. For example, in the primary care study the sampling fraction, that is the proportion of GPs sampled, varied between different practice types, and this had to be accounted for in any analysis that pooled data across these strata in order to ensure that practices were given the same weight that they had nationally.

In summary, it is possible to see sample weights, as applied after selection, as consisting of three elements: the base weight, which accounts for different probabilities of selection; the non-response adjustment, correcting for differences in collecting information on individuals in the population; and post-stratification, correcting for bias in the population representativeness of the frame or list.[5]

Drawing inferences

The central strength of probability sampling is the much greater confidence we have in drawing inferences about the population to which we wish these results to apply. Ideally, we should be in a position to draw conclusions that are both precise (there should be a narrow band around our estimates) and accurate (they should be close to the true value of the parameters in the population). The base case is one in which a simple random sample has been drawn with replacement and a single parameter, like a proportion or a mean, estimated. These are the conditions for the typical 'test of significance' using standard packages.

Once the sample design becomes more complex, and particularly if any weighting is required, a more elaborate approach is needed. In the case of sample designs that are more elaborate than the simple random sample, the 'design effect' captures the impact of this design complexity (Agarwal et al. 2005).

For instance, a design effect of four means that the standard error is twice that for a similarly sized simple random sample on the same population. A design effect of four means that the sample size needs to be four times that of a simple random sample in order to achieve the same accuracy (overcoming the extra burden of sampling error introduced by the more complex sample design). The consequence is that, in technical terms, the standard error needs to be twice that for a similarly sized simple random sample, on the same population. Rather than increasing the sample size four-fold – which would generally not be practical – the confidence interval would have to be doubled and the value of a statistical test would need to be increased before reaching significance.[6] In the dental health survey we estimated the impact of a multistage sample with clustering. We went further and determined how this design effect might vary according to the kind of item. Thus, very little adjustment was required in the case of gender, because of the uniform distribution of men and women across clusters, but the design effect was quite marked in the case of ethnicity as there was extensive clustering on this variable (Davis and Scott 1996).

Case study: Sampling in practice in primary health care

The National Primary Medical Care Survey (NatMedCa) was undertaken to describe primary health care in New Zealand, including the characteristics of providers and their practices, the patients they see, the problems presented and the treatment management proposed. Although the study covered community-governed organizations, Accident and Medical (A&M) Clinics and Emergency Departments, as well as private general practices with 'family doctors', this case study will concentrate on this last group.

A nationally representative, multistage sample of private GPs, stratified by place and practice type, was drawn. Each GP was asked to provide data on themselves and on their practice, and to report on a 25 per cent sample of patients in each of two week-long periods. A pad of forms, structured to select each fourth patient, was provided. On the first page the visits of four patients could be logged; on the second, a detailed record of the visit of the fourth patient was to be entered. The process was repeated on each subsequent pair of pages.

A sampling frame of all active GPs was generated from telephone White Pages listings. Other sources included the Medical Council Register and laboratory client lists. A comparison of the Medical Register with the White Pages listings showed a poor match. In particular, many individuals entered on the Medical Register did not appear to be in active practice in New Zealand. Conversely, some practitioners listed in the telephone book did not appear on the Medical Register. Another data source, the laboratory client list, was not freely available and only included practitioners receiving results electronically.

Seven strata were used in the sample selection of GPs for the National Medical Care Survey. While the first stratum covered those GPs working in community-governed practices, GPs in private practice were sampled through the strata 2–7 shown below. The strata for sample selection were defined as follows:

(Continued)

1   A single stratum of GPs working in community-governed non-profit organizations, who were sampled with certainty wherever they were located.
2   GPs who had participated in the earlier Waikato Medical Care (WaiMedCa) Survey study.
3   Independent GPs in metropolitan and city areas.
4   Independent Practitioner Association (IPA) GPs in metropolitan and city areas.
5   GPs paid on a per capita basis in metropolitan and city areas.
6   GPs in areas surrounding the big cities.
7   GPs in towns and rural areas.

In order to generate adequate, and approximately equal, numbers of GPs in strata 2–7, different sampling fractions were chosen. In the analysis presented below the results are weighted to compensate for the different likelihood of being sampled. It should be noted that the GPs in stratum 7, towns and rural areas, were sampled in two stages: (a) a representative 4 out of 11 areas were first selected on judgement criteria; (b) a sample of 59 GPs was selected randomly from these four areas. Account was taken of the two-stage sampling process in stratum 7 in the calculation of standard errors in all subsequent analyses.

In Table 9.2 the sampling probabilities used in weighting the results for all strata are shown (the weighting factor is the inverse of the sampling probability). It should be noted that for Auckland and the cities, the sampling probability differed by practice type, while for the towns and rural areas a single sampling probability was applied across types. The number sampled was calculated to allow for a 30 per cent refusal/ineligible rate.

Table 9.2   *Sample size and sampling percentage, all strata*

Stratum	Description	Population of GPs	Sample drawn	GP weights	GPs in sample
1	Community governed	66	63	1.00*	63
2	WaiMedCa	118	58	2.03	38
3	City independent	444	50	8.88	23
4	City IPA	886	72	12.31	51
5	City capitated	71	40	1.78	21
6	Areas around the big cities	367	55	6.67	33
7	Remaining towns and rural	831	59	14.08	33
Total		2,783	397		262

* Sampled with certainty.

(Continued)

(Continued)

Table 9.2 shows the GP weights associated with each stratum calculated as the inverse of the sampling probability. Visit weights were calculated as GP weight × 4 (where 4 is the inverse of the sampling probability of each patient visit). The weight for each practice was calculated approximately by multiplying the GP weight by the inverse of the number of GPs in the practice, to compensate for the increased likelihood of sampling large practices.

When attempts were made to contact a GP it was sometimes found that they were on sabbatical, had moved or had retired. In such cases, if a new practitioner had been appointed specifically to take on the departed person's workload, the new practitioner was asked to participate. Where there was no direct replacement, the sampled GP was marked ineligible. The other cause of ineligibility was the discovery that the individual was in speciality practice.

It was anticipated that additional practitioners who had not appeared on the sampling frame might be discovered when the practice of a sampled practitioner was approached. This might be because the practitioner was newly arrived or was an assistant, a trainee or a locum. When such people were identified they were added to the overall sample, and 13 per cent, matching the average sampling ratio, were requested to join the study.

Recruitment of selected practitioners included the following steps:

1 A letter from the project team requesting participation, accompanied by a letter of support from the local Professor of General Practice, were sent.
2 A telephone call was made by the Clinical Director or the Project Manager requesting an interview.
3 A practice visit was made, at which an information booklet was presented and, with agreement, a time for data collection was set; an estimate of weekly patient numbers was obtained and practitioners signed a consent form.
4 The visit record pad and other questionnaires were delivered by courier.
5 A telephone call was made to the practice early in the week of data collection as a reminder.
6 Follow-up telephone call(s) were made if the data pack was not returned.
7 A telephone call was made prior to the second week of data collection.
8 The second visit record pad was delivered by courier.

(Continued)

9 Follow-up telephone call(s) were made if the second data pack was not returned.
10 A short questionnaire was sent to GPs who felt unable to contribute to the research.

A small payment was made to practitioners based on the number of completed visit forms. This was seen as recognition of the opportunity cost of contributing to the research, and was based on an hourly rate similar to the after-cost earnings of GPs. The Royal New Zealand College of General Practitioners agreed to recognize participation as a practice review activity able to be submitted for postgraduate education credit (MOPS). All these features of the recruitment process probably contributed to the achievement of a relatively high response rate for surveys of this kind.

CONCLUSION

This chapter has outlined the basic principles of probability and non-probability sampling. Although non-probability sampling is the more reliable method in statistical terms as it is based on the theory of random numbers, the decision about how to sample will depend on a number of factors such as cost, convenience and whether a reliable sampling frame exists from which the researcher can draw a sample. Researchers who are developing their non-probability sampling skills should seek advice from a statistician if they are uncertain about how many subjects to sample, to make sure that their results are generalizable.

Whatever the choice of method, when writing up results the researcher should explain clearly in the text or a methodological appendix why they have chosen a particular approach, how the sample has been drawn and the limitations on the inferences that can be drawn from the findings. Further discussion on writing up research results is given in Chapter 21, while the next chapter deals with other aspects of survey research. An exercise for the reader follows on developing effective sampling strategies.

Exercise: Planning for health with a sampling strategy

Below are outlined three plausible scenarios of research settings in which a social scientist might be involved in helping to formulate a plan, an essential part of which would be the development of an effective sampling strategy. These scenarios (developed for teaching by Andrew Sporle) have been selected because they require engagement with communities and target populations that might be seen as outside the standard range for orthodox sampling theory and practice. Therefore, aside from the more conventional considerations of sample design, frame and coverage, sample size and distribution, and sampling and non-sampling error, you will also need to think about how to engage with key stakeholders and keep them supportive of your research goals.

- *Scenario A*: An industrial area has recently had a spate of cancers among residents in a nearby neighbourhood. Most of those affected had worked at a timber treatment plant, recently closed. Those living in the community are concerned that the cancers may be the result of chemical poisoning from the timber plant. They have approached you as a social researcher for help in investigating a possible association between the chemicals and the recently diagnosed cancers.
- *Scenario B*: Your market research firm has been approached to undertake a study for a large telecommunications company. This company is interested in exploring the potential for the expansion of the 'pink dollar' (gay and lesbian) sector of their market, due to its perceived high disposable income and lifestyle expenditure. A survey is proposed to assess how telecommunications are used by gay and lesbian people in order to target this market.
- *Scenario C*: You are a member of a research team that has developed a new type of follow-up and self-management plan for managing diabetes symptoms among those diagnosed as having chronic diabetes. This system has proved effective in the United Kingdom, but you are interested in implementing it in predominantly Maori, rural communities where diabetes is rife (or in the UK context in an area with a predominantly South Asian population). Your research team are interested in improving the management of diabetes in this group.

In each of these scenarios, develop a written plan, outlining the proposed sampling strategy.

NOTES

1   All four illustrative examples used in this chapter were funded either by the Health Research Council of New Zealand or by its predecessor, the Medical Research Council. We wish to thank Martin von Randow for his helpful research assistance.

2   A term that is also used to identify the same concept is 'study universe'. Population and universe are used interchangeably, and refer to the pool of elements from which the sample is drawn. A related, but distinct, term is that of 'survey population'. This is not universally applied in the literature, but can be a useful distinction. The survey population refers to that subset of the target population that has a chance of being selected into the sample. For very good practical reasons, it may be that not all units in the target population can be accessed. For example, if the survey involves telephone interviewing, then people in the target population who do not have telephones will have no chance of selection.

3   In both the dental health and partner relation surveys the sample size and precision calculations were made around a single parameter (mean and proportion respectively). It should be noted that for complex sample designs, the standard formula for the simple case will underestimate the required sample size. The most straightforward way to correct this is to calculate the so-called design effect and multiply the estimate for the simple case by this value.

4   This technique is used widely in the commercial world to correct for sampling shortcomings (for instance, quota selection and non-probability designs).

5   It should be noted that, although weighting may assist in correcting an overall potential bias, it is also inefficient because it wastes information on those units that are weighted downwards.

6   A further refinement occurs in the case of 'complex statistics'. These are parameters that are much less straightforward than a mean or proportion – for example, a regression coefficient or a difference between two means (or proportions). Again, the sample size will usually need to be greater to achieve the same level of precision as that attained for a simple parameter. This means that the confidence intervals and levels of significance have to be adjusted accordingly.

RECOMMENDED FURTHER READING

Aday, L.A. and Cornelius, L.J. (2006) *Designing and Conducting Health Surveys: A Comprehensive Guide*, 3rd edition. New York: Jossey-Bass.
This is a standard reference written with the non-technical user in mind, drawing substantially on recent methodological research on survey design and cognitive research on question and questionnaire design and presenting a total survey error framework.

Fowler, F.J. (2002) *Survey Research Methods*, 3rd edition. Thousand Oaks, CA: Sage.
This book provides a concise overview of the entire survey research process, using clear and easy-to-understand language.

Korn, E.L. and Graubard, B.I. (1999) *Analysis of Health Surveys*. New York: Wiley.
This is a more advanced book dealing with the technical aspects of the analysis of data from complex surveys, illustrated with many examples from real health surveys.

REFERENCES

Aday, L.A. and Cornelius, L.J. (2006) *Designing and Conducting Health Surveys: A Comprehensive Guide*, 3rd edition. New York: Jossey-Bass.

Agarwal, R., Girdhar, G., Awasthi, S. and Walter, S.D. (2005) 'Intra-class correlation estimates for assessment of Vitamin A intake in children', *Journal of Health and Population Nutrition*, 23 (1): 66–73.

Botman, S.L, Moore, T.F., Moriarity, C.L. and Parsons, V.L. (2000) *Design and Estimation for the National Health Interview Survey, 1995–2004*. Vital and Health Statistics, Series 2, No. 130. Hyattsville, MD: National Center for Health Statistics.

Cardozo, B.L., Bilukha, O.O., Crawford, C.A., Shaikh, I., Wolfe, M.I., Gerber, M.L. and Anderson, M. (2004) 'Mental health, social functioning, and disability in postwar Afghanistan', *Journal of the American Medical Association*, 292 (5): 575–84.

Cutress, T.W., Hunter, P.B.V., Davis, P.B., Beck, D.J. and Croxson, L.J. (1979) *Adult Oral Health and Attitudes to Dentistry in New Zealand 1976*. Wellington: Dental Research Unit, Medical Research Council of New Zealand.

Davis, P. and Scott, A. (1996) 'The effect of interviewer variance on domain comparisons', *Survey Methodology*, 21: 99–106.

Davis, P., Lay Yee, R., Chetwynd, J. and McMillan, N. (1993) 'The New Zealand Partner Relations Survey: methodological results of a national telephone survey', *AIDS*, 7: 1509–16.

Davis, P., Lay-Yee, R., Briant, R., Schug, S., Scott, A., Johnson, S. and Bingley, W. (2001) *Adverse Events in New Zealand Public Hospitals: Principal findings from a National Survey*, Occasional Paper No. 3. Wellington: Ministry of Health.

Diehr, P., Chen, L., Patrick, D., Feng, Z. and Yasui, Y. (2005) 'Reliability, effect size, and responsiveness of health status measures in the design of randomized and cluster-randomized trials', *Contemporary Clinical Trials*, 26: 45–58.

Goupille, P., Logeart, I. and Combe, B. (2003) 'Naturalistic survey on nonsteroidal anti-inflammatory treatment in patients with musculoskeletal pain', *Joint Bone Spine*, 70: 219–25.

Hosler, A.K. and Melnik, T.A. (2005) 'Population-based assessment of diabetes care and self-management among Puerto Rican adults in New York City', *Diabetes Educator*, 31 (3): 418–26.

Korn, E.L. and Graubard, B.I. (1999) *Analysis of Health Surveys*. New York: Wiley.

Liu, H., Hays, R.D., Adams, J.L., Chen, W.P., Tisnado, D., Mangione, C.M., Damberg, C.L. and Kahn, K.L. (2005) 'Imputation of SF-12 health scores for respondents with partially missing data', *Health Services Research*, 40 (3): 905–21.

Momartin, S., Silovec, D., Manicavasagar, V. and Steel, Z. (2003) 'Dimensions of trauma associated with posttraumatic stress disorder (PSTD) caseness, severity and functional impairment: a study of Bosnian refugees resettled in Australia', *Social Science and Medicine*, 57: 775–81.

Murphy, E. and Dingwall, R. (2003) *Qualitative Methods and Health Policy Research*. New York: Aldine de Gruyter.

Partin, M.R., Malone, M., Winnett, M., Slater, J., Bar-Cohen, A. and Caplan, L. (2003) 'The impact of survey non-response bias on conclusions drawn from a mammography intervention trial', *Journal of Clinical Epidemiology*, 56: 867–73.

Pyper, C., Amery, J., Watson, M. and Crook, C. (2004) 'Access to electronic health records in primary care – a survey of patients' views', *Medical Science Monitor*, 10 (11): SR17–22.

Raymont, A., Lay-Yee, R., Davis, P. and Scott, A. (2004) *Family Doctors: Methodology and Description of the Activity of Private GPs*, Occasional Paper No. 4. Wellington: Ministry of Health.

Statistics New Zealand (2001) *Introduction to the Census*. Wellington: Statistics New Zealand.

Vijayapushpam, T., Menon, K.K., Rao, D.R. and Antony, G.M. (2003) 'A qualitative assessment of nutrition knowledge levels and dietary intake of schoolchildren in Hyderabad', *Public Health Nutrition*, 6 (7): 683–8.

10

Quantitative Survey Methods in Health Research

MICHAEL CALNAN

INTRODUCTION

This chapter explores the use of survey methods in research into health and health care which are widely used in this and other fields of research (see, for example, Bryman 2004; Fowler 2001). It begins by defining and explaining what quantitative survey methodology is; describing the techniques and resources required for carrying out a survey; and discussing the role of theory. It then outlines the process of translating concepts into indicators and assesses the strengths and weaknesses of different survey techniques for collecting data, and identifies the major issues in managing a survey, and in analyzing and in presenting data. The chapter concludes with a description of how different survey methods are put into practice, illustrated through examples drawn from my own research.

Survey methods can be defined in a number of different ways but the most cogent is provided by De Vaus (2002), who argues that the two defining characteristics of a survey are how data are collected and the method of analysis used. In a survey, data should be collected on the basis of the same characteristics – such as social position, beliefs, attitudes and behaviours – from a number of cases or units of analysis to provide a structured data set. Analysis in survey methods involves a comparison of cases. This can be descriptive, for example by trying to identify amongst a group of people the level of satisfaction with health care, or it can be taken further analytically to locate cause. For instance, the level of public satisfaction with health has been systematically associated with age: older people have higher levels of satisfaction than younger people. Causal inferences may then be drawn by a careful comparison of the characteristics of cases to try to explain why age may affect public assessments of satisfaction. However, it is important to avoid the mistake of attributing a causal link between age and satisfaction. Showing that two variables are associated does not, in itself, provide sufficient evidence to prove a causal link.

TYPES OF SURVEY

Surveys can be of different types. An ad hoc survey is carried out for a one-off purpose such as a local survey of health care users to find out the level of satisfaction with a particular organization or service. Cross-sectional surveys are regular surveys that monitor trends over time, such as the British Social Attitudes Survey (Park et al. 2003). This national survey is carried out annually and consists of a set of core questions with new questions added that relate to a current problem area. These regular surveys are useful for monitoring general trends such as public satisfaction with the NHS and the various services it provides in the United Kingdom.

It should be stressed, though, that such surveys may not be able to identify certain aspects of change. For example, the British Social Attitudes Survey can show people's attitudes to private health care, the level of coverage and the level of subscriptions to private health insurance, and how these change over time. Thus, during the 1980s, this survey showed a gradual increase in the proportion of the population covered by private insurance. However, as the overall figure did not identify the proportion of lapsed subscribers, which in the case of private health insurance was high, the data could not show whether the increase reflected a large or small increase in new subscriptions (Calnan et al. 1993).

A longitudinal study, that is a survey repeated on the same cohort or population at different points of time, would show the proportion over time who took out a new subscription to private health insurance; the proportion who maintained their subscription to private health insurance; and the proportion that let their subscription lapse. So surveys carried out on a regular basis can be useful for measuring gross change but longitudinal designs, using cohort or panel studies, are more appropriate for understanding individual, and within-group net change.

Survey methods are often associated with the use of a questionnaire where data are collected through interview, face to face, by telephone, or are self-completed through postal or other means. However, surveys can draw on a wide range of techniques. They may, for instance, have a qualitative element when the interview schedule includes both open-ended and semi-structured questions, and some surveys include structured observation where specific activities are recorded. For example, if the aim is to explore practitioner–patient encounters, activities may be recorded in a hospital ward or general practice. Another technique for data collection is the structured record review where the researcher uses a specially created form to elicit information, for example from patients' medical records. Finally, qualitative data in a survey may be organized and analyzed quantitatively, using a content analysis method (Fink 2003). This might involve counting the frequency that topics occur in respondents' narratives as discussed in Chapter 4. Thus, a survey is not synonymous with using a questionnaire as various methods can be used to collect and analyze data as in other case study and experimental designs.

THE RATIONALE FOR EMPLOYING SURVEY METHODS

The previous discussion has hinted at the type of research question where it may be appropriate to employ quantitative survey methods. The sample survey using different data collection techniques can be used to address descriptive questions, such as what, who, when and how questions. It can also look at variations in the characteristics of different groups, as discussed above. Furthermore, surveys may be used for explanatory research to explore 'why?' questions where the aim is to try to impute cause, or consequence. In cross-sectional surveys information is collected at one point in time to take a 'snapshot' to explore such questions. However, this approach lacks a time dimension that can hinder the exploration of causal influences. Surveys that are repeated or that are repeated at intervals can better explore changes in relationships and the strength of interrelationships between variables. They will also identify naturally occurring variation, although it is generally difficult to pinpoint a specific cause of such variation and impossible to eliminate a range of confounding or contaminating factors. In these circumstances, an experimental or quasi-experimental design could attempt to control, or allow for, a range of possible confounding influences.

In summary, survey methods are distinguishable from other research methods, in terms of the form of data collection and methods of analysis adopted. However, surveys are not necessarily distinguished by the techniques of data collection that may also be used in other methods. Survey methods tend to address questions that are both descriptive and analytical, although they have limitations in relation to exploring specific causal influences.

THE TECHNIQUES AND RESOURCES REQUIRED FOR THE SURVEY METHOD IN PRACTICE

What resources are required in terms of time and money to carry out the survey method? Fink (2003) suggests that to estimate the resources necessary, the following questions should be addressed: What are the major tasks of the survey? What skills are needed to complete each task? How much time does each task take? How much time is available to complete the survey? Who can be recruited to perform each task? What are the costs of each task? What additional resources are needed?

These questions may be addressed by quantifying and listing basic information on the direct and indirect costs and expenses incurred by the survey:

- Decide on the number of days (or hours) that constitute a working year.
- Formulate survey tasks or activities in terms of the number of months it will take to complete each task.
- Estimate how long, in a number of days (or hours), you will need for each person to complete their assigned task.
- Decide on the daily (an hourly) rate for each person that will need to be paid.
- Decide on the cost of benefits (such as superannuation).
- Decide on other expenses that will be specifically incurred in the study, such as questionnaire piloting or focus groups.
- Decide on the indirect costs that will be incurred to keep the survey team going, such as overheads and accommodation.

TRANSLATING CONCEPTS INTO INDICATORS

Operationalizing concepts

Survey research should be informed by theory and the impact of theory, as with most other research methods, helps to focus questions and enhances the value of the findings. Once a theoretical framework is constructed, an important issue is deciding how concepts should be translated into questions or indicators. In other words, how theory can be operationalized in the survey. This, according to De Vaus (2002), involves three essential steps, which are: clarifying concepts, developing indicators and evaluating indicators. Concepts have been seen by De Vaus as abstract summaries of sets of behaviours, attitudes and characteristics that share something in common.

Three steps assist in the process of conceptual clarification. These are set out in Figure 10.1 which uses 'deprivation' to illustrate the different elements involved in operationalizing a concept. First, obtain a range of definitions. In the case of deprivation five different definitions are identified: physical, economic, social, political and psychic. Second, decide upon a particular definition, which in the case of deprivation might be the 'social' aspect. Third, the dimensions of the concept must be delineated. For deprivation, three have been identified: social isolation, the absence of socially valued roles and a lack of social skills.

The process of moving from abstract concepts to the point where they can be operationalized via a specific questionnaire item is called 'descending the ladder of abstraction'. Clarifying concepts involves descending this ladder.

How many indicators should be used?

There is no definite or clear-cut answer to the question of how many indicators should be used, but the following points provide a guideline for indicator development:

- Where there is no agreed way of measuring the concept, it is helpful to develop indicators for a range of definitions in order to see the effect on the results.
- If the concept is multidimensional, it is necessary to decide if there is interest in all, some, or any one of these dimensions.
- The researcher must be able to develop measures of key concepts.
- Complex concepts are best measured via a number of questions so as to capture the scope of the concept.
- Piloting indicators is an essential way of eliminating unnecessary questions.
- The number of items will be affected by pragmatic considerations (for example, the length of the questionnaire and the method of administration).

How should indicators be developed?

For certain concepts, it is simple to identify indicators as they are well established, as is the case with age or marital status. However, other more abstract concepts are more difficult, although there are a number of different ways of approaching the problem. First, a well-established measure from previous research may be used. This makes it possible for a direct comparison to be made between the results of the research and previous research findings. However, the danger of using an 'off-the-shelf' instrument is that it may not be tailored to measure the specific concept that one wishes to explore. A second approach, which is less convenient and more time consuming, is to use a qualitative method such as informal face-to-face interviews or focus groups initially to develop relevant questions. A third approach is to interview key informants or interest groups to provide clues or pointers to what the most appropriate questions might be.

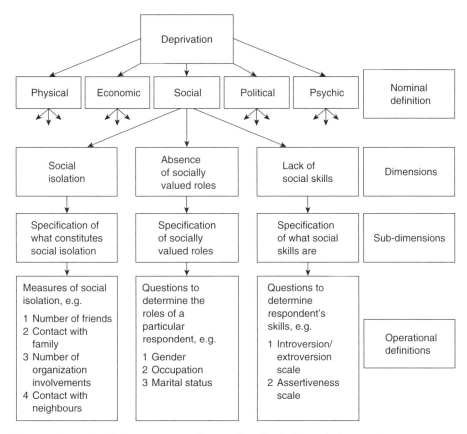

Figure 10.1   *Clarifying concepts: descending the ladder of abstraction*

Source: De Vaus (2002)

Figure 10.1 shows how the three dimensions of social deprivation might be operationalized. To assist further, see De Vaus (2002: 49) for a discussion of how the concept of social capital could be operationalized. Chapter 18 in this volume also describes an approach to conceptualizing ethnicity.

Evaluating indicators: Reliability and validity

How should indicators be evaluated to ensure that they are reliable and valid before the survey is conducted? Reliability is where a similar result is obtained in response to a particular question or indicator on repeated occasions. Sources of unreliability stem from a range of factors such as poorly worded, or ambiguous, questions and the effect of different interviewer characteristics or styles on responses. Reliability can be tested for single items by the method of test–retest and by item-to-item correlation for multiple item scales, which involves examining the strength of the statistical relationship between items. Using multi-item indicators and removing the unreliable item after testing should increase reliability. Other ways of improving reliability are through using well-tested questions, training interviewers prior to embarking on the research and reading and rereading questions, preferably with colleagues to find unambiguous wording for questions.

The question of validity is more complex and involves the extent to which the operationalized indicator is really measuring the concept it is intended to measure and whether it is a valid empirical indicator of the theoretical concept. There are various methods of judging validity but the four outlined here are the most common (see Litwin 1995; Fink 2003). The first is *content validity*. This refers to the extent to which a measure thoroughly and appropriately assesses the characteristics or skills it is intended to measure. A concept should be derived from a conceptual framework or set of theoretical ideas and the indicator should closely match the concept. The second is *face validity*, which refers to how a measure appears on the surface and whether all the required questions are framed in the appropriate language. In this case, it may not necessarily have been informed, at least explicitly, by theory. The third approach is *criterion validity*. This refers to the degree of convergence or divergence with a tried and tested indicator of the concept. Criterion validity may be concurrent or predictive. Concurrent refers to the validity of a measure, for example for current health status, while predictive validity is the extent to which a measure forecasts future health status: for example, a general health examination, or a particular indicator, may predict health status over the coming years. The final, and fourth, type of validity is *construct validity*. This refers to examining whether or not a proposition that is assumed to exist is actually confirmed when the new indicator is tested. For example, there is strong evidence of a positive relationship between health status and affluence/ deprivation. Thus, the development of an indicator of deprivation could have its validity tested by examining its relationship with a robust measure of health status.

STRENGTHS AND WEAKNESSES OF THE SURVEY METHOD

This section of the chapter evaluates the specific techniques used in surveys to elicit information. At a general level, as the earlier discussion suggested, survey methods are valuable in examining comparisons and variations between groups, particularly in large populations. Surveys can provide a broad overview of a social phenomenon and a general, if sometimes superficial, picture. What are the weaknesses? One possible weakness is that surveys are incapable of capturing the meanings and perceptions of social actors and the context in which action is taking place. Qualitative methods, such as informal interviews and observation, are more appropriate in addressing this type of research question. Surveys have also been seen to be tied to a more positivistic school of thought (see Chapter 2) which emphasizes the importance of structural forces or 'causes' and neglects the importance of human action or agency. Certainly, survey methodology is associated with measurement and not all social phenomena are measurable.

What then of the strengths and weaknesses of data collection techniques commonly used in surveys? The question will be addressed by first looking at the shortfalls of the most common forms of data collection through questionnaires administered by postal, telephone and face-to-face methods:

- Postal questionnaires are poor in avoiding response bias, do not tend to use open-ended questions, do not control question sequence, cannot motivate people to answer 'boring' questions and may not produce high-quality entries.
- Telephone interviews are more costly than postal surveys, are more difficult to implement and tend not to be useful for exploring sensitive topics.
- Face-to-face questionnaires are difficult to implement in that they are costly, slow and involve recruiting suitable staff. There may also be difficulties with the quality of the answers, particularly the distortion of response due to interviewer characteristics that may subvert the questions.

On the positive side, all three techniques can achieve good response rates. However, telephone surveys consistently have been found to produce significantly higher response rates than postal surveys, but lower response rates than face-to-face interview surveys (Bourque and Fielder 2003).

THE MANAGEMENT OF THE SURVEY AND SURVEY DATA

Data collection and fieldwork

The management of the survey and the fieldwork are important for the quality of the data collection and adherence to the proposed design. For example, the tasks involved with a telephone interview survey will include ensuring that all the questions are asked; the response rate at each follow-up is recorded; the interviewer stays within the time limit set; the interests of the respondents are respected; and the ethical guidelines are agreed prior to the interview. A crucial element in organizing an interview survey is ensuring that interviewers are well trained and that training is standardized.

Managing a postal survey places more responsibility on survey coordinators. The coordinators must develop identifiers and package the questionnaires to include self-addressed, prepaid envelopes for respondents for return. They must have a method for identifying and sending out follow-up letters or reminders to those who did not respond by the due date. It is important that the survey coordinators record the reason for non-response so that a distinction can be made between those who refused to take part and those who did not do so because they have moved away or were too ill. For surveys in general in the United Kingdom, it is becoming difficult to gain a high response rate and researchers increasingly use rewards and incentives to try to encourage respondent participation and therefore boost response rates. The survey coordinators may therefore manage the distribution of incentives such as prizes or shopping vouchers. A crucial element in organizing an interview survey is ensuring that interviewers are well trained and that training is standardized. This is generally the responsibility of the researcher or project manager.

Coding/Analysis of survey data

Data management begins when the first batch of survey questionnaires is returned, and a key task is developing the coding frame. The coding frame contains the definition of all the variables (such as age); the categories for each variable (for example, one way of dividing an age group up would be in 10-year intervals: 10 years or younger, 11–20 years, 21–30 years and so on); the location of the variables and their values (often expressed as numbers in columns). The development of the coding frame, as well as its operationalization, is the method whereby the data are translated from the respondent's answer to the survey questions to a database where aggregate data can be analyzed. The development of the coding frame is based on the questions asked. The complexity of the coder's task will depend on the extent to which the questions are pre-coded, that is codes have been allocated already in the questionnaire, or are open ended, with no pre-codes attached.

For some variables, such as marital status, educational qualifications, socio-economic status, sets of codes exist and where possible these may be used as they are well worked out and enable comparison with other studies. However, the open type of question requires the development of specific codes to accommodate the range of answers. This can be done by coding a sample of responses to identify the answer most frequently reported. The provisional coding categories can be refined if new categories emerge as the main body of the questionnaires are coded. Given the possibility of variation in interpretation of response, particularly to open-ended questions, it is important that those coding the questionnaires are well trained as the codes they enter represent the data. It is also important to double-code the data, or at least a sample of them, to test for reliability and consistency but also to identify problematic questions and possible variations in interpretation.

One common problem in surveys is that some questions are better answered than others and hence there are sometimes marked variations in the response rate to specific questions. Thus, the overall response rate to a questionnaire will not always reflect usable questions. Data entry is also a major activity in data management. Survey data can be entered into a computer spreadsheet or statistical program. Statistical programs can verify the accuracy, although it is important, once again, that those entering data are well trained and directed during the project. Data entry tends to be automatic with computer-assisted, online or scanned surveys that have used pre-coded, closed questions.

Issues of data analysis and presentation

The objectives of data analysis

The approach to data analysis will depend upon the specific research questions or objectives being examined. For example, the five objectives outlined below have different implications for data analysis (see Chapter 11 for further background to the points about statistical analysis made below).

One objective might be to describe the background of the respondents who took part in a 'satisfaction with health care' survey. It might be a matter of providing a frequency count or percentages of the proportion who were men or women; or who owned a car(s) or who did not (a possible indicator of deprivation).

A second objective might be to describe the responses to specific questions: for example, on average how many times did respondents consult their general practitioner (GP) in the past year? The average might have been 4 and the range between 0 and 20. This average refers to the measure of central tendency and the range refers to the measure of dispersion.

A third objective might be to determine the relationship between recent use of the GP and the level of satisfaction. This would involve estimating the relationship between level of use of GPs and level of satisfaction. One way of estimating the relationship between the two would be through the correlation. The expected result would be a positive relationship or correlation, with levels of satisfaction increasing with higher use.

The fourth objective might be to examine whether there were any differences between men and women, in terms of levels of satisfaction with care received in general practice. This would involve comparing the average satisfaction scores for men and women and using a test of statistical significance to see if any differences observed are statistically meaningful, rather than simply due to chance. The statistical test used will depend, at least in part, on whether the survey data being analyzed are nominal (that is, with no numerical preferential values), ordinal (the rate or order of a list of items) or numerical (numbers, such as age in years or height in metres).

The fifth objective might be to find out if gender, age or income predicts the level of satisfaction. To answer this question an appropriate design is needed, but a distinction also needs to be made between an independent and dependent variable. Independent variables are usually applied to explain or predict a result or outcome – in contrast to the dependent variable. In the case of our example of a patient satisfaction survey, the independent variables are gender, age or income and the dependent variable is level of satisfaction. However, to choose an appropriate statistical method of analysis it is necessary to specify the purpose of the analysis, and identify the number of independent and dependent variables and whether the data being analyzed are nominal, ordinal or numerical. Once these questions have been addressed, then a choice of a statistical method can be made. The appropriateness of choice of a statistical method depends on the extent to which the assumption about the characteristics and quality of data associated with the method can be met (Fink 2003).

Writing up and presenting survey findings

Survey findings can be written up in reports, articles and scientific/academic papers and in books or monographs. Whatever the medium of dissemination, it is important that the findings are clearly presented. However, if the aim is to publish a scientific or academic paper a number of points should be addressed. The paper format, at least for quantitative surveys, usually consists of an introduction, methods, results and discussion ending with a concluding paragraph – as is discussed in Chapter 21. The methods section should contain a concise rationale for the use of a particular method of data collection and why survey methods were used to address the research objectives. It should also contain details of the response rate and possible biases, particularly estimates of non-response bias and details of the statistical analysis and packages used, on which Chapter 11 further elaborates.

Chapter 11 on statistical methods also underlines that the presentation of an accurate report of the survey results is facilitated by the use of such aids as lists, charts and tables that are more fully described in this context. Lists are useful for stating survey objectives, methods and findings. Presenting data in the graphic form is becoming increasingly popular, perhaps because of the ease with which this can be undertaken electronically through word processing packages. Pie, bar and line charts provide different kinds of figures. Pie charts are useful for describing proportions or slices that make up the whole. Bar charts are common because they are relatively easy to read and interpret and useful for purposes of comparison. Figure 10.2 provides an example of data presentation using a bar chart. In order to address the question of whether GPs experience higher levels of job stress than other members of the health workforce, Calnan and Wainwright

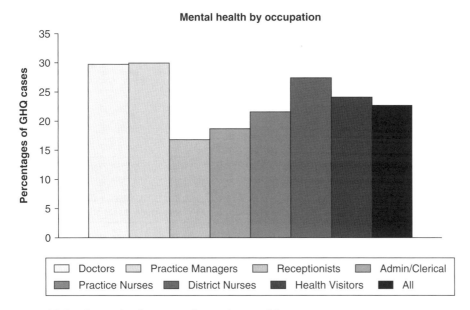

Figure 10.2 *Stress in the general practice workforce*

Source: Calnan and Wainwright (2002)

(2002) examined stress levels amongst various groups in a primary care setting, such as doctors, nurses, managers, administrators and clerical staff. The bar chart in the figure presents comparisons and shows that practice managers have the highest levels of stress, followed by GPs.

Line charts are helpful when plotting trends and changes over time. For example, Figure 10.3 examines changes in levels of public satisfaction and dissatisfaction with the NHS over the last 20 years. It shows that the differences have tended to decrease with levels of satisfaction generally falling and dissatisfaction generally increasing.

Tables can complement charts and are particularly useful for providing detailed information and the results of statistical analyses about patterns of findings which other researchers might wish to replicate. The number of tables presented will depend on the length of the article and are more commonly used in research reports. Charts, on the other hand, are useful in oral presentations for maximizing the visual impact. Finally, in terms of writing up, it is important for the discussion and conclusion to be based on the results presented and the limitations of the methods and design identified and accounted for, along with the interpretation and significance of the findings.

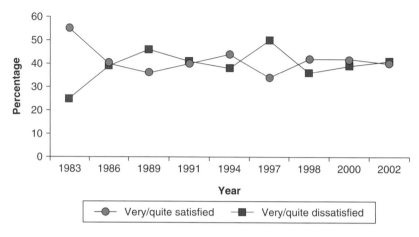

Figure 10.3 *Changes in levels of public satisfaction with the NHS*

Source: Appleby and Rosete (2003)

Case study: Examples of the use of different survey methods in practice

Examples of survey methods in the area of health and health care are numerous. The following examples illustrate different types of survey methods based primarily on the author's own research.

Postal surveys

In a national study, Calnan and Sanford (2004) aimed to examine how the public assess trust in health care in England and Wales. This formed part of an international study, including the Netherlands and Germany, to compare levels of trust in different health care systems. A postal survey was used because it was the most efficient means of eliciting information from a national sample. It contained a common core of structured questions derived from a survey instrument developed in the Netherlands that could assist international comparison. One of the problems with carrying out national surveys is finding an easily accessible, comprehensive and up-to-date sampling frame. One of the most popular, at least until recently, has been the Electoral Register. The Electoral Register provides an accessible and up-to-date source of information but is biased towards those who are more likely to register and under-represents those who do not register. Registers may also be out of date.

(Continued)

In the study in question, pilot work suggested it would be necessary to allow for at least 10 per cent inaccuracy when estimating sample size. There was also the added problem that no information was available from the Electoral Register about the non-respondents, so estimates could not be made of the representativeness of the respondents who participated in the survey. Thus, a comparison had to be made between the characteristics of the respondents and the national census data which showed that the survey under-represented the younger age groups and the healthy. This was particularly important, as the overall response rate was low (48%, *n* = 1,187) with 49 per cent of respondents not replying and 3 per cent refusing. Furthermore, the original sample of 2,777 was reduced to 2,489 as 288 had died or moved away. Respondents were sent three follow-up mailings in addition to the first mailing.

This study also illustrated a problem commonly found in international studies using survey methods (see Chapter 20 for a further discussion of the issues involved in comparative research). To enable comparison it is important to use common core questions, although these questions must be meaningful to respondents within different countries. For example, in the English survey the two terms 'confidence' (in the doctor's competence) and 'trust' (that the doctor worked in the patient's interest) could be distinguished, but no such semantic distinction is made between the terms in Dutch or German. To deal with this difference, confidence was used as equivalent to trust in the core questions, but when undertaking the survey in England and Wales, we asked additional questions about other aspects of trust (for example, whether respondents thought the practitioner works primarily in the interests of the patient or the organization) to see if they were associated with confidence in competence.

Postal surveys may combine various methods. For example, a survey can be preceded by a qualitative method, such as using focus groups as an antecedent. Focus groups may be used to identify the salient themes and to refine the questions for use in a postal survey aimed at collecting data from a wider population. Alternatively, postal surveys are sometimes used as precursors to qualitative methods to identify cases for follow-up with in-depth interviews.

An example where survey methods acted as a precursor to qualitative methods may be found in a study of sufferers with upper limb pain (Calnan et al. 2005). The study aimed to find out why people sought help and how symptoms were presented; how the problem was managed and

(Continued)

(Continued)

treated; and the implications for outcome of form of treatment. There were several design options considered, each with strengths and weaknesses. However, as the study aimed to obtain information from a broad range of informants, some of whom did not consult orthodox or non-orthodox care at all, the design consisted of a community-based screening survey followed by a case comparison study as set out in Figure 10.4. The sample for the screening survey was drawn from a population of patients registered with five general practices in the local area. A postal questionnaire, which included screening questions on upper limb pain taken from a previously validated instrument, was sent to a random sample of the working population, aged 25 to 64.

Figure 10.5 shows the overall response rate (56%) and illustrates the response to the two reminders both of which elicited around a 10 per cent response rate. The first reminder was a postcard to those who intended to take part. The second reminder was a letter, questionnaire and prepaid envelope (identical to the first mailing) aimed at persuading the 'hard core' of non-responders to participate.

For this study, one of the major aims of the initial screening survey was to identify 'cases' for follow-up. These cases were selected according to predefined inclusion criteria to encompass those who had experienced arm pain during the previous 12 months; had had arm pain for longer than a month or not (a measure of duration); the level of difficulty they had with activities (a measure of severity); had consulted a doctor or not; and who were in paid employment or not. For each group, informants were randomly selected from the survey sample. In all, 50 informants were contacted according to these criteria. It was only possible to interview 47 of the informants. Each had agreed to have their medical records examined and were invited to be examined by a nurse. Informants were asked to nominate a health care worker they had seen for their upper limb pain. This health worker was then approached for an interview. The interview with the practitioner focused on the informant's 'case' to begin with, and then expanded to general policies and practices. This example illustrates how postal surveys can be used as precursors to qualitative methods by identifying groups for follow-up.

In their study of stress in a random sample of general practices, Calnan and Wainwright (2002) used a similar two-stage methodology. A postal survey of general practices was used to identify those practices under stress at one end of the spectrum, and, at the other end, those that had lower levels of stress. The 10 practices (five at either end) were selected according to criteria based on data collected in the survey on mental distress (General Health Questionnaire score), job strain and

(Continued)

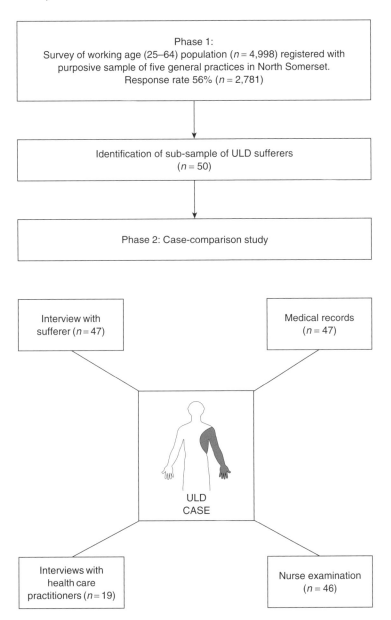

Figure 10.4   *Study design*

Source: Calnan et al. (2005)

(Continued)

(Continued)

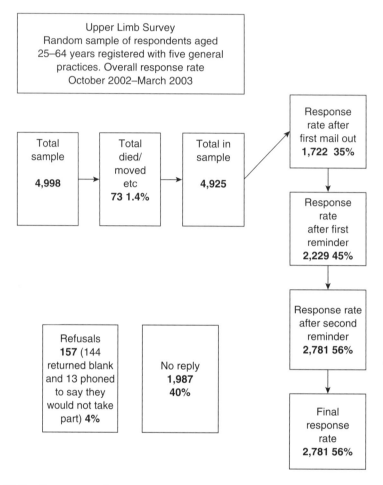

Figure 10.5 *Response rates*

Source: Calnan et al. (2005)

additional information about practice size and geographical location (see Figure 10.2). This was followed by in-depth interviews (*n* = 87) with members of the five practices who were stressed and the five who were not. However, analyzing this type of mixed-method database is not always

(Continued)

straightforward, as respondents' responses to a postal questionnaire are sometimes different from their accounts in the interview. The follow-up interviews showed that even amongst the 'high-stress' practices, work stress was not the major problem it initially appeared to be and the experience of work stress in general practice was more about low morale, dissatisfaction and negative affectivity rather than severe anxiety or psychological strain.

Interview surveys

Interview surveys take at least two forms, namely face-to-face interviews and telephone interviews. A typical example of an interview survey is the British Social Attitudes Survey referred to earlier in this chapter. This survey (Park et al. 2003) began in 1983 and has been conducted annually, except for 1988 and 1992. The survey is designed to produce annual measures of attitudinal shifts. One of its main objectives is to monitor patterns of continuity and change, and the relative rates at which attitudes, in respect of a range of social issues, change over time. It is a regular survey rather than a longitudinal study as it does not follow the same sample of people (a cohort) over time, but samples from a new population each year. The interview questionnaire contains a number of core questions covering major topic areas such as defence, the economy and the welfare state. The remainder of the questionnaire is devoted to a series of questions on a range of social, economic, political and moral issues. The questions are predominantly structured and closed. Each year the survey samples adults aged 18 and over, living in private households in Britain. It is based on a multistage stratified random sample. From 1993, the sample was drawn from the postcode address file, and for all years of the survey a weighting procedure is available to adjust for unequal selection probabilities. Sample sizes vary each year, and between 1983 and 2002 they ranged between 1,355 and 3,469.

One strength of the British Social Attitudes Survey is that it can be used to monitor changes in attitudes over time. This is clearly illustrated by attitudes to the NHS. A set of core questions have been included in the survey nearly every year since 1983. These consisted of a general question:

(Continued)

(Continued)

> All in all, how satisfied or dissatisfied would you say you are with the way in which the NHS runs nowadays?

And more specific questions:

> From your own experience, or from what you have heard, please say how satisfied or dissatisfied you are with the way in which each of these parts of the NHS runs nowadays: local doctors or GPs, being in hospital as an inpatient, attending hospital as an outpatient, and NHS dentists?

It is, therefore, possible to monitor changes in attitudes to the NHS and specific sectors of health care over time. As Table 10.1 shows, over the last two decades there is clear evidence of a decline in satisfaction with the NHS overall. While this trend was halted in the early 1990s, possibly due to reforms in the NHS introduced at that time, the trend has continued up until the present, although there was an increase in satisfaction during the early years of the Labour administration between 1997 and 1999. The British Social Attitudes Survey data have been shown to report higher levels of dissatisfaction than other surveys which in general record a high degree of satisfaction with health care (see Judge and Solomon 1993). This is believed to be due to the context in which the questions are asked. In the interview, the questions on satisfaction are next to questions about government priorities and public expenditure.

Table 10.1 *Satisfaction with the NHS, 1983–2002*

	1983	1986	1989	1991	1994	1997	1998	2000	2002
Very/quite satisfied	55	40	36	40	44	34	42	42	40
Neither satisfied nor dissatisfied	20	19	18	19	17	15	22	19	18
Very/quite dissatisfied	25	39	46	41	38	50	36	39	41
Net satisfaction (satisfaction minus dissatisfaction)	+20	+1	−10	−1	+6	−16	+6	+3	−1
Base	1,719	3,066	2,930	2,836	3,469	3,146	3,146	3,426	2,287

Source: Appleby and Rosete (2003)

(Continued)

Thus, the British Social Attitudes Survey questions may elicit a more political response, whereas other satisfaction surveys may be more firmly grounded in local knowledge. It has been suggested that general attitudes to the NHS tell us as much about government popularity as they do about the NHS per se (Appleby and Rosete 2003).

An increasingly popular method of collecting interview data is via the telephone. The high level of access to a telephone in the United Kingdom coupled with concerns about security make the telephone an increasingly acceptable medium for interview. Baeza and Calnan (1998) used telephone interviews in a national study to evaluate the new health promotion arrangements introduced into general practices in England and Wales in 1996. Once again a mixed-method design was employed, beginning with a national survey followed by a series of in-depth case studies using qualitative methods. The objective of the survey was to explore the extent and nature of health promotion activity being undertaken through a survey of all health authorities in England.

A postal survey was not appropriate because many of the questions were semi-structured and the interviewee was the person responsible for the health promotion scheme in the health authority. This could vary depending on the health authority and could be a manager, a health promotion worker, a medical adviser or public health consultant. A face-to-face interview survey was inappropriate due to resource constraints. In the event, the response rate to the telephone interview was high with 89 per cent ($n = 85$) of the 96 health authorities in England taking part. The interviews lasted, on average, an hour.

CONCLUSION

The survey is probably the most widely used and well-tested method for obtaining data from a selected population. If correct sampling techniques are used, then findings can be generalized to very large populations. As has been argued, the survey can be particularly effective when used to compare changes over time. However, surveys can also be carried out on a modest scale and telephone surveys in particular can be a useful technique for students and other researchers. Questionnaire design with critical reflection on what a question is aiming to find out and pilot testing of questions is a crucial aspect of conducting a survey. All surveys require careful planning and management and need to be underpinned by good administrative systems. If interviewers are being used, they should be properly trained and briefed prior to, and during, the course of a project. The unexpected often occurs during the course of the fieldwork or data collection phase and interviewers may require access to ongoing support and discussion with researcher leaders.

The examples set out in this chapter highlight how different survey methods have been used in practice in health research. However, the reader now has the opportunity to complete an exercise on translating concepts into indicators in the health field.

Exercise: Translating concepts of health into indicators

The final section of this chapter provides a problem-solving exercise which readers are invited to complete. It follows the discussion presented in an earlier section about how concepts can be operationalized into indicators by using a descending ladder of abstraction. The focus of the exercise is on translating concepts of health into indicators or questions to be used in a survey that aims to assess the health status of the adult population. Figure 10.6 provides a schema to encourage readers to break down the general abstract concept of health to various component parts. Reference back to Figure 10.1 may be helpful as a guide.

(Continued)

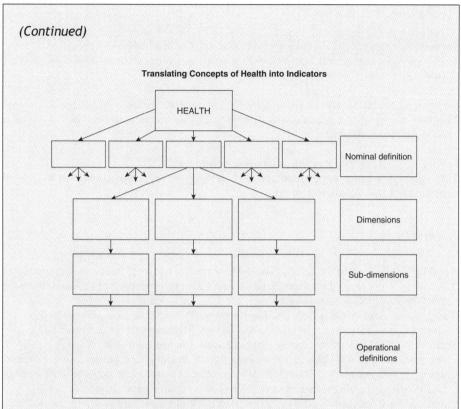

Figure 10.6   *Clarifying concepts: descending the ladder of abstraction*

Fill in the empty boxes in Figure 10:6 which provides the ladder of abstraction by:

1. Providing a number of different definitions of health
2. Choosing one definition to focus on
3. Identifying the dimensions and sub-dimensions which emerge from the chosen definition
4. Developing questions that would act as indicators of these dimensions and sub-dimensions in the sample survey of the adult population.

Once the exercise is completed readers might like to evaluate their indicators against a standardized instrument for measuring physical and mental health status – such as the SF-36 or the Nottingham Health Profile (Jenkinson 1994).

RECOMMENDED FURTHER READING

Bryman, A. (2004) *Social Research Methods*. Oxford: Oxford University Press.
This book provides useful complementary reading to this chapter, especially in Part Two.

De Vaus, D. (2002) *Surveys in Social Research*, 5th edition. London: Routledge.
This text covers all the main issues discussed in this chapter in more detail – and is strongly recommended.

Fowler, F. (2001) *Survey Research Methods*. London: Sage.
This again is a good supplementary text, setting survey methods within a general context of other research methods.

REFERENCES

Appleby, J. and Rosete, A. (2003) 'The NHS: keeping up with public expectations', in A Park., J. Curtice, K. Thomson, L. Jarvis and C. Bromley (eds), *British Social Attitudes: The 20th Report. Continuity and Change over Two Decades*. London: Sage.
Baeza, J. and Calnan, M. (1998) 'Beating the bands?', *Health Services Journal*, 26–27.
Bourque, L. and Fielder, E. (2003) *How to Conduct Telephone Surveys*. London: Sage.
Bryman, A. (2004) *Social Research Methods*. Oxford: Oxford University Press.
Calnan, M., Cant, S. and Gabe, J. (1993) *Going Private*. Buckingham: Open University Press.
Calnan, M., Wainwright, D., O'Neill, C., Winterbottom, A. and Watkins, A. (2005) 'Lay evaluation of health care: the case of upper limb pain', *Health Expectations*, 8 (2): 149–60.
Calnan, M. and Sanford, E. (2004) 'Public trust in health care: the system or the doctor?', *Quality and Safety in Health Care*, 13: 92–97.
Calnan, M. and Wainwright, D. (2002) 'Is general practice stressful?', *European Journal of General Practice*, 8 (1): 5–17.
De Vaus, D. (2002) *Surveys in Social Research*, 5th edition. London: Routledge.
Fink, A. (2003) *The Survey Handbook*, 2nd edition. London: Sage.
Fowler, F. (2001) *Survey Research Methods*. London: Sage.
Jenkinson, C. (ed.) (1994) *Measuring Health and Medical Outcomes*. London: UCL Press.
Judge, K. and Solomon, M. (1993) 'Public opinion and the National Health Service: patterns and perspectives in consumer satisfaction', *Journal of Social and Political Studies*, 22 (3): 299–322.
Litwin, M.S. (1995) *How to Measure Survey Reliability and Validity*. London: Sage.
Park, A., Curtice, J., Thomson, K., Jarvis, L. and Bromley, C. (eds) (2003) *British Social Attitudes: The 20th Report. Continuity and Change over Two Decades*. London: Sage.

Acknowledgments

Figure 10.3 reproduced by permission from Sage Publications.

11

Statistical Methods for Health Data Analysis

GEORGE ARGYROUS

INTRODUCTION

This chapter provides a basic introduction to statistics for analyzing health data. Although there are a number of more or less advanced texts on statistics for those involved in the health field (see, for example, Kirkwood and Sterne 2003; Mathers et al. 2000; Scott and Mazhindu 2005), the distinguishing feature of this chapter is its accessibility in introducing the subject of *data analysis* – what we do with quantitative research information once we have gathered it. More specifically, this chapter aims to help us to describe data more effectively. As such, it focuses on the first step in statistical analysis – straightforward statistical description – pointing the way to more advanced methods for those who wish to undertake further reading on the subject. For example, if we have collected measurements for the sex, age, amount of weekly exercise, smoking history and health status of patients visiting a clinic on a certain day, this chapter should help us to communicate this information more effectively, beyond simply listing the individual measurements that give the *distribution* for each of these variables.

Descriptive statistics are the numerical, graphical and tabular techniques for organizing, analyzing and presenting data. The major types of descriptive statistics are listed in Table 11.1.

Table 11.1 *Types of descriptive statistics*

Type	Function	Examples
Graphs	Provide a visual representation of the distribution of a variable or variables	Pie, bar, histogram, polygon (univariate) Clustered pie, clustered/stacked bar (bivariate,nominal/ordinal scales) Scatterplot (bivariate, interval/ratio scales)
Tables	Provide a frequency distribution for a variable or variables	Frequency table (univariate) Cross-tabulations (bivariate/multivariate)
Numerical measures	Mathematical operations used to quantify, in a single number, particular features of a distribution	Measures of central tendency (univariate) Measures of dispersion (univariate) Measures of association and correlation (bivariate/multivariate)

The great advantage of descriptive statistics is that they make a mass of research material easier to 'read' by reducing a large set of data into a few statistics, or into a graph or table.

LEVELS OF MEASUREMENT

The decision as to which descriptive statistic most effectively summarizes a set of data involves many considerations. One of the most important is the level at which each variable is measured. To illustrate what is meant by *levels of measurement* assume that the health status of the patients in our study is measured in three different ways, based on simplified measures used in the Australian Bureau of Statistics (2001):

- By classifying patients according to the organ of the body affected by their disease (for example, blood and blood-forming organs, the nervous system, the respiratory system).
- By classifying patients according to whether they rate themselves as Very Unhealthy, Unhealthy, Healthy or Very Healthy.
- By counting the number of times in the previous year a patient has consulted a doctor or other health professional.

Each of these scales provides a different amount of information about the variation in health status among patients. The first scale of measurement classifies patients according to the organ system where the disease is located. This scale only allows us to say that patients are qualitatively different according to the location of the disease, and as such is an example of a *nominal scale*: it classifies cases into categories that have no quantitative ordering.

Compare this to the second scale for measuring health status. The four categories that make up the scale have a logical order, starting with the lowest point, Very Unhealthy, and moving up to the highest point, Very Healthy. This scale allows us not only to talk about patients being different in terms of their health status, but also to say that the health status of individual patients is better or worse than others. This ability to *rank-order* cases according to the quantity or intensity of the variable expressed by each case makes this an *ordinal* scale. We cannot, however, measure how much healthier one person is relative to another.

The third scale for measuring health status does allow us to measure such differences. As with nominal and ordinal scales, measuring the number of times in the past year someone has consulted a health professional allows us to classify patients into different groups. As with ordinal (but not nominal) scales, we can rank patients according to their respective scores from lowest to highest. But unlike both nominal and ordinal scales, we can measure the differences – the intervals – between them. We now have a unit of measurement, number of consultations, which allows us to quantify the difference in health status. This is therefore an example of an *interval/ratio* scale (sometimes called a *metric* scale).

This example of measuring health status illustrates that any given variable can be measured at different levels, depending on the particular scale that is used. It is important to be clear about the level at which a variable has been measured, since the descriptive statistics that we calculate to express any variation across cases may be limited by this fact.

GRAPHS

Graphs or *charts* are the simplest, and often most striking, method for describing data, and there are some general rules that apply to their construction. Most importantly a graph should be a self-contained bundle of information. In order for a graph to be a self-contained description of the data we need to:

- Give the graph a clear title indicating the variable displayed and the cases that make up the study.
- Clearly identify the categories or values of the variable.
- Indicate, for interval/ratio data, the units of measurement.
- Indicate the total number of cases.

- Explain why there is a difference if the total in the graph is less than the total number of cases in the study.
- Indicate the source of the data.

Pie charts

The pie graph drawn from a patient survey in Figure 11.1 illustrates these rules of presentation. A *pie graph* presents the distribution of cases in the form of a circle. The relative size of each slice of the pie is equal to the proportion of cases within the category represented by the slice. Pie charts can be constructed for all levels of measurement and their main function is to emphasize the relative importance of a particular category to the total. They are therefore mainly used to highlight distributions where cases are concentrated in only one or two categories. For example, the pie chart in Figure 11.1 highlights the heavy concentration of patients who have a disease of the respiratory system.

Pie graphs begin to look a bit clumsy when there are too many categories for the variable. As a rule of thumb, there should be no more than five slices to the pie. Thus the pie chart in Figure 11.1 has grouped together a number of categories with low frequencies into an 'Other' category.

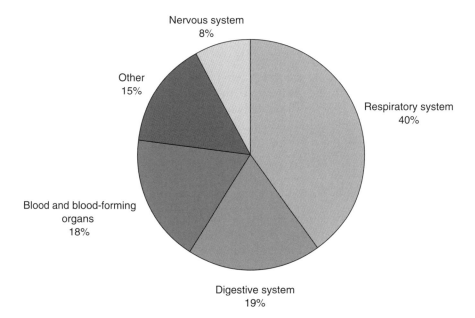

Figure 11.1 *Pie graph: main organ affected by disease for a sample of patients (n = 200)*

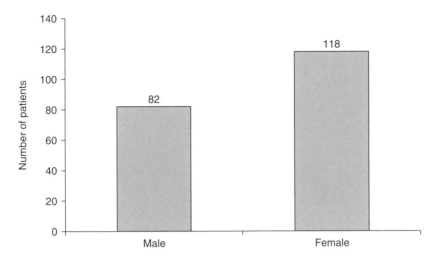

Figure 11.2   *Bar graph: sex of patients*

Bar graphs and histograms

Bar graphs and *histograms* emphasize the frequency of cases in each category relative to each other. Along one axis of graphs are the categories or values of the scale. This axis is called the *abscissa*, and is usually the horizontal base of the graph. Along the other axis are the *frequencies*, expressed either as the raw count or as percentages of the total number of cases. This axis is known as the *ordinate*. This is usually the left, vertical axis. A rectangle is erected over each point on the abscissa, with the area of each rectangle being proportional to the frequency of the value in the overall distribution.

The difference between bar graphs and histograms is that bar graphs are constructed for discrete variables, such as the sex of patients, which are usually measured on a nominal or ordinal scale, as illustrated by Figure 11.2.

With bar graphs there are always gaps between each of the bars: there is no gradation between male and female, for example. A person's age, on the other hand, is a continuous variable, in the sense that it progressively increases. As a result, the bars on the histogram for age in Figure 11.3 are 'pushed together'.

As an alternative to a histogram, Figure 11.3 also presents the distribution for age of patients in the form of a *frequency polygon*, which is a continuous line formed by plotting the values in a distribution against the frequency for each value.

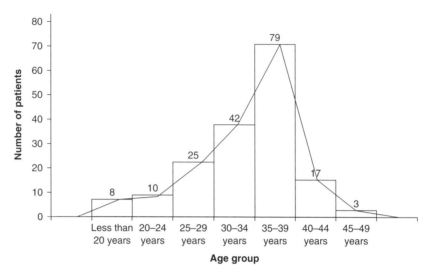

Figure 11.3 *Histogram: age of patients*

Interpreting graphs

Once we have constructed the relevant graph we then need to interpret it. When we look at a graph, we generally try to identify one or more of the following four aspects of the distribution it represents:

- The shape
- The centre
- The spread
- The existence of outliers.

There are certain common *shapes* that appear in research. For example, the histogram for age in Figure 11.3 is 'bell shaped' or 'mound shaped'. For a distribution that has this 'bell shape', we also describe its *skewness*. If the curve has a long tail to the right, it is *positively skewed*, or, as is the case with the age distribution of patients, a long tail to the left indicates a *negatively skewed* distribution.

To gauge the *centre* of a distribution, imagine that the bars of the histogram are lead weights sitting on a balance beam. Where would we have to locate a balance point along the bottom edge of the graph to prevent it from tipping either to the left or right? This, in a loose fashion, identifies the average or typical score. In the example in Figure 11.3 we might say that the average age of patients is around 35–39 years of age.

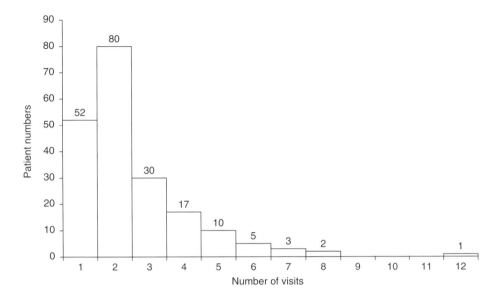

Figure 11.4 *Number of visits to a health professional in the past year*

We can also observe how tightly clustered our measurements are around the central point. Do the scores *spread* very wide across the range of possible values (that is, the distribution is *heterogeneous*) or are most similar to each other (that is, the distribution is *homogeneous*)?

Lastly, we can also note the existence of any *outliers* that are not just at the upper or lower end of the tails, but are disconnected from the rest of the group. Figure 11.4 for example presents the annual frequency of visiting a health professional. We can immediately see an outlier with 12 visits to a health professional in the previous year. Where we identify such an outlier we isolate the reason why it appears (data entry error or real case), and exclude it from further analysis so that it does not distort other statistics.

FREQUENCY TABLES

The power of graphs is their simplicity; the visual impact of a graph can convey a message better than the most advanced statistics. The simplicity of graphs can also be their weakness. We often do want to 'dig deeper' to extract more precise understandings of the data than can be gleaned from a chart. Obtaining

Table 11.2   *Number of visits to doctor or other health professional in the previous year*

Number of visits	Frequency	Per cent*	Cumulative frequency	Cumulative per cent
1	52	26	52	26
2	80	40	132	66
3	30	15	162	81
4	17	9	172	86
5	10	5	182	95
6	5	3	187	97
7	3	2	197	99
8	2	1	199	99
More than 8	1	<1	200	100
Total	200	100		

* Does not sum to 100% due to rounding error.

a more detailed breakdown of a distribution usually begins with the construction of *frequency tables*. At the very least a frequency table tallies the number of times (f) each value of the variable appears in a distribution. Such a table has in the first column the name of the variable displayed in the title row, followed by the categories or values of the variable down the subsequent rows of the first column. The second column then presents the frequencies for each category or value. Table 11.2 presents the same distribution as Figure 11.4, but provides much more detail about the frequency of cases across the range of scores.

Frequency tables follow the same rules of presentation that we listed above for graphs, with the addition of the following points:

- Arrange the values of ordinal and interval/ratio scales so that the lowest score in the distribution appears in the first row and the scale then increases down the page. Thus in Table 11.2, which presents the distribution of an interval/ratio scale, we have as the first row those who visited a health professional only once.
- Arrange the categories of nominal scales so that the category with the highest frequency (referred to below as the mode) is the first row. The category with the second highest frequency is the second row, and so on. The modal category is often of specific interest when analyzing the distribution of a nominal variable, and therefore it is convenient to present it first.

Table 11.2 also provides the *relative frequencies*, which express the number of cases within each value of a variable as a percentage or proportion of the total number of cases. *Percentages* are statistics that standardize the total number of cases to a base value of 100, whereas *proportions* standardize the total to a base of 1. The formulae for calculating a percentage or proportion respectively are:

$$\% = \frac{f}{n} \times 100$$

$$p = \frac{f}{n}$$

where f is the frequency of cases in a particular category and n is the total number of cases.

Notice that the column of percentages in Table 11.2 should add up to 100 per cent, since all cases must fall into one classification or another. The actual percentages listed in the table, however, sum to 101 per cent, as the numbers have been 'rounded off'. Where this occurs, a footnote should be added to the table that states 'Does not sum to 100 due to rounding error', or words to that effect, as is done in Table 11.2.

With ordinal and interval/ratio data one further extension to the simple frequency table can be made, which is also illustrated in Table 11.2. This is the addition of columns providing *cumulative frequencies* and *cumulative relative frequencies*. Since ordinal and interval/ratio scales allow us to rank-order cases from lowest to highest, it is sometimes interesting to know the number, and/or percentage, of cases that fall above or below a certain point on the scale. For example, in Table 11.2 we can see that 162 patients (81%) visited a health professional three times or less, which is the sum of the frequencies in the first three rows of the table. By implication this means that 19 per cent of patients visited a health professional more than three times in the last year. Cumulative frequencies are not appropriate where we have a nominal scale, as the ordering of the categories is not fixed, or where there are only two categories, as the simple frequencies and cumulative frequencies will be the same.

One additional point needs to be made about tabulating interval/ratio data: we often use *class intervals* rather than individual values to construct a frequency distribution. A *class interval* groups together a range of values for presentation and analysis. We use class intervals if the range of values that appears in the distribution is so large that it makes presentation and analysis difficult. For example, if we have many individual ages for the patients in our study we may first group them into five-year intervals, such as 1–5 years, 6–10 years, and so on, before constructing the table or graph. Generally, class intervals should have the same width, although at the lower and upper end of the data range we often have open-ended class intervals, such as '60 years or over'. The exception is the value of 0, which is usually listed separately. It is common for readers of tables to be specifically interested in the number of cases that have a zero value for a particular variable. The actual width of class intervals depends on the particular situation, especially the amount of information required. The wider the class intervals, the easier it is to 'read' the table, since this will reduce the number of rows. However, this increase in 'readability' comes at the cost of information, and therefore should not be undertaken if the data are already in a few, easily presented, values.

MEASURES OF CENTRAL TENDENCY

We mentioned above that graphs and tables give us a quick visual sense of key features of a distribution. But we sometimes want to be more precise about the centre of a distribution. For instance, rather than stating that 'the scores tend to centre around an average of 35–39 years' we may need to be more precise about the average score. *Measures of central tendency* indicate the typical or average value for a distribution.

There are three common measures of central tendency: mode, median and mean. Each measure embodies a different notion of average and choosing the measure to calculate on a given set of data is restricted by the level at which a variable is measured.

The mode

The *mode* (M_o) is the simplest measure of central tendency, and can be calculated for all levels of measurement. The mode is the value in a distribution that has the highest frequency. The great advantage of the mode over other measures of centre is that it is very easy to calculate. A simple inspection of a frequency table is enough to determine the mode. In Table 11.2, for example, we can see that the most frequent number of times a patient visited a health professional is 2, which accounts for 80 patients. However, the mode has one major limitation that arises especially when it is used to describe interval/ratio data that have many values. Take, for example, the following scores that represent the time in seconds for a drug to take effect on a sample of patients, arranged in rank order:

36, 36, 81, 82, 84, 85, 86, 89, 91, 95, 97, 98

It is clear to the naked eye that the data are 'centred' somewhere in the range of 80–90 seconds. Yet the mode is 36 seconds since this appears twice in the distribution, whereas every other score only appears once. The mode is not really reflecting the central tendency of this distribution. We should either use other measures of central tendency, such as those we are about to discuss, or else organize the data into suitable class intervals, and report the modal class interval, rather than the individual modal score.

The mean and median

With interval/ratio data, the *mean* and *median* can be calculated as measures of central tendency rather than the mode. The mean is the sum of all scores in a distribution divided by the total number of cases. The actual formula we use to calculate the mean depends on whether we have the data in listed form or in a frequency table. If we have the raw data with each individual score listed separately the equations for the mean of the population and the mean of a sample respectively are:

$$\mu = \frac{\sum X_i}{N}, \quad \overline{X} = \frac{\sum X_i}{n}$$

where μ (pronounced 'mu') is the mean for an entire population, N is the size of the population, $\overline{X}$ (pronounced 'X-bar') is the mean for a sample, n is the size of the sample, and X_i is each score in a distribution. The symbol Σ (pronounced 'sigma') means 'the sum of' (or 'the total from the addition of'), so we read these equations in the following way: 'the mean equals the sum of all scores divided by the number of cases'.

Alternatively, where the scores are already grouped into a frequency table such as in Table 11.2, the relevant formula for a sample is:

$$\overline{X} = \frac{\sum fX_i}{n}$$

This formula instructs us to multiply each score by the frequency with which it appears in the table and to sum these products before dividing by the number of cases. For Table 11.2 the calculations will be:

$$\overline{X} = \frac{\sum fX_i}{n}$$

$$= \frac{(1 \times 52) + (2 \times 80) + (3 \times 30) + (4 \times 17) + (5 \times 10) + (6 \times 5) + (3 \times 7) + (2 \times 8)}{199}$$

$$= \frac{487}{199}$$

$$= 2.4 \text{ visits}$$

The mean has two major limitations, both of which derive from the fact that it is calculated using every score in the distribution. The first limitation is that it is affected by the presence of outliers, and therefore we generally exclude outliers from the calculation of the mean. Thus, when calculating the mean number of visits to a health professional, we exclude the one 'outlier' who visited a health professional more than eight times. When presenting a 'trimmed' mean as the centre of the distribution it should be noted to the reader that such 'trimming' has occurred.

The other limitation to the use of the mean as a measure of central tendency, even where outliers are excluded, is that its value is pulled away from the centre of a distribution that is skewed. For example, in Figure 11.4 we can see that the spread of scores for number of health visits is skewed to the right and this has produced a value for the mean that is higher than that we might expect from a quick visual inspection (even after we exclude outliers).

An alternative measure of central tendency to the mean, especially where a distribution is heavily skewed, is the *median* (M_d). If all the cases in a distribution are ranked from lowest to highest, the median is the score in the middle of the sequence. The actual calculation of the median will differ according to whether we have an odd or even number of scores. For an odd number of rank-ordered cases, the median is the middle score. For an even number of rank-ordered cases, the median is the mean of the two middle scores. Thus if I lined up the 200 patients in my study according to the frequency with which they visited a doctor in the previous year, starting with patients that attended a health professional only once, the middle scores in this line-up are those for the 100th and 101st patients, both of which have a value of 2 visits. We have an even number of cases, so the median is the mean of these two middle scores, which is 2.

If a cumulative relative frequency table such as Table 11.2 has been generated, an easier way to calculate the median is to identify the value at which the cumulative per cent first passes 50 (i.e. 2 visits). We can see that the median depends solely on the value of these scores in the middle, and is not 'pulled' in one direction or another by the long tail of a skewed distribution or the presence of any outliers, factors which we have seen affect the value of the mean.

MEASURES OF DISPERSION

Measures of dispersion are descriptive statistics that indicate the spread or variety of scores in a distribution, and most of these require interval/ratio-level measurement (a measure for nominal scales, the Index of Qualitative Variation, is not covered here, but further details can be found in Argyrous 2005: 141). The simplest measure of dispersion is the *range*, which is the difference between the lowest score and highest score. This is an easily calculated measure of dispersion, because it involves a straightforward subtraction of one score from another. This advantage of the range is also its major limitation: it only uses the extreme scores, and therefore changes with the values of the two extreme scores.

The *inter-quartile range* (IQR) overcomes this problem with the simple range by ignoring the extreme scores of a distribution. The IQR is the range for the middle 50 per cent of cases in a rank-ordered series: the difference between the upper limits of the first quartile and the third quartile. Unlike the simple range, the IQR will not change dramatically if we add one or two cases to either end of the distribution.

The *standard deviation* is a more complex measure of spread, the value of which captures the average distance each score is away from the mean, and is calculated for a sample and population respectively by the following equations:

$$s = \sqrt{\frac{\sum (X_i - \bar{X})^2}{n - 1}} \text{ (sample)}, \ \sigma = \sqrt{\frac{\sum (X_i - \mu)^2}{N}} \text{ (population)}$$

where s represents the standard deviation for a sample, and σ (pronounced 'sigma') represents the standard deviation for a population.

A close look at these equations indicates how they capture the notion that the standard deviation is the average distance that each score is from the mean. The numerator is the difference between each score and the mean, and the denominator adjusts those differences by the number of cases. Unfortunately, we cannot simply add all the *positive deviations* (scores above the mean) with all the *negative deviations* (scores below the mean), since by definition these will sum to zero. This is why the equation for the standard deviation squares the differences: it thereby turns all the deviations into positive numbers, so that the larger the differences, the greater the value of the standard deviation. But the general idea is clear. Distributions that are more spread out will have many scores that are different from the mean, producing numerous large deviations and thereby a high value for the standard deviation. Another set of scores may have the same mean, but with the scores more tightly clustered around it. In this case, the deviations between each score and the mean will thereby generally be small, producing a lower value for the standard deviation.

BIVARIATE DESCRIPTIVE STATISTICS: SIMPLE COMPARISONS

The previous section looked at methods for describing the distribution of a single variable. This *univariate analysis* can help address simple questions such as 'what is the age distribution of patients?' or 'what is the health status of patients visiting a clinic?' This simple analysis may only be a precursor to more complex analysis that asks whether the health status of patients is related to another variable, such as their smoking history. A question that addresses the possible *relationship* between two variables requires *bivariate statistical analysis*.

Probably everyone has a common-sense notion of what it means for two variables to be 'related to' each other. We know that as children grow older they also get taller: age and height are related. This example expresses a general concept for which we have an intuitive feel: as the value of one variable changes, the value of the other variable also changes. If we do believe two variables such as health status and smoking are related, we need to express this relationship in the form of a *theoretical model* before we undertake bivariate analysis to measure the relationship. A theoretical model is an abstract depiction of the possible relationships among variables. For this example, the model is easy to depict. If there is a relationship, it is because a patient's smoking history affects their health level. It is not possible for the relationship to 'run in the other direction' – a patient's smoking history will not change as a result of a change in their health level. In this instance we say that smoking history is the *independent variable* and health status is the *dependent variable*.

Once we have specified the model that we believe underpins any relationship between two variables, we can then generate appropriate statistics to see if such a relationship does in fact appear in the data we collect. There are two ways we can assess whether a relationship exists between two variables:

- For each of the groups defined by the independent variable, calculate univariate descriptive statistics to summarize the dependent variable and compare the differences.
- Calculate measures of association and correlation.

The first method is the simpler since we generate the univariate statistics we have already discussed, but rather than doing so for the whole data set, we generate these statistics for each of the groups defined by the independent variable. For example, if I wished to see whether health status is affected by smoking history, I would calculate summary statistics for health status, but I would do so separately for smokers and for non-smokers. This is illustrated by the *stacked bar chart* in Figure 11.5. The same comparison between smokers and non-smokers is also made using the *bivariate table* in Table 11.3 (also known as a *contingency table* or *cross-tabulation* or 'cross-tab' for short).

It should be noted that with cross-tabs we follow these two rules for arranging the information:

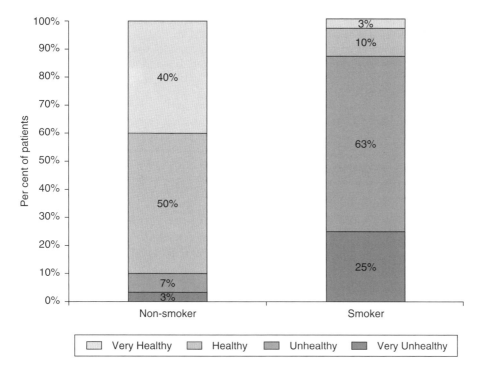

Figure 11.5   *Stacked bar chart: health rating by smoking history of clinic patients*

Table 11.3   *Health rating by smoking history of clinic patients*

Health rating	Smoking history		
	Non-smoker	Smoker	Total
Very Unhealthy	3%	25%	12%
Unhealthy	7%	63%	29%
Healthy	50%	10%	34%
Very Healthy	40%	3%	25%
Total	100%	100%	100%
	(120)	(80)	(200)

- Place the appropriate variables in the rows and columns. If there is reason to believe that one of the variables is dependent on the other, the independent variable should be arranged across the columns and the dependent variable down the rows. In this example we have specified that smoking history is the independent (column) variable and health status is the dependent (row) variable.

- For scales that can be ranked, ensure the scale increases down the rows/across the columns. Notice that one of the variables, 'Health rating', is ordinal. Thus the categories that make up this scale can be ordered from lowest to highest. We therefore place the lowest point on the scale, the 'Very Unhealthy' category on the first row, so that the scale increases down the page until we reach the highest point on the scale, which is the 'Very Healthy' category.

To help us compare the difference in the health levels of smokers and non-smokers, the cross-tab presents the *column percentages*. For example, we can see that of all 120 non-smokers in the study, 3% were Very Unhealthy. This compares with the 25% of all 80 smokers who were Very Unhealthy. Figure 11.5 similarly presents the breakdown of each group's health status as a percentage of the total number of cases in that group, rather than the actual number of people that are Very Unhealthy, Unhealthy, Healthy or Very Healthy. In both the cross-tab and the bar chart, these percentages adjust for the different total number of smokers and non-smokers in the data and thereby allow for a more valid comparison than just using the raw counts.

Where the dependent variable is measured on an interval/ratio scale, we can also compare the groups defined by the categories of the independent variable in terms of summary statistics such as the mean, as illustrated in Table 11.4.

Table 11.4 *Mean annual number of visits to health professional by smoking history of clinic patients*

	Non-smoker	Smoker
Mean number of visits to health professional	1.2	3.1

Once we have generated graphs, tables or summary statistics such as a mean to compare the relevant groups, the task is then to interpret the differences. We must assess whether they reveal a relationship between the two variables. When comparing differences between the relevant groups, we look at the *pattern* and *strength* of any relationship that such differences reveal. For example, the cross-tab in Table 11.3 shows that the health status of smokers is lower than for non-smokers and smokers are more heavily concentrated in the Unhealthy category than non-smokers. We can thus say that there is a relationship between these variables and that the relationship is negative: a higher level of smoking is associated with lower health status.

BIVARIATE DESCRIPTIVE STATISTICS: MEASURES OF ASSOCIATION AND CORRELATION

In the previous section, we detected a relationship between smoking and health status by observing a difference in the set of percentages in each column of a cross-tab. The next step is to ask: what is the *strength* of this relationship? We can make an arbitrary assessment of a relationship's strength by arguing that the two sets of column percentages are very different from each other and therefore suggest a moderate-to-strong relationship. We can, alternatively, arrive at a more precise and objective measure of the strength of a relationship by calculating numerical *measures of association and correlation*. These measures are descriptive statistics that quantify a relationship between two variables. Table 11.5 lists the most common measures.

Table 11.5   *Measures of association and correlation*

Measure	Data consideration
Lambda	At least one variable nominal
Goodman and Kruskal tau	At least one variable nominal
Eta	Suitable where independent variable is nominal and dependent variable is interval/ratio
Somer's *d*	Both variables at least ordinal
Gamma	Both variables at least ordinal
Kendall's tau-*b*	Both variables at least ordinal
Kendall's tau-*c*	Both variables at least ordinal
Spearman's rho	Both variables at least ordinal with many points on the scale
Pearson's *r*	Both variables interval/ratio with many points on the scale
Kappa	Both variables at least ordinal and measured on the same scale

Detailing the logic of each of these measures and the methods for calculating them is beyond the scope of this chapter, but for a comprehensive guide see Liebetrau (1983). We should note here, however, that as with most other statistics, the appropriate choice is affected by the level at which the variables under analysis have been measured, as indicated in Table 11.5.

The general point to note about these measures is that they give a precise value on a scale from 0 to 1 indicating the *strength* of any relationship observed

Table 11.6 *Interpreting values for measures of association and correlation*

Range (±)	Relative strength
0	No relationship
0 >–0.2	Very weak, negligible relationship
0.2–0.4	Weak, low association
0.4–0.7	Moderate association
0.7–0.9	Strong, high, marked association
0.9–<1	Very high, very strong relationship
1	Perfect association

between two variables. We can then interpret the value according to the terminology suggested in Table 11.6. Rather than just relying on a visual impression of a cross-tab or graph, measures of association thereby provide a single figure to show the strength of association. In addition, where both variables are measured at least at the ordinal level, a + or − sign also indicates the *direction* of association: whether an increase in the quantity of one variable is associated with an increase (positive association) or decrease (negative association) in the quantity of the other variable. For instance, in the previous part of the chapter we observed that the health level decreases as the smoking level increases, and therefore we observe a negative relationship between them.

It is important to remember that the measures only detect a *statistical association*; they do not necessarily show whether one variable causes a change in another. We may suspect theoretically that one variable causes a change in the other, but the measures listed in Table 11.5 cannot prove causation. They only provide supporting evidence for a theoretical model. For example, a relationship between the number of storks in an area and the birth rate in that area has been observed, and we may calculate a measure that quantifies this statistical relationship. However, we cannot go from this statistical regularity to the conclusion that the presence of storks determines the birth rate!

DESCRIPTIVE STATISTICS: ADVANCED METHODSFOR ANALYZING MANY VARIABLES

The simple statistical techniques we have discussed above can take us a long way into data analysis and help answer many of the research questions we wish to answer. However, there are many more, and more complicated, methods of analysis that are available to the researcher willing to learn and use them. One such technique readers may frequently encounter is *regression analysis*, which seeks to depict the relationship between an independent variable and

Table 11.7 *Types of multivariate analysis*

Multivariate technique	Data considerations
Multiple regression	Interval/ratio independent and dependent variables. Categorical independent variables can be included as dummy variables
Logistic regression	Dependent variable is categorical and independent variables are interval/ratio
Loglinear analysis	All variables are categorical

one or more dependent variables in the form of a *regression equation*. For example, we may have data for the number of minutes of weekly exercise undertaken by a sample of people along with their respective rested pulse rates. To see whether these two variables are related we use regression analysis to yield the following equation:

$$\text{Rested pulse rate} = 89 - 0.3(\text{Minutes of weekly exercise})$$

This equation allows us to estimate what any given individual's rested pulse rate might be given their respective exercise level. For example, where the amount of weekly exercise is 0, we expect the rested pulse rate to be 89 beats per minute (bpm). For every minute of weekly exercise above 0, we expect the rested pulse rate to decrease by 0.3. Thus for someone who exercises for 30 minutes per week, we predict their pulse rate to be:

$$\text{Rested pulse rate} = 89 - 0.3(30) = 89 - 9 = 80 \text{ bpm}$$

Regression analysis can be extended to take into account even more complex relationships involving three or more variables. For example, the relationship between regular exercise and pulse rate may be affected by a person's sex and also their age in years, and *multiple regression analysis* produces a single equation that will measure the extent to which each of these variables affects rested pulse rate.

Table 11.7 lists the main techniques for such *multivariate analysis*. To detail these choices for undertaking multivariate analysis would take us beyond the limits of this chapter, but see Argyrous (2005) for a more detailed introduction.

INFERENTIAL STATISTICS

We have discussed at some length various ways of describing our data. These data often come from a sample rather than from the whole population, so that we are faced with a problem: are the sample statistics 'representative' of the population from which the sample is drawn? The operation of *sampling error* may cause the sample to be 'off'. Sampling error is simply the fact that despite our best efforts at drawing a representative sample, random factors can cause us to include in our sample members of the population that have relatively low or high scores for the variable we are investigating, and this then causes the overall sample statistics to be different from those we would have obtained if we did study the whole population. Given that sampling error is an inevitable possibility, on what basis can we make a valid generalization from the sample to the population?

We address this problem with *inferential statistics*. Inferential statistics are the numerical techniques for making conclusions about a population based on the information obtained from a random sample drawn from that population. The nature of inferential statistics can be illustrated by an example. Assume that we have randomly selected 200 people who perform regular weekly exercise and we find that this sample has a mean resting pulse rate of 60 bpm, and standard deviation of 10 bpm. What can we infer about the population of all people who regularly exercise?

We may have information that the general population has a mean rested pulse rate of 72 bpm. On the basis of the sample result, can we say that the *population* of all people who regularly exercise is lower than that for the general population? Maybe it is not, and our sample of 200 has produced a relatively low mean rested pulse rate as a result of sampling error. Alternatively, maybe the population of regular exercisers does have a lower mean rested pulse rate and the sample of 200 reflects this. The process of *hypothesis testing* helps us decide between these inferences by calculating the *statistical significance* of the sample result (also called the *p*-value). Statistical significance is the probability that the sample did indeed come from a population of regular exercisers whose mean rested pulse rate is the same as that for the general population, and that the low sample mean is due to sampling error alone.

Another way of making an inference from a sample result to the population is to ask from what kind of population is it reasonable to assume the sample was derived? If the sample mean is within the 'normal' bounds of sampling error, what range of values can we confidently believe includes the population mean? Answering this type of question involves the calculation of *confidence intervals*. In our example, we may calculate the confidence interval to be 60 ± 1.4 bpm. In other words, if we assume that the sample is not greatly affected by sampling error, the population from which it is drawn has a mean rested pulse rate between 58.6 and 61.4 bpm. Underlying the calculation of such a confidence interval is the simple logic that random samples will only rarely produce a result that is very different from the value for the population from which they are drawn.

This section gives some general idea about the role of inferential statistics in quantitative analysis, but the issues and calculations involved in the application of inferential statistics are far more complex than we can discuss here. The recommended further reading at the end of the chapter should be consulted as a starting point for those wishing to grapple with these issues.

TOOLS FOR ANALYZING QUANTITATIVE DATA

It was not long ago that statistical analysis was normally undertaken 'by hand' using pen and paper (and a calculator). Since the development of affordable desktop computers, and the Internet that connects them, hand calculations are the exception rather than the rule. There are four broad classes of alternatives to hand calculations:

- *Spreadsheet data management programs*: Practically every computer has an 'office' suite of software designed to handle various tasks such as word processing and data management. Examples include Microsoft Excel, which is part of Microsoft Office, OpenOffice, AppleWorks and Gnumeric. Such programs can generate graphs, tables and most of the statistical analysis that we require. Their advantage is their ubiquity. Their disadvantage is that they do not perform more complicated statistical analysis, or if they do it is often through the use of complicated equations that have to be precisely entered.
- *Comprehensive commercial programs*: There are many commercial programs such as SPSS, GB-Stat, InStat, JMP, Minitab, SAS and StatA. A full list of such packages is available at statistics.com/content/commsoft/fulllist.php3. These packages often have the appearance of spreadsheet data management programs, but are specifically designed for statistical analysis, so that they have a more complete range of options, and also the type of analysis desired can be selected from a menu of options rather than by entering equations on the spreadsheet.
- *Free comprehensive programs:* An exciting development in recent years is the availability of free software, and this includes some useful statistical analysis software. A list of such software is available at freestatistics.altervista.org/stat.php and members.aol.com/johnp71/javasta2.html. Of these, Epi Info developed by the US Center for Disease Control (www.cdc.gov/epiinfo) is particularly worth mentioning as a tool for health researchers. An open-source version of Epi Info, called OpenEpi, which runs on all platforms and in a web browser, is available from www.openepi.com.
- *Calculation pages for specific statistical pages*: These are web pages that provide tools for conducting specific analysis. A general listing of these pages is available at the web page members.aol.com/johnp71/javastat.html or Stat Pages.net.

CONCLUSION

The chapter has covered a wide range of tools for quantitative data analysis. A key element determining which of these tools are appropriate is the way in which our variables of interest have been measured. In particular, we need first to determine whether our variables have been measured at the nominal, ordinal or interval/ratio levels.

We then introduced three broad classes of statistical techniques that help us describe the data that we collect, namely graphs, tables and numerical calculations, and within each of these broad groups we have further choices. For example, we saw that there are different classes of numerical calculations depending on whether we are trying to identify the central tendency of a distribution or the amount of dispersion it contains. The choices also depend on how complicated the analysis is that we wish to undertake – whether we are interested in describing the distribution of a single variable, or the relationship between two variables, or indeed the relationship among many variables.

The chapter concludes with an exercise in which the reader is invited to apply some of the statistical methods outlined to the health data set out in Table 11.8.

Exercise: Statistical tests on a health data set

Table 11.8   *Health data set*

ID	Height	Weight	Age	Sex	Smokes	Exercise	Pulse
1	180	77	18	F	No	15	47
2	186	87	23	M	No	12	49
3	188	87	20	M	No	14	50
4	171	71	41	M	No	15	52
5	173	64	20	F	No	12	55
6	182	63	20	M	No	8	56
7	169	68	19	M	No	12	58
8	175	75	20	M	No	10	59
9	175	65	19	M	No	11	60
10	182	85	20	M	No	14	60
11	170	54	20	F	No	8	60
12	175	54	18	F	No	10	61

Table 11.8   *(Continued)*

ID	Height	Weight	Age	Sex	Smokes	Exercise	Pulse
13	170	60	18	M	No	11	62
14	183	73	20	M	No	5	63
15	164	78	28	F	No	5	64
16	173	70	20	M	No	9	64
17	170	56	19	M	No	9	64
18	170	62	20	F	No	4	64
19	165	58	23	F	No	8	64
20	180	75	20	M	No	4	65
21	184	65	21	M	No	8	65
22	167	75	20	F	No	10	65
23	174	60	19	F	No	8	66
24	162	60	19	F	No	8	66
25	175	66	20	M	No	11	66
26	158	51	18	F	No	8	68
27	180	85	19	M	Yes	10	68
28	191	78	19	M	No	8	68
29	164	56	19	F	No	5	68
30	176	59	19	M	No	6	68
31	162	57	20	F	No	7	68
32	170	65	18	M	No	10	69
33	180	72	18	M	No	4	69
34	157	41	20	F	No	11	70
35	177	74	18	F	No	5	70
36	140	50	34	F	No	6	70
37	163	55	20	F	No	7	70
38	163	51	18	F	No	10	70
39	182	85	20	M	Yes	2	70
40	170	68	22	M	No	5	70
41	178	62	21	M	No	1	70
42	163	47	23	F	No	4	71
43	195	84	18	M	No	4	71
44	169	55	18	F	No	1	71
45	175	57	20	F	No	2	72
46	172	53	20	M	No	5	72
47	167	63	28	M	No	2	72
48	164	66	23	F	No	1	74
49	168	55	24	F	No	3	74
50	180	76	21	M	No	2	74
51	189	88	45	M	No	5	74
52	178	58	19	M	No	6	74
53	160	57	19	F	No	4	75
54	185	85	19	M	No	2	75
55	194	110	25	M	No	1	75

(Continued)

Table 11.8   *(Continued)*

ID	Height	Weight	Age	Sex	Smokes	Exercise	Pulse
56	170	75	20	M	No	5	76
57	166	50	19	F	Yes	2	76
58	182	98	19	M	No	3	76
59	179	80	20	M	No	2	76
60	180	102	20	M	No	1	76
61	190	82	19	M	Yes	0	76
62	171	67	18	F	No	1	76
63	171	70	26	F	No	1	76
64	178	86	21	M	Yes	4	76
65	185	110	22	M	No	0	77
66	172	59	18	F	No	5	78
67	186	96	19	M	No	6	78
68	184	74	22	M	No	2	78
69	189	60	19	M	No	1	78
70	163	55	20	F	Yes	0	78
71	155	50	19	F	No	3	78
72	187	59	18	M	No	4	78
73	185	90	18	M	No	1	80
74	180	70	18	M	No	0	80
75	160	49	19	F	No	0	80
76	192	105	21	M	No	1	80
77	182	75	26	M	Yes	1	80
78	164	54	18	F	No	0	80
79	170	60	19	F	No	2	80
80	180	80	21	M	No	2	80
81	170	59	20	M	No	2	80
82	172	60	21	F	Yes	3	81
83	179	58	19	F	No	1	82
84	155	55	20	F	No	0	82
85	166	56	21	F	Yes	0	83
86	165	48	19	F	No	2	83
87	194	95	18	M	No	1	84
88	165	63	18	F	No	1	84
89	178	63	23	M	No	3	84
90	151	42	22	F	No	4	85
91	175	79	19	M	No	0	85
92	178	56	21	F	No	1	86
93	182	60	22	M	Yes	0	86
94	173	57	18	F	No	2	86
95	165	60	19	F	Yes	3	88
96	68	63	19	M	No	4	88
97	180	65	20	M	No	0	88
98	168	60	23	M	No	1	88
99	175	60	19	M	No	2	88

Table 11.8   *(Continued)*

ID	Height	Weight	Age	Sex	Smokes	Exercise	Pulse
100	162	50	19	F	Yes	1	90
101	170	58	21	M	Yes	1	90
102	173	64	18	F	Yes	1	90
103	161	43	19	F	No	1	90
104	170	63	20	F	No	0	92
105	167	70	22	M	Yes	0	92
106	167	62	18	F	Yes	2	96
107	155	49	18	F	No	1	104
108	164	46	18	F	Yes	0	104
109	155	65	19	F	Yes	0	119
110	179	80	20	M	Yes	2	145

The data in Table 11.8 are the results from a random sample of 110 people. The rested pulse rate of each person is measured and also their height in centimetres, weight in kilograms, age in years, sex, whether each considers themself a regular smoker, and the amount of regular exercise each undertakes in hours.

Either consider the data directly or enter them into a computer program of your choice, or download the data in various formats at http://ftp2.arts.unsw.edu.au/argyrous/otherdatasets/chapter11.htm. Then complete the following questions:

1   What is the level of measurement for each variable?
2   Produce appropriate descriptive statistics to assess the distribution of rested pulse rate. Your statistics should allow you to analyze the shape, centre and spread of the distribution, as well as the existence of any outliers. How might you explain any outliers and how should they be handled in further analysis?
3   Compare the mean pulse rate for smokers and non-smokers. In this analysis, which variable is the independent variable and which is the dependent? What is the appropriate measure of association?

RECOMMENDED FURTHER READING

Argyrous, G. (2005) *Statistics for Research*. London: Sage.
This book provides reasonably comprehensive coverage of the descriptive statistics introduced in this chapter, as well as an entry point for the more advanced measures of association and inferential statistics that have only been briefly outlined here.

Liebetrau, A.M. (1983) *Measures of Association*. Beverly Hills, CA: Sage.
This is a definitive and accessible presentation of measures of association, including their calculation and respective limitations.

Sterne, J.A.C. and Smith, G.D. (2001) 'Sifting the evidence – what's wrong with significance tests?', *British Medical Journal*, 322: 226–31.
This is a short and cogent discussion of the logic and history of hypothesis testing, and its limitations.

REFERENCES

Argyrous, G. (2005) *Statistics for Research*. London: Sage.
Australian Bureau of Statistics (2001) *National Health Survey*. Cat. No. 4364.0.
Kirkwood, B. and Sterne, J. (2003) *Essential Medical Statistics*, 2nd edition. Oxford: Blackwell.
Liebetrau, A.M. (1983) *Measures of Association*. Beverly Hills, CA: Sage.
Mathers, N., Williams, M. and Hancock, B. (eds) (2000) *Statistical Analysis in Primary Care*. Oxford: Radcliffe Medical Press.
Scott, I. and Mazhindu, D. (2005) *Statistics for Health Care Professionals: An Introduction*. London: Sage.

12

Randomized Controlled Trials

GEORGE LEWITH AND PAUL LITTLE

INTRODUCTION

This chapter will focus on the underlying principles and concepts that govern all randomized controlled trials (RCTs) and will define their place within clinical research. It will also examine the different types of RCT and the practical issues that arise when carrying out a trial in a clinical setting. In the main, examples will be drawn from complementary and alternative medicine (CAM), not only because this is the first author's area of expertise, but also because some philosophical and ethical issues occur in this setting in particularly stark form.

RCTs can be used in a number of different contexts, although they are used mostly in laboratory or clinical settings. For instance, the performance of two pieces of machine or device that claim to perform the same function can be compared. A trial, holding other factors constant, can be run to compare performance on a number of criteria, such as: Which device uses the least energy? Which is the cheapest or which is the most cost effective? Although it is much more difficult to control for variables and extraneous influences, trials can also be conducted in social care or educational settings where an outcome of an intervention can be compared with a control group to find the most appropriate solution to a particular problem. Examples have been the therapeutic benefits of 'regular good-neighbour visits' to elderly people in terms of improving their sense of well-being or the outcome of a new reading scheme compared with an existing scheme comparing two similar groups of 6 year olds. The fundamental principles of RCTs remain the same in whichever context they are applied and this chapter aims to outline the steps that are fundamental to setting up a RCT and meeting the requirements of a research protocol.

HOW TO APPROACH SETTING UP A RANDOMIZED CONTROLLED TRIAL

The historical and philosophical origin of the RCT centres on a desire to find an answer to a very specific question. It sets out to evaluate the effects of a particular treatment or management strategy in a population where an intervention is introduced, by comparing the outcome with a control group where no intervention has been made. The population must be well defined, and carefully selected.

A number of implicit assumptions underpin the RCT as follows (adapted from Vickers et al. 1997):

- We have an incomplete understanding of the world and knowledge evolves and develops. It is contingent and never definitive.
- Research methods evolve and change as we continue to learn about the world – thus any trial will be as good as we can make it at the time and the knowledge gained is likely to be modest and incremental.
- Logically, cause precedes effect, or put another way, A leads to B.
- Beliefs cannot influence random events.
- In a well-designed study, the researcher's beliefs cannot influence the outcome.
- Good research aims to minimize the effects of bias, chance variation and confounding.
- Research that investigates whether treatments do more good than harm must be a priority.

These tenets lead to the claim that the RCT provides the 'gold standard' for research. It is the best means of attributing clinical real cause and effect and therefore adds to the stock of knowledge. Not all researchers necessarily believe all of these assumptions (see, for example, Frank and Frank 1991; Ronsenzweig 1936), but they provide a sound framework for conducting a RCT.

REFINING THE RESEARCH QUESTION

Setting up a RCT is a challenging task and researchers contemplating a trial must ask themselves:

- What is a good question?
- How can questions be matched to the research design?
- What is the best strategic approach to the research?
- How can an appropriate interpretation of the results be made and an inappropriate interpretation avoided?

The first prerequisite for refining a research question is to carry out a thorough literature search, as described in more detail in Chapter 3. A literature search is an iterative and developmental process that will contribute directly and indirectly to protocol development. It will help to identify whether the question one wants to ask has already been asked and also point out the strengths and weakness of previous research in addressing and answering the question.

A question is likely to be answerable if it is explicit, focused and feasible. In other words, it should be possible to link the effect of an intervention explicitly to a specific outcome. The research should be focused. There should be a very clear, simple primary question and a research method that will provide an answer – the trick is not to ask too many primary questions simultaneously even in a complex study. If there are multiple questions, then the primary research question must be given priority. The primary research question must be framed so that it is both possible and practical to answer the question. Some examples of questions are given in Table 12.1. The findings must be achievable within a reasonable period of time and within the bounds of the scientific and financial resources available. Factors that may allow for the misinterpretation of the study's findings, such as 'bias' and 'confounding', must be considered at an early stage and the research questions then modified, so that an appropriate trial design eventually emerges. These are considered further below.

WAYS TO DEVELOP A VIABLE RANDOMIZED CONTROLLED TRIAL

Clinical research evolves slowly, but for many therapies it is best not to try and solve too many questions simultaneously. A study's design is primarily predicated by the question it is designed to answer. The specificity and rigour of high-quality clinical trial design means that while a specific question may be asked, it is impossible to answer all the relevant questions that may surround a particular illness or a specific therapy. It is wise to recognize this at the outset when considering the details of a trial design. The study structure, rationale and design will have largely been formulated on the evidence provided in the background section of a protocol. If there is little solid RCT evidence for a particular intervention, then a feasibility or pilot study will almost certainly be required. This may be a RCT, or it may be an observational study that could be

Table 12.1 *Different types of research question and their suitability for a RCT*

Category of question	Examples	Suitable for RCT
Attributing cause and clinical effect	Does homoeopathically prepared grass pollen reduce symptoms of hay fever more than a non-active (placebo) treatment?	Y
	Is polypharmacy more effective than a single remedy approach in the homoeopathic treatment of chronic hay fever?	Y
What happens in clinical practice?	What is the cost-effectiveness of adding homoeopathic treatment to a standard care package in hay fever?	Y
	What are the patterns of cross-referral between conventional and CAM practitioners in a multidisciplinary pain clinic?	N
	How common are serious neurological complications following chiropractic cervical manipulation?	N
What do people do?	How many people visit practitioners of CAM each year?	N
	What do patients tell their primary care physician about usage of CAM?	N
	How many nurses practice complementary medicine?	N
What do people believe and how do they explain it?	What do nurses believe about therapeutic touch? What is the patient's experience of the acupuncture consultation?	N
By what mechanisms does a therapy work?	What are the effects of needling the Hoku point on the production of endogenous opiates?	Y
Does something proposed in a therapy actually exist?	Does peppermint oil reduce histamine-induced contractions of tracheal smooth muscle?	Y
	Does homoeopathically prepared copper ameliorate the effects of copper poisoning in a plant model?	Y
	Can an acupuncture point be distinguished from non-acupuncture points by measuring the electrical resistance of the skin?	N
Is a diagnostic or prognostic test accurate?	How sensitive and specific is detection of gall bladder disease by examining photos of the iris?	N
	Is tongue diagnosis reliable?	N

Source: Vickers et al. (1997)

designed to evaluate recruitment and treatment effect size. The study structure will need to be appropriate to the illness and intervention. The planning stages of any clinical trial are vital.

Some tips for a successful project

First, based on our experience of conducting research using RCTs, we have found that working in a group with colleagues that meets on a regular basis provides an opportunity for supportive yet critical ongoing review of projects. It helps to avoid making definitive decisions too rapidly and protect against mistakes.

Second, we believe that it is essential to carry out a thorough and ongoing literature review for each project (see Chapter 3). Data on references should be stored in a secure way but accessible to colleagues working on a project. Regular attendance at academic meetings, reading journals and reviewing Internet sources regularly will help to keep the researcher abreast of developments in the field.

Third, carrying out an initial pilot, or feasibility, study is often useful in testing out whether a properly constructed RCT study is worthwhile. This can help to refine the research question, develop hypotheses to be tested and check whether a project is feasible. Pilot projects allow students to test out their ideas without incurring large costs in money and time. Although the findings of small-scale studies may not be generalizable as they are likely to be underpowered (see Chapter 9), questions can be tested out. Some questions suitable for further investigation were listed in Table 12.1.

Fourth, it is essential to ensure that a pilot study or RCT will be feasible. For example, researchers should make sure that it is or will be possible to recruit an adequate number of patients with disease X or in situation Y in the time frame they have in mind, and also make sure that the volunteers or patients/clients will be able to complete the instruments that have been designed to measure outcomes. The latter should not be too burdensome for participants and, most importantly, the information sheet given to participants to give their consent to the research should be written in clear and non-technical language so it is easy for them to understand what is expected of them and makes them fully aware of any risks, costs and the time involved.

Fifth, in relation to the technical aspects of the project, researchers should make sure that the process of randomization and blinding is feasible in the context of the study. It is particularly important to ensure that if a placebo is being used, it is appropriate for the control group concerned (Vincent and Lewith 1995; White et al. 2003).

Finally, the degree of variance in the main outcome measure should be calculated as this can inform decisions on the appropriate sample size for a further study.

Nowadays, for all but the most simple, small and straightforward study, clinical research is usually best conducted in teams. The sophistication of the research process – given the complexity of clinical governance, ethics, requirements for trial design and protocols, trial management, data handling and statistical analysis – is often simply too much for the lone researcher. Even for teams, advice is needed from collaborators who are experts in particular areas and have a variety of expertise which will supplement and help develop the principal investigator's and the team's initial ideas and the development of a research protocol. However, both pilot studies and moderate-sized trials are well within the remit of undergraduate and postgraduate students working within a team and can provide an important learning opportunity.

COMMON METHODOLOGICAL PROBLEMS

A number of decisions and dilemmas must be faced by those carrying out a trial. First, while research is usually feasible and necessary, it may not be ethical (for example, it would be unethical to carry out a RCT on the benefits of antibiotics in the treatment of meningitis because the benefits of antibiotics are known and these could not therefore be withheld from a control group). Second, some research may be important, but not practical. Third, research rarely provides unequivocal answers: there is often room for reasonable people to disagree about the interpretation of the findings.

Avoiding bias

Bias can occur in many stages of a trial and, unless recognized and countered, this will lead to false estimates of the effect of an intervention. There may be:

- *Recruitment bias*: A population may be selected for recruitment that does not represent the key population of interest — in consequence, the results of the study will only apply to the specific population recruited.
- *Selection bias*: This occurs where the intervention and control patient groups are not comparable.
- *Performance bias*: This occurs when groups within the intervention arm, for example in a multicentre study, may receive different kinds of treatment.
- *Detection bias*: This refers to systematic differences in the outcome assessment between groups.
- *Attrition bias*: This occurs when withdrawals from the study distort the symmetry of the initial selection process and therefore the results — so there must be proper reporting of those who withdraw from a trial in order to avoid distortion (Feinstein 1985), as considered below.
- *Researcher/participant bias*: This occurs when the behaviour or response of those involved in a trial is affected positively or negatively by the knowledge that they are in the intervention or control group. This is sometimes referred to as the Hawthorne effect. In order to offset this, a trial may be 'blinded'. Here the researcher does not know which group the research participant is in and/or a participant may be given a placebo.

Assessing confounding factors

Confounding occurs when there is an association between an exposure to an intervention and the outcome as a consequence of an intervening variable – a third unknown factor. The control of confounding in the case of both known and anticipated and unknown confounders can be achieved through randomization, which is a major advantage of the RCT. With the randomization of those selected for trials, potential confounders can be equally distributed between groups and the effect neutralized. This is the main reason why the RCT is advocated as the best source of evidence of therapeutic benefit. An example of this is the following: a greater proportion of males over 60 die of lung cancer than males under 40. It might be incorrectly assumed that lung cancer is predominantly associated with age. However, an important intervening variable is smoking history. A history must be taken so that both age and smoking can be allowed for in interpreting trends as they can both be measured. Randomization is discussed further below.

By definition, unknown confounders cannot be measured. A RCT that selects randomly for an appropriate size of population (statistical advice will be needed for how large that population should be for a particular trial) is a good way to attribute cause because it can allow for unknown confounding variables in, for example, attributing a therapeutic effect to a particular drug intervention. It may also be valuable in the context of a health economic evaluation. However, it is unlikely to be valuable in understanding people's activities, beliefs or the accuracy of a prognostic or diagnostic test.

PHASES WITHIN A CLASSIC RANDOMIZED CONTROLLED TRIAL

The classic clinical trial process was designed around testing the efficacy of drugs rather than for use in surgical or manual interventions such as physiotherapy or osteopathy. It is essentially a prospective study. It looks forward in time. More recently, clinical trials have been divided into four main phases which represent vital progressive steps in testing the efficacy of modern pharmaceutical agents. These are pre-clinical trials and Phase I, II and III trials.

In pharmaceutical development, before a *pre-clinical trial* is launched there will have been many years of very careful testing carried out both *in vivo* and *in vitro* to minimize the risk to humans of taking a particular drug and to maximize the potential therapeutic benefit. The primary aim of these studies is to assess the absorption of a drug, its distribution through the body, the effect on metabolism and the extent of excretion – collectively known as the ADME of a drug.

In *Phase I* clinical trials the population is not randomized into two groups and are usually carried out in individuals who have a pre-existing pathology. The aim of these studies is two-fold:

- To establish the maximum tolerated dose by very cautiously increasing the dose of the medication in patients with real pathology and to look for side effects.
- To assess whether the medication is effective.

The criteria used to define the 'maximum tolerated dose' and 'treatment efficacy' vary significantly depending on the illness. For instance, patients with terminal cancer may give consent to a trial even if there are uncomfortable side effects because they wish to help future patients or because they believe the drug will be effective. This is less likely in the case of patients with an intermittent benign illness such as migraine.

Phase II studies are carried out in patients with a known illness and usually involve four treatment groups recruited to a prospective RCT. While a Phase I study may estimate the likely doses of a potential therapeutic agent, a Phase II study carries this work further, usually looking at three different therapeutic doses in three different arms of the trial with a placebo in the fourth arm. With most conventional pharmaceutical agents, therapeutic benefit increases with the size of the dose, but so does the potential risk of adverse reactions. The aim is to find a dose that provides the best clinical effect with the lowest level of adverse reaction. Typically, in one arm of the trial patients will receive what is thought to be the therapeutic dose; a second arm will be given half that dose and a third arm double the optimal dose, while the fourth arm receives a placebo. The specific treatment efficacy will be evaluated by comparing the balance of therapeutic benefit and adverse reaction with the active agent versus a placebo.

A *Phase III* clinical trial mirrors most closely the classic RCT. It is usually a study that involves two groups (arms) and compares the optimal dose of active treatment with a placebo over a period of time and uses outcome measures that will allow researchers to conclude that any effects observed will be the specific effect of the drug or intervention being evaluated.

The commonest trial designs used within a Phase III RCT are two armed comparative trials designed to evaluate the difference between a specific intervention and a comparative placebo or control intervention with clearly defined primary and secondary outcomes. In some instances, particularly for chronic conditions, various adaptations on this central scheme may be applied. For instance, a run-in period may be used to establish baseline symptoms prior to trial entry. This allows for the general improvement that may occur as a 'trial effect' will become apparent as patients record their symptoms over a period of a week or a month (Lewith et al. 2002a; White et al. 2004b). It may also protect against a ceiling effect as some presentation of symptoms is necessary to demonstrate a clinical improvement has occurred as a consequence of the intervention.

THE PROCESS OF PROTOCOL DEVELOPMENT

The process of protocol development forms the foundation of any RCT. It provides a road map or process for a trial setting out the aims and rationale, a detailed methods section covering recruitment, the process of the research over time, the end points for measurement, any risks to patients, the statistical advice received and concludes with a patient consent form. This explains the research project in lay language and must be signed by the patient and retained by the patient. As suggested above, protocol development is generally a group activity with input required from clinicians, research methodologists, statisticians and, where appropriate, health economists, social scientists and, often, users and consumers.

Protocols are designed first to clarify the researcher's thoughts, but more importantly to convey the scientific essence of the research proposal to others through a peer review process. A protocol must have clarity and focus with a logical flow that justifies the researcher's plan of investigation. It will form the basis for all relevant research applications for ethics and governance committees, external or internal funding, as well as any subsequent publications. Research protocol forms are usually obtained from the institution sponsoring the research. Forms may differ in detail, but generally cover broadly similar areas as described below.

The background section

The aim of the background section is to show that the researcher has a complete understanding of the problem they wish to investigate. It provides the argument for why a particular research question is both important and relevant within the specific field. It should be clearly and concisely written, concluding with a focused research question in the context of existing knowledge. The researcher should demonstrate an understanding of the disease process in question and its natural history and give a clear description of issues that might impact on the disease outcome. For example, a study of one of the authors on stroke and the use of acupuncture (Hopwood et al. 2006) required an understanding of stroke and its physiological and emotional impact on functioning that might affect the outcome of the evaluation of acupuncture.

A thorough review of research is required so that the research question is appropriate and logical, filling a gap in knowledge in the existing literature.

The quantity of previous studies does not rule out the need for another study. For example, many studies have evaluated the use of acupuncture for back pain (White et al. 2002; White et al. 2004b; Manheimer et al. 2005). However, in some of these the methodology has been flawed. Arguably, there is still a need for a large, rigorous trial.

Developing a hypothesis

The design of a research project will be influenced by the primary hypothesis, or the proposition to be tested. This can be briefly stated but must be firmly based on the research question, and is frequently a null hypothesis – that is, a proposition that suggests that statistically it is unlikely that the treatment will be shown to have an effect (see Chapter 11 on statistics). A Phase III clinical trial will inevitably have one main hypothesis, although there will almost certainly be a number of secondary research questions.

Outcomes expected and their measurement: Validity and reliability

The research protocol will require a statement of how the effect of an intervention will be measured. This may be done by stating clinical measures such as blood pressure levels, air flow or exercise tests, or quality of life measures or patient questionnaires. There are advantages in using existing well-validated and reliable primary outcome measures. The concept of validity has a number of dimensions as follows:

- *Face validity*: On the 'face' of it, the outcome measure is relevant to the study questions.
- *Content validity*: The outcome measure includes the range of issues considered important by patients and experts in the field.
- *Construct validity*: The outcome measure used in previous studies behaves in an appropriate manner which is relevant to the factors that it is measuring based on previous literature or theories — for example, a knowledge outcome should relate to training.
- *Criterion validity*: The outcome measure is congruent with an acknowledged 'gold standard' measure.

It is also important that the outcome being measured gives reliable results. This can be demonstrated by:

- *Test–retest reliability*: Measures show the same result when repeated after a short interval, such as two weeks in a stable condition.

- *Internal reliability*: This refers to the degree of rigour or consistency as a measure. For example, where questionnaire items are combined in a scale or subscale, individual questionnaire items should relate well to each other and to the scale total (Streiner and Norman 1995).
- *Outcome sensitivity*: An outcome should be sensitive to change.

New outcome measures may be developed in the context of a clinical trial providing they are or can be compared and validated with a standard measure in the same group of patients. For example, in a study where acupuncture was used to treat neck pain, the primary outcomes used were well-validated scales measuring the quality of life perceptions of pain in a group of patients suffering from chronic, mechanical neck pain (White et al. 2004a). A further process of 'scale validation' was developed and therefore was a secondary outcome from the study. It is usual, particularly in large clinical trials, to have both primary and secondary outcomes. For instance, a study on acupuncture and pain may have a visual analogue of pain as its primary outcome, with secondary outcomes relating to quality of life and range of movement measures.

It is important to specify a primary outcome in a research study so that a Type I error, that is an error due to chance findings, can be avoided. For example, if 20 outcome measures were used in one clinical trial, it is likely that one of these would show a significant difference between an active and placebo treatment at the 5 per cent level (that is, 1:20 times), and consequently this might be considered a significant outcome. It is, in fact, likely to be simply a random event if all the other 19 outcomes show no difference between the active and the placebo treatment. The choice of primary outcome will be determined by the type of trial: thus in a pragmatic trial where the beliefs and behaviour of the participants are as natural as possible, with minimal interference, then patient-based outcomes may be developed for use rather than objective measurement of outcomes by independent observers.

It is also important to consider, measure and control, if necessary by stratification (see below), what may predict or confound an outcome. For example, if patients are receiving either acupuncture or physiotherapy for their neck pain, then outcomes may be predicted by the attitudes and beliefs that trial participants hold about a particular intervention. If possible, these attitudes should be established in the initial part of the study (White 2003).

Ideally, outcomes should be measured independently of the investigator and if possible blind to the group to minimize outcome assessment bias (see 'blinding' above). Outcomes should also be measured in the same way in each group to avoid bias as the manner and timing of a measurement may affect that measurement. For example, in the British Family Heart Study blood pressure was measured in the intervention group at the beginning and the end, but only at the end in the control group. One finding was that a fall in blood pressure was observed in the intervention group. However, it was not possible to say whether this was due to the intervention alone, or also due to the effect of measurement that was repeated (Family Heart Study Group 1994). Poor trial design led to measurement bias. In sum, both the measurement and placebo arm of a trial should be subject to the same set of measures.

The selection of research participants: Inclusion and exclusion criteria

The decision about who to include in, and who to exclude from, a trial is of key importance. An effect of an intervention is most likely to be found with a homogeneous group of patients and those who are most likely to benefit, if this can be predicted from previous research. If too varied a group is included, then the higher variance in the primary outcome measure will limit the ability of the treatment to show an effect, and may obscure real and important benefit. The weakness of using a highly selected group is that treatment effects observed in highly selected groups may not apply to a broader group generally seen in the community. If, for instance, a study is conducted involving a new intervention for chronic obstructive pulmonary disease (COPD), but excludes all patients taking oral steroids, then how relevant is such a conclusion to general practice where many patients with COPD are likely to be on long-term oral steroids? Thus, there is a continuing tension within any clinical trial between reducing variability by selecting patients with clearly defined clinical and social characteristics, and providing evidence that is generalizable to the population managed in everyday practice. Inclusion and exclusion criteria require careful thought with respect to this balance.

The recruitment process

The recruitment process involved in a clinical trial will affect the generalizability of findings. For instance, a group of volunteers selected via the Web may be an entirely different population from those invited to participate in a clinical trial via a general practice. As a consequence, it is vital to keep information on the flow of patient recruitment (Brien et al. 2003; Moher et al. 2001). A good clinical trial will have a pre-specified mechanism for recording and handling the data and it is important to track missing data from patients who drop out. The most important guiding principle is that once a patient has been entered into a clinical trial and randomized, then they must be followed up throughout the study. It is important to try and achieve a follow-up of at least 80 per cent or above, otherwise attrition bias may seriously compromise the validity of the results. If patients are rejected during a baseline recording period because they do not ultimately fulfil the entry criteria for a study (Lewith et al. 2002a) or have not otherwise entered the trial process, they do not need to be followed up throughout the study. Those who are eligible but decline to take part should be documented and reported as part of the CONSORT trial flow diagram, which is the standard mechanism for reporting the flow of patient recruitment for clinical trials.

During the development of a protocol, the sample size calculation forms the basis of the numbers that will need to be recruited to a trial in order to answer the trial's primary and secondary hypotheses, and provides the foundation for costing and development within the context of a clinical trial.

Figure 12.1 illustrates patient recruitment in a study involving homoeopathic proving. It records the number of people who were contacted about the study; those included in the initial baseline screening and those subsequently randomized within the study; and those who dropped out. This helps to highlight the generalizability of findings and sources of bias.

Randomization and related issues

Randomization is one of the most important ways of removing confounding within a RCT. The initial aim is to select a homogeneous group of patients, while identifying within the introductory or background section to a protocol the important factors (potential confounders) that may independently predict outcome. The method of randomization should separate whoever generates the randomization codes from the person carrying out the randomization to minimize any possibility that the clinician managing the patient could have any influence on the choice of group. In a placebo-controlled trial this is accomplished by an independent pharmacy making up randomization packs containing active drug or placebo, and for an open trial this is best accomplished using an external telephone randomization line.

Stratification

In small single-centre clinical trials, great attention must be paid to understanding both the illness and the effect of interventions, along with potential predictive factors that may independently influence treatment outcome. This is because, for very large trials, confounders will be equally distributed between groups. For smaller trials, particularly where some variables strongly predict outcome, it is important to make sure that such variables are balanced between groups by 'stratification'. For instance, in our asthma study, we were aware that initial asthma severity and the presence of smokers would need to be balanced between the two treatment groups, as both these factors might significantly influence outcome. As a consequence, we randomized the first 10 patients using sealed opaque envelopes to receive either real homoeopathy or placebo, and then

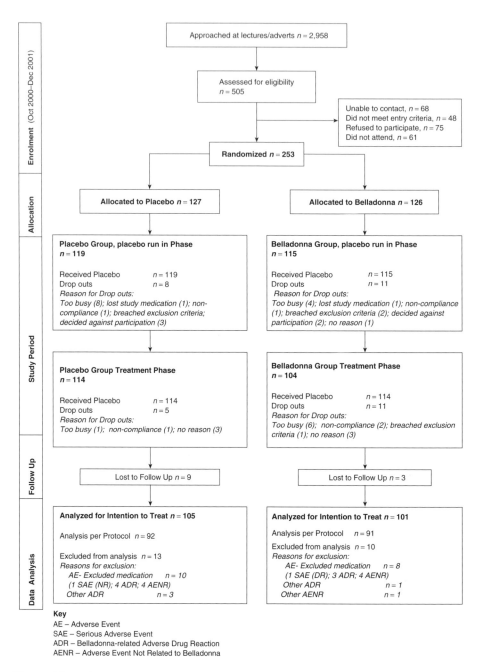

Figure 12.1 *Patient recruitment in a study of homoeopathic proving*

Source: Brien et al. (2003)

subsequently used a minimization programme. This allocates patients so that with each randomization, any difference between groups for the potential confounding variables is minimized. The two treatment groups were therefore balanced for all major known potential predictors of outcome (Lewith et al. 2002b).

In other studies, for instance with stroke, it was known that stroke severity would predict outcome irrespective of treatment. We therefore stratified patients so that the treatment groups were clearly balanced with similar numbers of patients with relatively severe and relatively mild stroke (Hopwood et al. 2006). Specific responses to particular therapies and/or therapists are important and must be considered when defining the process of randomization in a two-armed trial, or the order of treatment in a cross-over study (White et al. 2003).

Clustering

Randomization in multicentre trials can present a variety of different problems. The same treatments may not be delivered in the same way at every centre, or treatments may be delivered at some centres and not others, so the outcomes found might be centre dependent with treatment effects 'clustered' in consequence. Every effort should be made to standardize for recruitment, sample size and any analysis should allow for possible clustering. Those interested in multicentre trials should refer to Campbell and Machin (1999).

The statistical analysis plan

Whatever the protocol and however the study is designed, a clear plan for data analysis must be presented at the protocol stage (see Chapter 11 on statistics). An important principle in analysis is that the primary analysis should generally be an 'intention to treat' analysis – that is, where all patients, whether they complied with the intervention or not, are included in the analysis according to their original study group. This is important because, to estimate the average effect patients can expect to receive from a treatment, the results should include both patients where it has worked and those where it has not worked or who have had to stop the treatment for whatever reason. This mirrors what is likely to happen in the real world. Most studies usually also perform a so-called 'per protocol' analysis where only those patients who have complied with the intervention are assessed; this will give an estimate of the effect of the intervention in ideal circumstances.

Ethics and governance

The process of ethics and governance has changed radically with the introduction of the new European Union clinical trial directive in April 2004. This is dealt with elsewhere in this book in Chapter 15, but it is important to recognize that it is an essential part of a protocol and requires careful consideration, particularly with respect to data protection, obtaining fully informed consent and following good clinical practice. Great care should be taken in drafting the patient consent form so that the research is comprehensible in lay terms. Research ethics committees are often most critical of this aspect of a research protocol.

METHODOLOGICAL ISSUES

The replicability of research

The essence of any scientific experiment is to describe, within the methods section, an experimental procedure that can be completely duplicated by any other interested and properly trained researcher. This requires that the intervention made is described specifically and exactly. In the case of a drug trial, the exact medication used must be defined, along with its specific manufacture, dosage and delivery method. In studies involving surgical or manual intervention, such as physiotherapy, a methodological prerequisite is to describe all the interventions in all arms to a high level of specificity. A study should be capable of replication so that any other researcher would be able to carry out the same study using the same interventions and, hopefully, come to the same conclusions.

Blinding and its problems

The process of blinding is designed to remove bias and retain patient equipoise. It is used to detect the specific effects of an intervention by removing any prior 'expectation' that the researcher or participant may have of the trial results from the active or placebo treatment. It is usually possible to blind a medicinal intervention. A placebo can almost always be made to look, taste, feel and present as indistinguishable from the active treatment. However, blinding with respect to a surgical intervention or pragmatic intervention such as physiotherapy, exercise prescription or reflexology is more difficult. While it may have been ethical to blind patients as to whether they had or had not received a real surgical intervention in the mid-1950s (Beecher 1955), it is no longer thought reasonable or ethical to do so. Within the context of a clinical trial, patients must consent to receive, or not to receive, medication, surgery or spinal manipulation.

A very pragmatic definition of a double-blind trial is where both the investigating researchers and the trial participants (volunteers/patients) are unaware whether they are receiving or delivering active or placebo treatment. Both parties are blind to the nature of the intervention, hence expectation is removed and equivalence created with respect to treatment outcome.

A single-blind trial is where the therapist delivering the intervention knows which is the placebo and which is the active treatment, but the patient or volunteer thinks that both interventions are equally likely to be therapeutically effective. This has been achieved with some acupuncture studies (Wood and Lewith 1998). This is also the case where the primary outcome measure is achieved through, for example, a patient self-assessment questionnaire, a visual analogue scale or Short Form 36 (SF-36) or a generic quality of life measure; then a patient can remain in equipoise, with an equal belief in the active and placebo treatment although the groups receive two distinctly different treatments. Outcomes assessed either by themselves or by an entirely objective or independent source (a blood test or a blinded third party) may also mean that a study can be legitimately described as a single-blind trial.

It has been estimated that approximately 70 per cent of clinical trials fail to report the details of blinding (Schulz and Grimes 2002). Schultz argues that the removal of bias is the foundation upon which causal associations can be derived within clinical research. He points out that many conventional clinical trials fail to report the blinding and randomization process adequately and indeed a proportion of researchers may have deliberately subverted the process (Grimes and Schulz 2002). However, it is possible to minimize the effect of open (unblinded) interventions by generating a placebo effect in each group, using the therapist/physician as a placebo – for example, in an open pragmatic trial of prescribing strategies for a sore throat where the placebo effect of prescribing antibiotics was abolished, using structured advice sheets to support management in each group (Little et al. 1997).

When carrying out a trial, researchers should aim to detach themselves from reconceptions about the efficacy of a therapy. This is particularly essential during the data interpretation. The Jadad score (Jadad et al. 1996) and other such scores are widely used among systematic reviewers as the basis of summarizing major sources of bias in relation to blinding, randomization and the reporting of results (internal validity). However, such quality scores rarely assess generalizability to the community of individuals suffering from the illness.

COMMON USED VARIATIONS WITHIN THE RANDOMIZED CONTROLLED TRIAL

It has been argued above that the classic RCT is demanding on staff and resources and is often beyond the scope of the lone researcher. There are some variations that are less resource intensive and still contribute to knowledge.

Cross-over studies

A cross-over study is a study that involves one treatment in a first phase, a washout period with no treatment and then a second randomized treatment with a control group in a further phase. Every individual takes part in both phases, but the order of treatments is randomized. The advantage of a cross-over design is that it minimizes variation. Each individual becomes their own control and so the inter-individual variation is minimized, and thus smaller numbers are needed. Cross-over designs are only appropriate for a stable disease and a therapy that has relatively short-term effects, such as an H_2 blocker in the treatment of gastro-oesophageal reflux. However, it is unlikely, for example, to be the approach of choice for the treatment of mild depression in the community, largely because modern antidepressants take time to work and usually require at least a two- or three-month prescription. At the end of this period, the patient may no longer be depressed. Similarly, as interventions such as acupuncture have unpredictable long-term effects, a cross-over is not appropriate either (Lewith et al. 2002a).

Variations in control mechanisms and pragmatic studies

Some studies may attempt to control for an intervention by having an 'attention' control. This is where some patients simply spend time with a therapist without the therapist providing a specific therapy. The methods section may give information about the intervention, as was the case in a trial to assess the effect of exercise classes for the relief of fibromyalgia. The disadvantage of such studies is that the total effects of an intervention may involve both specific and non-specific effects, although it is often this combined effect that the patient will experience in real life. Furthermore, cost-effectiveness cannot be estimated in studies which use an attention control as this would not occur in actual practice.

Pragmatic studies are defined simply as studies that look at what happens in practice. Thus, patients with chronic low-back pain go to their conventional doctor to receive an analgesic or an anti-inflammatory and may also simultaneously visit an acupuncturist. As a consequence, a pragmatic trial of acupuncture would involve the randomization of patients to receive acupuncture plus conventional care as compared with those simply receiving conventional care. Such a trial suffers from the disadvantage of being unable to define the specific effect of acupuncture, but it has the great advantage of being generalizable in a real-world context (Thomas et al. 1999; Thomas et al. 2005).

Case study: Factorial design in the evaluation of the Alexander Technique

It is generally the case that it is preferable to answer one question at a time. However, sometimes it will be important to ask more than one question. Factorial designs provide an excellent and efficient framework for asking several questions simultaneously and to illustrate this, a case study is provided. For instance, in our current study which evaluates the use of the Alexander Technique in chronic back pain, we have eight groups within our clinical trial (Deyo et al. 1998). The Alexander Technique is a hands-on approach where the teacher through both gentle touch and explanation helps pupils to release harmful muscle tensions, and improve muscle use and coordination. The questions asked in this trial are:

- What is the effectiveness of introductory or longer courses of the Alexander Technique and of massage therapy in restoring normal activities which have been restricted by back pain? (This is the primary research question.)
- What is the effectiveness of general practitioner exercise prescription with a nurse follow-up appointment in restoring normal activities which have been restricted by back pain?
- What is the cost-effectiveness of these treatments compared with normal care?

We wanted to evaluate whether it was necessary to give a prolonged course (24 teaching sessions) of the Alexander Technique or whether 6 sessions could achieve the same clinical outcome. We did this as we believed that 6 sessions might be acceptable for NHS funding if the Alexander Technique proved to be cost effective, but 24 sessions might not. However, we wished to retain the clinical assumptions prevalent among Alexander teachers and evaluate the best possible intervention, and therefore considered that our trial would be completely inadequate if one group did not receive complete (24 sessions) Alexander lessons.

Second, we wished to assess whether the educational element of the Alexander Technique was the key factor to improvement or whether this was simply due to a hands-on approach. For this we had one group of patients who received massage, where there was a hands-on treatment) but no education as usually given in the Alexander Technique. The massage

(Continued)

(Continued)

group was also useful to assess whether massage per se is helpful. A normal care group was required as the basic comparator for all groups. Without a normal care group, it would be difficult to estimate differences in resource use between the groups and therefore difficult to estimate cost-effectiveness.

Thus for one 'factor' we have four groups: longer Alexander Technique (24 lessons), shorter Alexander Technique (6 lessons), massage (6 sessions) and normal care. Each of these groups was split (with random assignment of subjects to two sub-groups). One of these had additional exercise and the other did not. Designing the trial with the presence or absence of exercise in all four groups allows us to compare the Alexander Technique with standard conventional treatment plus exercise, which many recent studies suggest is an effective and indeed cost-effective approach to the management of chronic low-back pain (Frost et al. 2004).

The advantage of this factorial design is that several questions may be asked simultaneously. The statistical calculations associated with this design meant that a number of questions could be asked with slightly fewer trial participants. Inevitably multifactorial studies are complex, difficult to execute and require considerable research expertise.

CONCLUSION

This chapter describes an iterative process to enable and understand the development of RCTs. It centres around the protocol and how best to consider study development with respect to the essential issues that emerge during clinical trial development. The advent of the RCT is both a blessing and a curse. Undoubtedly, it has improved the evidence base to inform the delivery of clinical care, but inevitably any RCT by its nature is limited in its scope. Furthermore, good science and clinical relevance do not always go hand in hand and attempting to achieve both simultaneously requires clear thinking and the ability to work within a team. To underline the themes of this chapter the reader is invited to engage in the short exercise set out below on evaluating the use of lavender essence as an alternative therapy.

Exercise: The evaluation of lavender essence using a randomized controlled trial

It has been suggested that *Lavandula augustifolia* (lavender essence) may be of assistance in treating insomnia. Quite a number of people just put a few drops of lavender on their pillow when they are having difficulty sleeping and say that it 'works a treat'. Insomnia affects 20 per cent of the British population, but many conventional drugs used to treat it have the potential to become addictive.

Consider the issues that you would need to take into account if you wanted to evaluate the use of *Lavandula augustifolia* using a RCT.

Some of the issues you might wish to consider might include:

- How would you search the literature to find out what has already been published?
- How would you construct a study to evaluate this?
- If you were going to use a placebo, how might you provide a convincing one?

RECOMMENDED FURTHER READING

Grimes, D. and Schulz, K. (2002) A series of articles in the *Lancet* on research design (359: 57–61; 145–9; 248–52; 341–5; 515–19; 614–18; 781–5; 881–4; 966–70).
These articles in the epidemiology series give a wonderfully concise introduction to research design.

Lewith, G.T., Walach, H. and Jonas, W.B. (eds) (2002) *Clinical Research in Complementary Therapies*. Edinburgh: Churchill Livingstone.
This book draws on the best of conventional research methods, including randomized controlled trials, and adapts them to the needs of complementary and alternative medicine.

REFERENCES

Beecher, H. (1955) 'The powerful placebo', *Journal of the American Medical Association*, 159: 1602–1606.
Brien, S., Lewith, G.T. and Bryant, T. (2003) 'Ultramolecular homoeopathy has no observable clinical effects. A randomized, double-blind, placebo-controlled proving trial of Belladonna C30', *British Journal of Clinical Pharmacology*, 56: 562–68.

Campbell, M. and Machin, D. (1999) *Medical Statistics. A Commonsense Approach*. Chichester: Wiley.

Deyo, R., Battie, M., Beurskens, A.J., Bombardier, C., Croft, P. and Koes, B. (1998) 'Outcome measures for low back pain research. A proposal for standardized use', *Spine* 23 (18): 2003–13.

Family Heart Study Group (1994) 'Randomised controlled trial evaluating cardiovascular screening and intervention in general practice: principal results of British Family Heart Study', *British Medical Journal*, 308: 313–20.

Feinstein, A.R. (1985) *Clinical Epidemiology: The Architecture of Clinical Research*. Philadelphia: Saunders.

Frank, J.D. and Frank, J.B. (1991) *Persuasion and Healing: A Comparative Study of Psychotherapy*. Baltimore, MD: Johns Hopkins University Press.

Frost, H., Lamb, S.E., Doll, H.A., Taffe Carver, P. and Stewart-Brown, S. (2004) 'Randomised controlled trial of physiotherapy compared with advice for low back pain', *British Medical Journal*, 329: 708–14.

Grimes, D.A. and Schulz, K.F. (2002) 'Bias and causal associations in observational research', *Lancet*, 359: 248–52.

Hopwood, V., Lewith, G.T. and Prescott, P. (2006) 'A single-blind, randomised, placebo controlled study of acupuncture for stroke', *Journal of Neurology* (in submission).

Jadad, A.R., Moore, R.A., Carroll, D., Jenkinson, C., Reynolds, D.J. and Gavaghan, D.J. (1996) 'Assessing the quality of reports of randomized clinical trials: is blinding necessary?', *Control Clinical Trials*, 17: 1–12.

Lewith, G.T., Watkins, A., Hyland, M.E., Shaw, S., Broomfield, J. and Dolan, G. (2002a) 'A double-blind, randomised, controlled clinical trial of ultramolecular potencies of house dust mite in asthmatic patients', *British Medical Journal*, 324: 520–23.

Lewith, G.T., Walach, H. and Jonas, W.B. (2002b) 'Balanced research strategies for complementary and alternative medicine', in G.T. Lewith, W.B. Jonas and H. Walach (eds), *Clinical Research in Complementary Therapies*. Edinburgh: Churchill Livingstone.

Little, P.S., Williamson, I., Warner, G., Gould, C., Gantley, M. and Kinmonth, A.L. (1997) 'An open randomised trial of prescribing strategies for sore throat', *British Medical Journal*, 314: 722–27.

Manheimer, M.S., White, A., Berman, B., Forys, K. and Ernst, E. (2005) 'Meta-analysis: acupuncture for low back pain', *Annals of Internal Medicine*, 142 (8): 651–63.

Moher, D., Schulz, K.F. and Altman, D.G. (2001) 'The CONSORT Statement: revised recommendations for improving the quality of reports of parallel-group randomized trials', *Explore*, 1: 40–45.

Ronsenzweig, S. (1936) 'Some implicit common factors in diverse methods of psychotherapy', *American Journal of Orthopsychiatry*, 6: 412–15.

Schulz, K.F. and Grimes, D.A. (2002) 'Blinding in randomised trials: hiding who got what', *Lancet* 359: 696–700.

Streiner, D.L. and Norman, G.R. (1995) *Health Measurement Scales: A Practical Guide to their Development and Use*. Oxford: Oxford Medical Publications.

Thomas, K.J., Fitter, M., Brazier, J., MacPherson, H., Campbell, M. and Nicholl, P. (1999) 'Longer term clinical and economic benefits of offering acupuncture to patients with chronic low back pain assessed as suitable for primary care management', *Complementary Therapies in Medicine*, 7: 91–100.

Thomas, K., MacPherson, H., Thorpe, L., Brazier, J., Fitter, M., Campbell, M., Roman, M., Walters, S. and Nicholl, J. (2005) *Longer Term Clinical and Economic Benefits of Offering Acupuncture to Patients with Chronic Low Back Pain*. Final Report to NHS Health Technology Assessment Programme.

Vickers, A., Cassileth, B., Ernst, E., Fisher, P., Goldman, P., Jonas, W., Kang, S., Lewith, G., Schulz, K. and Silagy, C. (1997) 'How should we research unconventional therapies?', *International Journal of Technology Assessment in Health Care*, 13 (1): 111–21.

Vincent, C. and Lewith, G.T. (1995) 'Placebo controls for acupuncture studies', *Journal of the Royal Society of Medicine*, 88: 199–202.

White, P. (2003) 'Attitude and outcome: is there a link in complementary medicine?', *American Journal of Public Health*, 93: 1038.

White, P., Lewith, G.T., Berman, B. and Birch, S. (2002) 'Reviews of acupuncture for chronic neck pain: pitfalls in conducting systematic reviews', *Rheumatology*, 41: 1224–31.

White, P., Lewith, G.T., Hopwood, V. and Prescott, P. (2003) 'The placebo needle, is it a valid and convincing placebo for use in acupuncture trials? A randomised, single blind, cross-over trial', *Pain*, 106: 401–409.

White, P., Lewith, G.T. and Prescott, P. (2004a) 'The core outcomes for neck pain – validation of a new outcome measure', *Spine*, 29: 1923–30.

White, P., Lewith, G.T., Prescott, P. and Conway, J. (2004b) 'Acupuncture versus placebo for the treatment of chronic mechanical neck pain. A randomised, controlled trial', *Annals of Internal Medicine*, 141: 911–20.

Wood, R. and Lewith, G.T. (1998) 'The credibility of placebo controls in acupuncture studies', *Complementary Therapies in Medicine*, 6: 79–82.

Acknowledgment

Figure 12.1: Brien, S., Lewith, G. and Bryant, T. 'Ultramolecular homeopathy has no observable clinical effects. A randomized double-blind, placebo-controlled proving trail of Belladonna 30C'. *British Journal of Clinical Pharmacology*. 2003; 56: 562–568. Blackwell Publishing. Reprinted with permission.

13

Experimental Methods in Health Research

A. NIROSHAN SIRIWARDENA

INTRODUCTION

This chapter provides an overview of experimental and quasi-experimental methods with a particular focus on experimental techniques that provide alternatives to the randomized controlled trial (RCT) described in the previous chapter. The RCT is a particular form of experimental method and in a double-blind controlled trial that ranks highest in the hierarchy of evidence described in Chapter 3, randomization can control for confounding variables and double blinding can reduce certain types of bias. However, it is not always possible to conduct a RCT for the methodological, practical and ethical reasons that are discussed below. What are broadly termed experimental methods, an umbrella term that includes a wide variety of particular techniques, aim to maintain scientific rigour in situations where it is not possible to set up controls. The chapter will explain the language of experimentation and discuss the advantages and disadvantages, as well as how such methods should be applied. A range of experimental research designs based on published or unpublished studies are described to illustrate the use of this method in practice.

THE EXPERIMENTAL METHOD

The key feature of an experiment is that it assesses the effect of introducing a change where the relationship between two or more things are investigated by deliberately prompting a change in one of them and observing the change in the other (Robson 1973). A change based on a hypothesis of cause is introduced in one variable (the independent variable), which may lead to a corresponding change, or effect, in another (the dependent) variable. The prediction of cause and effect (A leads to B) is the hypothesis. Experiments test hypotheses whereas other types of quantitative study test the strength of associations (A is associated with B). Experiments based on the scientific method of testing changes to establish a relationship between cause and effect have advantages over other methods in their ability to test hypotheses, reduce bias and limit confounding. Arguably, they are also more robust in determining the true size of the effect of an intervention. The effect size is the estimate of the magnitude of a change and may be calculated statistically.

There are a number of sub-types of experimental method that it is not possible to describe fully here: for example, case–control studies where the aim is to compare the characteristics of a particular phenomenon in the group of interest to a control or reference group – thus, the health of one group of people exposed to a risk factor, such as low-level radiation, may be compared with another group that has not been exposed. Cohort studies are where a selected population may be studied over time to investigate the effect of a particular variable on health outcomes.

Experimental methods should be distinguished from observational methods that are based on the method of an external observer noting behaviour, as for example in psychological studies. In turn, observational methods should not be confused with the participant observer or ethnographic methods used in qualitative research and described in Chapter 6.

NON-RANDOMIZED EXPERIMENTAL DESIGNS

Experimental methods have a particular value in assessing the effect of innovative interventions in health care. However, health care practitioners or organizations, sometimes purposefully and sometimes inadvertently, introduce new health technologies or services, which once applied are difficult to reverse from either an ethical or practical perspective. Once a new service is introduced or an intervention is established there are limited possibilities for more structured experimental designs to determine effectiveness or cost-effectiveness. In this situation non-randomized experimental designs may provide the only possibility for evaluation, and they may be the only option in this and a number of other situations. For example, randomization may not be possible due to factors, either intrinsic or extrinsic to the study, particularly in area-wide changes or organization-based interventions or because of external constraints such as a policy decision to introduce a new service or some other imposed or natural change across a geographical region.

Non-randomized experimental methods include a range of study types summarized in Figure 13.1 with a single intervention group only, or with an intervention group and non-randomized comparison or control group. These

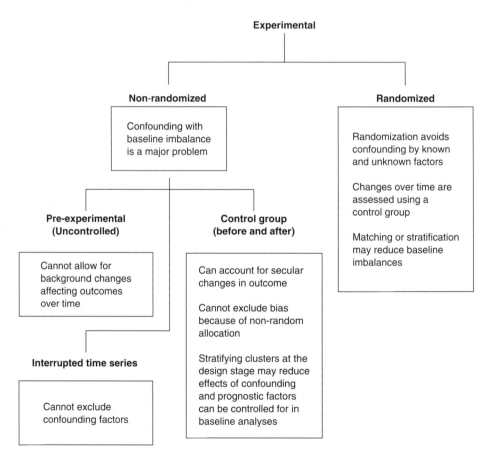

Figure 13.1 *A classification of experimental study designs*
Source: Adapted from Ukoumunne et al. (1999: 9)

methods may also classified into pre-experimental and quasi-experimental designs on the basis that the former are not likely to provide valid evidence for effectiveness of an intervention whereas the latter may do so in certain circumstances (Campbell and Stanley 1963; Cook and Campbell 1979).

PRE-EXPERIMENTAL DESIGNS

Pre-experimental designs are non-randomized experiments where a particular outcome of interest is measured, sometimes with a non-randomized control group for comparison in the intervention group. These include the so-called single-group post-intervention design (with or without controls) and the single-group pre- and post-intervention design when the outcome is measured before, and after, the intervention. Such designs are often used for evaluations of educational interventions, an example being an educational programme to improve the recognition of psychological illness in general practice (Hannaford et al. 1996) or when researchers wish to evaluate the impact of large-scale changes. One such study examined the effect on general practitioner (GP) workload (in terms of hours spent on general practice work per week and time spent per patient in consultations) of the introduction of a new contract for GPs in 1990 (Hannay et al. 1992).

Case study: **Performance of general practitioner trainers in an applied knowledge test**

CASE STUDY

Another example of a pre-experimental design was used in a recent study aimed at investigating the perceptions and performance of GPs in the multiple-choice paper taken as part of the membership examination of the Royal College of General Practitioners (MRCGP). The aim of the study was to assess whether the multiple-choice examination was a valid test of current applied knowledge in general practice using the knowledge of GP trainers as a proxy.

In this study, a self-administered questionnaire and written knowledge test was applied to volunteer GP trainers in the Northern, Wessex, Surrey and Northwest deaneries of the United Kingdom. The trainers completed a shortened version of a sample MRCGP paper under examination conditions and also provided feedback on their perceptions of the assessment (Dixon et al. 2007). It could be argued that the 'intervention' in this case was the experience of being a practising GP.

(Continued)

Table 13.1 Comparison of candidates' versus trainers' scores for total score, medicine, research and administration

		N	Mean	Standard deviation	95% confidence interval for mean		Minimum	Maximum	P (ANOVA)
					Lower bound	Upper bound			
Total score	Candidates	865	73.88	10.49	73.18	74.58	25.96	95.19	0.002
	Trainers	86	77.60	9.20	75.63	79.58	39.42	94.23	
Medicine	Candidates	865	74.80	10.28	74.11	75.49	26.32	96.05	0.014
	Trainers	86	77.63	8.79	75.75	79.52	39.47	92.11	
Research	Candidates	865	76.03	23.00	74.49	77.56	.00	100.00	0.90
	Trainers	86	75.69	21.17	71.15	80.23	.00	100.00	
Administration	Candidates	865	68.40	15.41	67.37	69.43	5.88	100.00	<0.001
	Trainers	86	78.73	12.57	76.03	81.42	41.18	100.00	

Source: Dixon et al. (2007)

(Continued)

The scores for 86 trainers were then compared with the scores in identical questions for the 865 candidates who had sat the paper, as set out in Table 13.1. Trainers were significantly better than candidates in their overall score (p = 0.002), as well as in answering questions on medical knowledge related to general practice (p = 0.014) and practice administration (p < 0.001). They scored less well on critical appraisal skills and research methods (p = 0.9). All trainers would have passed the test if their scores in the shortened paper were extrapolated to the full paper. Time was not a problem for trainers in the shortened test with most (74 or 91 per cent) believing that they had sufficient time to complete the paper. Most of the participating GP trainers believed that the paper assessed knowledge of common or important topics relevant to general practice, and that the majority of questions were clear.

A number of criticisms could be made of the study. The deaneries chosen were those in which the researchers were known and had access to trainer groups. This may therefore have increased the likelihood of trainer participation, but still only 45 per cent of GP trainers invited to participate did so. Those participating were volunteers and therefore may not have been representative of all trainers. They may also have been more positive, more confident and more knowledgeable than their colleagues. The assurance of confidentiality may not have been sufficient to persuade some trainers to participate and a lower than ideal response rate was anticipated given the anxiety and fear of failure any assessment can generate.

GP trainers perceived the examination to be a valid test of applied knowledge of current general practice. Lending further support to this was the fact that practising GP trainers normally did better in the applied knowledge test than doctors (mainly those in training) who took the examination. They performed more strongly on questions on medical aspects of general practice and practice administration. This was perhaps not surprising, as the trainers were all partners in general practice.

The weaknesses of pre-experimental designs

These designs suffer from a serious and often fatal flaw. It is virtually impossible to determine whether the outcome is due to the intervention or to another confounding factor noted in Figure 13.1. Such factors include an unpredicted external influence or the effect of changes that occur naturally over time in the process of health care, such as increased awareness of new technologies or processes, local and national influences or demographic factors. These may be referred to as the impact of secular trends. There may also be changes in the behaviour of study participants directly as a result of being observed, termed the Hawthorne effect (see Chapter 6), or due to regression to the mean, that is the tendency of outlying variables to move towards mean values. In addition, the possibility of generalizing from these studies may be severely compromised by selection bias. There may be a tendency for the researcher to select the objects of study where it is more likely that there will be factors present that bias the results.

However, such pre-experimental designs may have a place, particularly in quality improvement studies, where interventions are used in an attempt to improve the quality of care in a specific setting. Blenkiron (2001), for example, developed a pre-experimental design in a pilot study of the efficacy of a self-help audio cassette in coping with depression. He compared patient agreement with key messages on the audio tape before and after use and found improvement in attitudes and knowledge following its use. Pre-experimental studies may also be useful as a precursor to a randomized controlled study to evaluate a complex intervention, where two or more interventions are combined in a single study. This is often the case in interventions designed to implement innovations in health care as there is increasing evidence that multiple interventions may be more effective (Grimshaw et al. 2001; Wensing et al. 1998). An example is provided in the case study given at the end of this chapter.

QUASI-EXPERIMENTAL DESIGNS

Quasi-experimental designs include two main types of study. These are the non-randomized control group before and after study, and the interrupted time series design.

Non-randomized control group before and after studies

The method for the non-randomized control group before and after study involves one or more intervention groups with one or more non-equivalent comparator groups to act as controls with measurements of outcomes taken before and after the intervention. An example of a before and after study in relation to evaluating policy innovation is a study of the impact of legislation to ban smoking in public places in the Republic of Ireland. A before and after non-randomized control group design found a decrease in to reduce passive smoking and respiratory illness in bar workers (Allwright et al. 2005).

Another study, this time based in the United Kingdom, found that the introduction of legislation restricting pack sizes of analgesics led to reductions in pack sizes on pharmacy shelves. This study found that associated with this change were reductions in analgesic overdoses. It also found that the severity of the overdoses that did occur was also reduced and so were other sequelae, such as the level of suicide deaths and of liver transplantation (Hawton et al. 2004).

Studies using an interrupted time series design

In the second type of study, repeated measurements of the outcome of interest are taken from the population beginning before the intervention and continuing afterwards. Measurements are taken to assess whether there is any change over and above that which would have been expected from the secular trend prior to the intervention. Measurements for time series studies may be taken from a whole population or by sampling from a cohort of the population, or alternatively by using repeated cross-sectional samples from the whole population. This method need not necessarily involve a control group, but does benefit from a control in accounting for confounding external influences on the outcome of interest. Cohort designs, although offering greater statistical power, are more likely over longer periods of time to lead to bias due to non-response; a loss to follow-up, sometimes referred to as attrition; Hawthorne effects; maturation effects where individual ageing may be a factor; and contamination. A study can be 'contaminated' when the change that is intended for the intervention group is inadvertently introduced to the control group. This can occur, for example, due to staff moving between health facilities, an unexpected movement of patients or the introduction of a parallel intervention, which could skew the outcomes being measured.

The main sources of bias in this type of study include external effects on outcome and secular (time-related) changes unrelated to the intervention. Although this source of bias can be minimized by having a control group, this may not be possible because of limited funding or because a new policy is introduced. Some studies have shown the unwanted effects of media coverage of certain subjects. An example is an episode in *Casualty*, a BBC television drama, which portrayed the effect of a drug overdose (Hawton et al. 1999). Although a control group in a time series design may not be possible, research using this method can nevertheless provide useful findings. This is exemplified by a recent study on the implementation of the National Institute of Health and Clinical Excellence (NICE) guidelines (Sheldon et al. 2004), which showed variable adoption of guidance across departments.

Case study: A demonstration project to implement influenza vaccination through Medicare

An example of a non-randomized control group before and after design was employed in a very large so-called demonstration project designed to study methods of improving influenza vaccination in the United States from 1988 to 1992 as part of a million-dollar-funded study across nine states (Barker et al. 1999). Monroe County, New York State, was one of the nine original sites for the Medicare Influenza Vaccine Demonstration or 'McFlu' project. Area-wide systems were implemented in Monroe County for promoting and documenting influenza vaccine delivery to those aged 65 years or over, funded through Medicare (the system of limited health insurance available for certain categories of citizen), with an objective of achieving vaccine coverage of greater than 60 per cent. Systems were also established for conducting laboratory-based influenza surveillance in Monroe County and in neighbouring Onondaga County, the latter serving as a non-randomized control site where there was initially no Medicare coverage for influenza vaccination.

Vaccination uptake and virological surveillance data were collected from doctors' practices, hospitals and nursing homes, and showed rates of influenza and other viral infections in the community during the study period. The public health department, university medical centre and local physicians coordinated various providers, including public agencies, private providers, hospital outpatient facilities, nursing homes and insurance providers, to develop a variety of methods to increase vaccine uptake in the target group. The new systems included central claims processing (to claim funding through Medicare), vaccine distribution and promotion, and an educational programme for both patients and providers. Other approaches including a financial-target-driven incentive scheme for family doctors were also implemented and evaluated. As a result of the programme, influenza vaccination rates among elderly people aged 65 years of age or over increased from 41 per cent to over 74 per cent in Monroe County compared with an increase from 46 per cent to 57 per cent in Onondaga County. This increase occurred in almost 90,000 Medicare patients over a three-year period. The project subsequently led to annual influenza vaccination being covered by Medicare throughout the United States. The main features of the study are summarized in Figure 13.2.

(Continued)

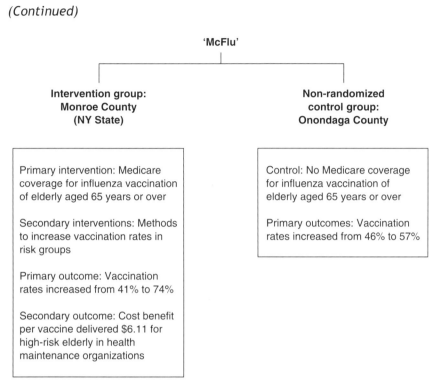

Figure 13.2   *Example of a non-randomized control group study: 'McFlu'*

Source: Adapted from Barker et al. (1999)

THE ADVANTAGES OF NON-RANDOMIZATION

The ethical case

The key advantage of non-randomization is that randomization need not be undertaken in situations where it would not be ethical or acceptable to clients or other stakeholders to do so. Non-randomized studies may also be the only ethical option. For example, in relation to an educational intervention versus no intervention or access to treatment versus no treatment, it can be argued that the educational intervention or the treatment may lead to some positive change and therefore access should not be denied to the control group. In a non-randomized educational intervention study to investigate the effect of introducing decision rules for referral for x-ray in suspected ankle and foot fractures (the so-called Ottawa ankle rules), it was decided that it was inappropriate to have a control group. The results were that reductions in requests for x-ray, waiting times and costs occurred with no increase in missed fractures following an educational programme (Stiell et al. 1995). It can be assumed that, pending further research, this was due to the education effect.

Although it is widely accepted that randomization in trials reduces some types of systematic error that may interfere with the results, it has also been argued that in certain circumstances there may be an advantage in allowing patients' preferences to play a part in determining which arm of a trial they enter even if this leads to some loss in assessing the therapeutic treatment effect. One reason for allowing patient preferences to be taken into account is that some patients may have such strong preferences that they may refuse randomization, leading to selection bias. In studies where there are difficulties in recruiting patients, there may be advantages in following preferences even if this motivation may skew the results.

It could equally be argued that, where it is not possible to disguise which treatment arm patients are in, the results may also be skewed by low motivation. Furthermore, certain interventions require the active engagement of participants – as, for example, where self-monitoring or self-medication is required, where rehabilitation or programmes for de-institutionalization are being assessed, and where behavioural or cognitive treatments for anxiety and depression are being compared with each other, or with treatments using drug medication. In these situations, comparisons may only work if participants have no preferences, which may be an unlikely scenario. One solution to this problem has been to distinguish between patients who have no preferences and apply a randomization method in their case. Thus, a trial with two interventions will have four groups: randomized to A and prefer A; randomized to B and prefer B. An example of this type of study was conducted by Chilvers and colleagues (2001) on the use of antidepressant drugs and generic counselling for the treatment of major depression in primary care.

The evaluation of innovation

Evaluation is most useful where an innovative practice is being introduced in a single or a limited number of sites for an evaluation period or to assess the effect of legislative or policy changes. An example is where non-randomized experimental methods were used to evaluate the impact of introducing an open-access walk-in centre for people needing first-line primary care. The Department of Health favoured the introduction of open-access walk-in clinics to reduce the pressure on Accident and Emergency Departments and general practices introduced this facility in certain localities in England. In order to estimate the effect in one locality, a study using a controlled before and after design was used for an evaluation of an open-access clinic on the use of Accident and Emergency Departments and general practices (Hsu et al. 2003). In another study, this time with a control group, a mental health facilitator was employed in six general practices to train GPs to recognize and treat postnatal depression (Holden et al. 1989). The results were compared with six control practices where there was no facilitator. In this study, there were demonstrable improvements in terms of the identification of mental illness by GPs but not in its management or outcomes.

The methodological challenge of non-randomized control group studies

There are a number of methodological problems with maintaining the comparison between the case and control groups. For instance, sometimes innovations are taken up inconsistently and comparisons can only be made between those that implement change and those that maintain the status quo. An example of this was a non-randomized control group study comparing the effect of prescribing practices of fundholding with non-fundholding general practices (Bradlow and Coulter 1993). In this case, it was only possible to compare practices that took up the initiative with those that did not. It was found that fundholding practices were more likely to remain within their 'indicative' budget, but there may have been other intervening or confounding variables to explain the behaviour.

RANDOMIZED AND NON-RANDOMIZED EXPERIMENTAL DESIGNS COMPARED

It is important for health care researchers to appreciate the advantages and disadvantages of the different types of study design. Large, well-designed and conducted randomized controlled studies ensure that intervention and control groups have a baseline of comparability and that differences in outcomes are therefore due to the intervention alone. Explanations for differences other than the intervention, or confounding factors, should be balanced equally between the intervention and control groups through randomization. Beyond these factors, both types of study have strengths and weaknesses.

The methodological flaws of randomized ontrolled trials

The use of RCTs, despite their 'gold standard' epithet, can be hampered by a number of problems, for example:

- There may be such strong evidence for an intervention that a placebo group may be unethical.
- Randomization may be impossible because clinicians or organizations may advocate strongly one particular approach over another. In this situation, there is a lack of clinical equipoise, without true clinical equivalence between the intervention and control. A strong preference for either effectively prevents random allocation.
- Educational or other interventions when active participation of subjects is required for the intervention to be effective may render randomization inappropriate or impossible.
- Randomized controlled studies may be ruled out on cost terms. They are more complex and costly than non-randomized designs (Black 1996).

RCTs are also subject to a number of possible design flaws. For example, when allocation to groups is not blinded, this can lead to an inflation of effect size. Moreover, participants in RCTs are often atypical and this selection bias can affect outcomes. Only a small proportion of patients with a given condition can be included in a trial, either directly through selection and exclusion criteria, or indirectly through a greater likelihood of inclusion of certain types of patient, such as those attending academic centres. Women, elderly people, children and those with co-morbidities or very severe illness are less likely to be subjects in trials. This tends to increase the treatment effects and to reduce the generalizability of a study. In treatment trials, there is a bias towards the inclusion of people who are less well-off and less well educated, whereas in the case of preventative interventions, participants tend to be healthier, wealthier and better educated. The so-called 'healthy user' bias tends to increase effect size on proxy outcomes because of better compliance, but conversely to reduce effect sizes on true outcomes because of a ceiling effect as better baseline measures have less capacity to improve.

Other types of experimental study can suffer from similar problems but usually tend to be less restrictive in terms of inclusion and exclusion criteria and therefore exhibit better external validity and generalizability. There is also no evidence that non-randomized studies have greater effect sizes than RCTs. The potential for subjects, whether individuals or organizations, to benefit from an intervention, and their similarity to the reference population of subjects, is for this reason more critical to the internal and external validity of an experimental study (Britton et al. 1998). Laboratory methods often involve experimental methods too. However, these involve a variety of methods of investigation and analysis that are outside the scope of this chapter.

Phases in the design process

In practice, a combination of methods may be used in a research project as part of the overall design. The Medical Research Council framework for the design and evaluation of complex interventions is often used as the basis for the development of designs that may eventually lead to the classic RCT (Medical Research Council 2000). In this framework, a phased approach involving pre-clinical (theoretical) modelling in Phase I, and an exploratory study or studies in Phase II, is the suggested approach before undertaking a definitive trial in Phase III. These initial phases could involve a qualitative study such as a case study or interviews, a before and after experimental study or a combination of these.

Case study: Introducing an influenza and pneumococcal vaccination procedure in a general practice setting

Such an approach was taken in a series of studies to develop a trial of an educational intervention to implement an influenza and pneumococcal vaccination procedure in a general practice setting (Siriwardena et al. 2002). In the pre-clinical phase, evidence was obtained from the literature review that these interventions might be effective. A pilot study formed the modelling phase. This used an action research methodology in a single general practice to establish the components of the intervention, how it could be managed and the possible barriers to change (Siriwardena 1999).

The main findings and experience gained from the pilot phase were applied to two further uncontrolled before and after studies. Initially, two multipractice audits using an uncontrolled before and after design were undertaken to investigate the feasibility of improving influenza and pneumococcal vaccination rates across a range of general practices using audit, feedback and written guidance. These tested outcome measures helped to define the control intervention, and allowed an estimate to be made of the effect size. This was later used for a power calculation in the subsequent RCT. The first multipractice audit was conducted in volunteer practices as part of a county-wide initiative.

The results are set out in Table 13.2 (for a fuller account see Siriwardena et al. 2003a). Mean values for vaccination uptake are shown for the two phases of the audit for practices that completed the audit cycle. Performance was compared with standards that practices set themselves (expressed as median standards set for each phase). Fourteen practices undertook both phases of the audit for coronary heart disease and splenectomy and 21 practices did so for diabetes. Improvements in vaccination uptake occurred in coronary heart disease, diabetic and post-splenectomy patients for both vaccinations. There were

(Continued)

Table 13.2 *Improvements in influenza and pneumococcal vaccination uptake*

Vaccine and risk group (number of practices)	Vaccination uptake		Median standard (Phase 1, Phase 2)	Mean improvement (95% CI)	Significance (p-value, two-tailed t-test)
	Phase 1 (%)	Phase 2 (%)			
Influenza vaccine uptake in CHD (n = 14)	63.6	74.4	80, 80	10.8 (5.3 to 16.1)	0.001
Pneumococcal vaccine uptake in CHD (n = 14)	31.1	58.6	68, 75	27.5 (13.6 to 42.3)	0.002
Influenza vaccine uptake in diabetes (n = 21)	62.1	70.6	80, 80	8.6 (1.5 to 15.7)	0.02
Pneumococcal vaccine uptake in diabetes (n = 21)	35.2	64.0	75, 80	28.8 (17.2 to 40.3)	<0.001
Influenza vaccine uptake for splenectomy patients (n = 14)	66.1	83.4	90, 100	17.3 (4.8 to 29.8)	0.01
Pneumococcal vaccine uptake for splenectomy patients (n = 14)	79.6	95.6	95, 100	15.9 (1.8 to 30.1)	0.03

Source: Siriwardena et al. (2003a)

a number of sources of potential bias. It was likely that those practices that did take part were more motivated to change (volunteer bias). Although those practices that took part comprised rural, suburban and inner city practices, including those serving areas of deprivation, it was possible that non-participating practices may have differed in terms of deprivation or case mix where the need for immunization may have been greater. The method could not account for secular trends or the Hawthorne effect. One could only conclude that the study demonstrated the capability and extent to which participating practices were able to improve performance with the aid of audit, feedback and written guidance rather than suppose that these interventions were the sole reason for the increase in vaccination rates.

The methodology was refined and applied to a multipractice audit undertaken as part of a clinical governance programme in a large primary health care oraganization (Siriwardena et al. 2003b). These preliminary investigations prepared the way for a cluster randomized study that included an educational outreach intervention for primary health care teams to use multiple methods to improve influenza and pneumococca; vaccination take-up (Siriwardena et al. 2002).

CONCLUSION

In this chapter it has been shown why and how experimental designs in health research extend beyond traditional RCTs. A number of pre-experimental, quasi-experimental and experimental designs have important potential applications for assessing and evaluating health technologies, interventions and services and for modelling prior to conducting RCTs, particularly where complex interventions are planned. These designs have been illustrated in this chapter, in a manner which attests to their value as a research method, notwithstanding their limitations as described. An exercise is now set out for the reader to complete in which experimental methods are applied to the ambulance service.

Exercise: Experimental methods and the ambulance service

In the United Kingdom Healthcare Commission Report in 2004 on ambulance services a majority of patients (four out of five) said they had suffered pain from their presenting condition while in the ambulance. Although 81 per cent

(Continued)

(Continued)

felt that the ambulance crew did everything they could to control pain, one in five wanted more pain relief; 14 per cent said the crew did this to some extent and 5 per cent said that the crew did not do everything they could to control their pain.

As a result of this report you are asked to design and implement a quality improvement process for improving the assessment and control of pain in an ambulance service in which you are working. Pain control is assessed in adults (aged 16 and over) using a verbal pain rating scale from 0 (no pain) to 10 (the most severe pain) and should be recorded for all patients. The trust's board is keen to see improvements across the service and both you and they consider a randomized controlled study to be neither ethical nor feasible.

In your report address the following questions:

1 Which patients or patient groups would you study in relation to pain? Who would you exclude, and why?
2 What outcome measures could you use for your evaluation?
3 What methods could you use to improve pain control and why?
4 Consider which other experimental methods could be used in this situation. Which of these would you prefer to use and why?
5 Where would you find a control group for your study?
6 Describe any sources of bias and confounding factors in your preferred study. How might you address these?

RECOMMENDED FURTHER READING

Shadish, W.R., Cook, T.D. and Campbell, D.T. (2002) *Experimental and Quasi-experimental Designs for Generalized Causal Inference*. Boston, MA: Houghton-Mifflin.
This is an updated version of a classic text, in which experts in the field of quasi-experimentation discuss in comprehensive fashion key issues relating to the theory and practice of experimental and quasi-experimental designs.

Trochim, W.M. *Research Methods Knowledge Base*, 2nd edition. Available at: http://www.socialresearchmethods.net/kb/
This excellent site provides a very readable and accessible account of quasi-experimental methods, written by an expert in quasi-experimental research methods.

Ukoumunne, O.C., Gulliford, M.C., Chinn, S., Sterne, J.A.C. and Burney, P.G.J. (1999) 'Methods for evaluating area-wide and organisation-based interventions in health and healthcare: a systematic review', *Health Technology Assessment*, 3 (5): 9.

This report is a systematic review of methods for cluster-based interventions and evaluations covering issues of design and analysis of complex organizational-level interventions and including key recommendations for those employing non-randomized approaches.

REFERENCES

Allwright, S., Paul, G., Greiner, B., Mullally, B.J., Pursell, L., Kelly, A., Bonner, B., D'Eath, M., McConnell, B., McLaughlin, J.P., O'Donovan, D., O'Kane, E. and Perry, I.J. (2005) 'Legislation for smoke-free workplaces and health of bar workers in Ireland: before and after study', *British Medical Journal*, 331: 1117.

Barker, W.H., Bennett, N.M., LaForce, F.M., Waltz, E.C. and Weiner, L.B. (1999) 'McFlu. The Monroe County, New York, Medicare vaccine demonstration', *American Journal of Preventive Medicine*, 16 (3): 118–27.

Black, N. (1996) 'Why we need observational studies to evaluate the effectiveness of health care', *British Medical Journal*, 312: 1215–18.

Blenkiron, P. (2001) 'Coping with depression: a pilot study to assess the efficacy of a self-help audio cassette', *British Journal of General Practice*, 51: 366–70.

Bradlow, J. and Coulter, A. (1993) 'Effect of fundholding and indicative prescribing schemes on general practitioners' prescribing costs', *British Medical Journal*, 307: 1186–89.

Britton, A., McKee, M., Black, N., McPherson, K., Sanderson, C. and Bain, C. (1998) 'Choosing between randomised and non-randomised studies: a systematic review', *Health Technology Assessment*, 2 (13): 3.

Campbell, D.T. and Stanley, J.C. (1963) *Experimental and Quasi-Experimental Designs for Research*. Chicago: Rand McNally College Publishing.

Chilvers, C., Dewey, M., Fielding, K., Gretton, V., Miller, P., Palmer, B., Weller, D., Churchill, R., Williams, I., Bedi, N., Duggan, C., Lee, A. and Harrison, G. (2001) 'Antidepressant drugs and generic counselling for treatment of major depression in primary care: randomized trial with patient preference arms', *British Medical Journal*, 322: 772–75.

Cook, T.D. and Campbell, D.T. (1979) *Quasi-experimentation. Design and Analysis Issues for Field Settings*. Chicago: Rand McNally College Publishing.

Dixon, H., Blow, C., Irish, W., Milne, P. and Siriwardena, A.N. (2007) 'Evaluation of a postgraduate examination for primary care: perceptions and performance of general practitioner trainers in the multiple choice paper of the Membership Examination of the Royal College of General Practitioneers', *Education for Primary Care* (in press).

Grimshaw, J.M., Shirran, L., Thomas, R., Mowatt, G., Fraser, C., Bero, L., Grilli, R., Harvey, E., Oxman, A. and O'Brien, M.A. (2001) 'Changing provider behavior: an overview of systematic reviews of interventions', *Medical Care*, 39 (8): 112–45.

Hannaford, P.C., Thompson, C. and Simpson, M. (1996) 'Evaluation of an educational programme to improve the recognition of psychological illness by general practitioners', *British Journal of General Practice*, 46: 333–37.

Hannay, D., Usherwood, T. and Platts, M. (1992) 'Workload of general practitioners before and after the new contract', *British Medical Journal*, 304: 615–18.

Hawton, K., Simkin, S., Deeks, J.J., O'Connor, S., Keen, A., Altman, D.G., Philo, G. and Bulstrode, C. (1999) 'Effects of a drug overdose in a television drama on presentations to hospital for self poisoning: time series and questionnaire study', *British Medical Journal*, 318: 972–77.

Hawton, K., Simkin, S., Deeks, J., Cooper, J., Johnston, A., Waters, K., Arundel, M., Bernal, W., Gunson, B., Hudson, M., Suri, D. and Simpson, K. (2004) 'UK legislation on analgesic packs: before and after study of long term effect on poisonings', *British Medical Journal*, 329: 1076.

Holden, J.M., Sagovsky, R. and Cox, J.L. (1989) 'Counselling in a general practice setting: controlled study of health visitor intervention in treatment of postnatal depression', *British Medical Journal*, 298: 223–26.

Hsu, R.T., Lambert, P.C., Woods, M. and Kurinczuk, J.J. (2003) 'Effect of NHS walk-in centre on local primary healthcare services: before and after observational study', *British Medical Journal*, 326: 530.

Medical Research Council (2000) *A Framework for Development and Evaluation of RCTs for Complex Interventions to Improve Health*. London: MRC.

Robson, C. (1973) *Design and Statistics in Psychology*. Harmondsworth: Penguin.

Sheldon, T.A., Cullum, N., Dawson, D., Lankshear, A., Lowson, K., Watt, I., West, P., Wright, D. and Wright, J. (2004) 'What's the evidence that NICE guidance has been implemented? Results from a national evaluation using time series analysis, audit of patients' notes, and interviews', *British Medical Journal*, 329: 999.

Siriwardena, A.N. (1999) 'Targeting pneumococcal vaccination to high-risk groups: a feasibility study in one general practice', *Postgraduate Medical Journal*, 75: 208–12.

Siriwardena, A.N., Rashid, A., Johnson, M.R.D. and Dewey, M.E. (2002) 'Cluster randomised controlled trial of an educational outreach visit to improve influenza and pneumococcal immunisation rates in primary care', *British Journal of General Practice*, 52: 735–40.

Siriwardena, A.N., Hazelwood, L., Wilburn, T., Johnson, M.R.D. and Rashid, A. (2003a) 'Improving influenza and pneumococcal vaccination uptake in high risk groups in Lincolnshire: a quality improvement report from a large rural county', *Quality in Primary Care*, 11 (1): 19–28.

Siriwardena, A.N., Wilburn, T. and Hazelwood, L. (2003b) 'Increasing influenza and pneumococcal vaccination rates in high risk groups in one primary care trust', *Clinical Governance: An International Journal*, 8 (3): 200–207.

Stiell, I., Wells, G., Laupacis, A., Brison, R., Verbeek, R., Vandemheen, K. and Naylor, C.D. (1995) 'Multicentre trial to introduce the Ottawa ankle rules for use of radiography in acute ankle injuries. Multicentre Ankle Rule Study Group', *British Medical Journal*, 311: 594–97.

Ukoumunne, O.C., Gulliford, M.C., Chinn, S., Sterne, J.A.C. and Burney, P.G.J. (1999) 'Methods for evaluating area-wide and organisation-based interventions in health and healthcare: a systematic review', *Health Technology Assessment*, 3 (5): 9.

Wensing, M., van der Weijden, T. and Grol, R. (1998) 'Implementing guidelines and innovations in general practice: which interventions are effective?', *British Journal of General Practice*, 48: 991–97.

14

The Use of Economics in Health Research

ALAN MAYNARD

INTRODUCTION

All societies face the twin problems of the inevitability of death and the scarcity of resources. These problems impose difficult choices on decision makers whether they are prime ministers, nurses, doctors or patients. Every choice has an opportunity cost: a value forgone. A decision to use the drug Herceptin to treat primary breast cancers consumes scarce resources that could be used to replace diseased and painful hips or treat patients with Alzheimer's disease. Every diagnostic or treatment choice made by a doctor or nurse uses resources and deprives other patients of care from which they could benefit. The scarcity of resources makes rationing in health care inevitable. The issue is what principles should determine who will receive care and who will be deprived of care and be left in avoidable pain and discomfort, and perhaps to die? The policy issue is not whether to ration but how to do so. A number of economic techniques have been used to develop principles and to evaluate the costs and benefits of different treatments. In this chapter, the rationale for economic evaluation is considered; the techniques for economic evaluation to prioritize treatments described and their limitations discussed; the different types of economic evaluation are outlined; and a case study is provided to illustrate the process in practice.

THE RATIONALE FOR ECONOMIC EVALUATION

In the NHS and the other publicly funded health care systems around the world, society has rejected the use of the price mechanism and the willingness and ability of people to pay as the means by which access to health care is determined. In these systems the dominant access criterion is 'need' but this concept has to be defined carefully.

Rationing access to health care in the face of scarcity involves depriving some patients of care from which they could benefit and they wish to have. Given that the demand for care usually exceeds supply, some argue that we should deliver those interventions that 'work', but this raises another definitional problem – how should this clinical effectiveness be defined? For instance, with a hip replacement, the major benefits are the removal of pain and improved mobility. With some cancer care, the focus of doctors is on survival rates of perhaps months or years, often with little attention being paid to the quality of life during this period. Identifying and agreeing the 'end point', that is what outcomes should be evaluated and how should they be measured in clinical trials, is never easy and makes economic evaluation challenging as we will see later.

DILEMMAS OF ECONOMIC ASSESSMENT

However, the crucial issue at this juncture is whether determining clinical effectiveness, as the criterion for access to care, is necessary and sufficient. The economic argument is that clinical effectiveness is a *necessary* characteristic for rationing access to care but is not *sufficient*. As argued in Maynard (1997), what is clinically effective may not be cost effective and what is cost effective is always clinically effective. Economists have developed a measure for clinical effectiveness in terms of the number of Quality Adjusted Life Years (QALYs) that can be expected from a particular treatment (Williams 1985). All these words require definition but put briefly, a QALY is one added year of perfect health. This measure must be set against the costs of treatment to assess clinical cost-effectiveness. QALYs provide the basis for comparing one treatment with another as described in the example in Box 14.1.

Box 14.1   *An example of the dilemmas of economic assessment*

Let us assume that there is a limited budget of £70,000 and that the costs of the alternative procedures, X and Y, for the particular disease that you will treat are known. Furthermore let us assume that the benefits of each procedure are known and measured in QALYs, where a QALY is one year of perfect health.

If therapy X produces 5 QALYs and therapy Y produces 10 QALYs, on the basis of clinical effectiveness, Y is superior and will be preferred by the patient and their physician who, motivated by the individualistic Hippocratic Oath, wishes to do the best for the patient.

But what if therapy X costs £1,500 and therapy Y costs £7,000? Therapy X produces a QALY at an average cost of £300, while therapy Y produces a QALY for £700. Therapy Y produces an additional 5 QALYs for an additional cost of £5,500 (£7,000 minus £1,500). The marginal cost of producing a QALY using Y is £1,100 (£5,500 divided by 5).

Therapy X is superior in terms of cost-effectiveness as it produces health QALYs at least cost, while therapy Y is clinically superior as it produces more QALYs. From the individualistic perspective of the patient and their agent, the doctor, therapy Y is preferred. However, from the social perspective of the economist and public health physician, therapy X is preferred as it produces the greatest health gain from a fixed budget. Thus, if a clinic had a fixed budget of £70,000, using therapy Y it would produce 100 QALYs of health gain, but if it uses therapy X it will produce more than twice as many QALYs.

This example highlights that society's goal is to get the maximum health gain from its finite health care budget. Indeed, the necessary and sufficient condition for resource allocation and determining access to health care is the *relative* cost-effectiveness of competing interventions. Those interventions that are cost effective give the 'biggest health care bang for the NHS buck'. Decision makers in the National Institute for Clinical Effectiveness (NICE) use this criterion to determine access to the new technologies they evaluate (www.nice.gov.uk). Internationally, this approach is gradually challenging and eroding the narrow clinical perspective and the individualistic ethic reflected in the Hippocratic Oath.

While the techniques of economic evaluation are increasingly used to prioritize interventions competing for funding in the NHS, the actual practice of both clinical and economic evaluation could be said to be flawed as many studies are inadequately designed. Despite this, studies with basic methodological and design faults are often reported and published in highly prestigious journals (Freemantle and Maynard 1994). Consequently, it is important for practitioners of the 'dark arts' of economic evaluation and the patients and carers who use services to be able to deconstruct and appraise studies using QALYs. To facilitate this, there are checklists of good practice and these provide a useful way of elaborating the component parts of an economic evaluation. An economic evaluation checklist developed by Williams (1976) and given in Box 14.2 is a very pragmatic, but provides an extremely useful start from which to explore any study.

Box 14.2 *Economic evaluation checklist*

Checklist for economic evaluations of costs and benefits of treatments

- What precisely is the question which the study was trying to answer?
- What is the question that it has actually answered?
- What are the assumed objectives of the activity studied?
- By what measures are these represented?
- How are they weighted?
- Do they enable us to tell whether the objectives are being attained?
- What range of options was considered?
- What other options might there have been?
- Were they rejected, or not considered, for good reasons?
- Would their inclusion have been likely to change the results?
- Is anyone likely to be affected who has not been considered in the analysis?
- If so, why are they excluded?
- Does the cost go wider or deeper than the expenditure of the agency concerned?
- If not, is it clear that these expenditures cover all the resources used and accurately represent their value if released for other uses?
- If so, is the line drawn so as to include all potential beneficiaries and losers and are resources costed at their value in their best alternative use?
- Is the differential timing of the items in the streams of benefits and costs suitably taken care of (for example, by discounting, and, if so, at what rate)?
- Where there is uncertainty, or there are known margins of error, is it made clear how sensitive the outcome is to these elements?
- Are the results, on balance, good enough for the job in hand?
- Has anyone else done better?

Source: Williams (1976)

Over the three decades since the Williams questions were posed, guidelines have been refined and differentiated by a range of authors – for example, by Maynard (1990), Drummond and the British Medical Journal Economic Evaluation Working Party (1996) and Drummond et al. (2005).

The list in the box can be divided into a number of categories that raise particular questions and are elaborated below.

Technical questions

What is the role of the particular service or treatment intervention and what would be the consequence of doing nothing? In all evaluations, the option of 'doing nothing' may be the one that is most cost effective!

What is the comparator? Any new service has to be compared with an alternative. The study description should not only define the alternatives being compared but also explain the choice of alternatives. Sometimes in drug evaluations a placebo, or dummy drug, is used. This is usually insufficient as we need to know not just whether the new treatment has an effect compared with using a dummy tablet, but whether it is better than the accepted 'best available' treatment being used now. Whatever the alternative selected, its selection should be explicit and explained.

Identifying costs

Are all the costs of the new service or treatment identified, measured and valued? The range of costs that are evaluated has to be clearly stated and defended. These should include operating or current costs, as well as capital costs. There should also be consideration of system costs (for example, the opportunity cost of resources denied to others) and the costs to patients (for instance, travel time costs) and other agencies such as local authority social services.

Identifying benefits

Are all the benefits identified, measured and valued? There are a number of important issues to be considered here: in particular the nature of the clinical trial method; the measurement of the 'end point' or benefit; and the valuation of the benefit or end point.

First, the randomized controlled trial is generally regarded as the best way of measuring clinical effectiveness. The Cochrane Collaboration (www.cochrane.org) is an international collaboration that has established good practice in the evaluation of 'what works' in clinical practice and is discussed further in relation to involving consumers in Chapter 19. Its website and related ones such as the National Electronic Library for Health (www.nelh.nhs.uk) and the NHS Centre for Reviews and Dissemination Database of Abstracts of Reviews of Effects (www.york.ac.uk/darefaq.htm) provide a starting place for identifying previous work, showing not only what works but also what is in use but unproven. The Cochrane criteria of validity and robustness should be used to guide you through these minefields. This is facilitated by systematic reviews that collect data from trials and then filter out those of poor quality to give an unbiased view of what works (NHS Centre for Reviews and Dissemination 2001).

Second, any review of a clinical area will immediately highlight the issue of the selection of the end point or benefit from trial interventions. The health economist prefers to use direct evidence of improvement in the length and quality of life. However, trials often use intermediate or incomplete 'end points'. For instance, in cancer the principle focus is often on survival or additional months or years of life, with the quality of survival being ignored. An end point such as myocardial infarctions (heart attacks) avoided begs the question of how long survival is enhanced and with what quality of life. Economic evaluations build on the clinical evidence base. If practitioners are not cautious, their work can be undermined by poor practice in clinical trials.

The final complex issue in outcome measurement and evaluation is the assignment of preferences and the valuation given to them. Ideally, we would like a benefit indicator that incorporates increased length and quality of life in a composite measure. However, patients themselves experience many health attributes including things such as physical and mental functioning and pain. Such attributes of the health effects of interventions can be explored by generic quality of life measures using, for example, Short Form 36. This asks patients to self-assess their health state before and after treatment. Whilst SF-36 can provide a patient profile of quality of life over time, it provides no insight into how a particular patient would trade off different health attributes. Consequently, for economic evaluations, efforts are made to measure the utility or value of particular combinations of health outcomes.

This is done using either 'the standard gamble' or 'time trade-off' approach. The former is regarded as the best option and involves an individual being asked to choose between the certainty of one health state and a gamble between the probability (p) of surviving for the same period with no disability or a probability $(1 - p)$ of immediate death. The value of p is changed until the individual is indifferent between the certain option and the gamble. This probability measure defines the utility for that particular person of the health state being considered, on a scale of 0 (death) to 1 (perfect health). The method and the simpler alternative, the time trade-off approach, are detailed in texts such as Drummond et al. (2005).

This preference-based, multi-attribute, health status measurement is epitomized by the EQ5D (EuroQoL Group 1991). EQ5D has five dimensions (mobility, self-care, usual activities, pain/discomfort and anxiety/depression – see www.euroqol.org). The scores from EQ5D can be used as a 'weighted health index' that gives a numerical value for quality of life in a given health state. Such scores can be used in the calculation of QALYs, which are discussed below in the cost–utility evaluation section of this chapter. (See also for further explanation Drummond et al. 2005; Jefferson et al. 2000.)

The timing of costs and benefits

In terms of health benefits, an investment now may produce health benefits over decades. An example is that if you are persuaded to stop smoking, this will add years to your life and quality to those years in the future as you avoid premature heart disease, cancer and other ailments. For an individual, the treatment of hypertension involves costs for the rest of that person's life. So the question can be asked, what is the opportunity cost of a pound spent now compared with a pound spent in 10 years' time on this treatment? In these cases it is expected that you will prefer gain now and loss in the future. To cope with the time preferences of individuals and of a society, streams of benefits and costs are adjusted in a process called discounting. Good economic evaluations should include this process (Drummond and the British Medical Journal Economic Evaluation Working Party 1995).

Sensitivity analysis

Inevitably there will be uncertainty about both the estimated stream of benefits and costs. A good study will carry out sensitivity analysis and this will involve, for instance, re-estimating the results if costs are 5 and 10 per cent higher and benefits are 5 and 10 per cent less. Sensitivity analysis using such variations in assumptions tests the robustness of the results in a world where the estimates of clinical effectiveness and cost-effectiveness are inevitably somewhat imprecise.

Decision analysis

Increasingly, the uncertainty surrounding cost and benefit data is leading to the use of decision analysis. Decision analysis is a clearly defined, systematic approach to decision making when there is uncertainty. Uncertainty is common in medicine as diagnostic tests may generate false positives and false negatives. Patients vary, treatments are never certain in their effects and may generate differing side effects. Furthermore, the costs of treatments alter over time. Such uncertainty can be dealt with by quantifying it in terms of probabilities. For example, if an antibiotic has a 0.80 probability of removing a bacterial infection, there is a 0.20 probability that it will not. In this case, probability represents the strength of the belief an individual has, as a result of their knowledge and experience. Thus, data from clinical trails can be supplemented or even supplanted by eliciting expert opinions. Decision trees can be constructed that make the alternative costs and benefits explicit and assign probabilities to them. A checklist for such analysis has been published in Philips et al. (2004) and this approach is also discussed in Drummond et al. (2005).

When scrutinizing economic evaluations the issues discussed above need to be studied with care. While such checklists have been available for three decades, practice continues to fall short. Studies to evaluate the costs and benefits of particular treatments continue to fall short in terms or rigour and quality. The aim of research studies should be to inform the clinical evidence base in an unbiased fashion.

TYPES OF ECONOMIC EVALUATION

The terms 'economic evaluation' and 'cost–benefit analysis' can be confusing if they are used loosely and without precision. In effect, there are several types of economic evaluation, of which the cost–benefit analysis discussed so far is just one. The following five types of economic evaluation can be found in the literature and are explored further below:

- Costing studies
- Cost minimization analysis
- Cost-effective analysis
- Cost and utility analysis
- Cost benefit analysis.

Costing studies

The first study type listed is costing studies (CS). These are common but are not economic evaluations, as alternatives are not compared. They are useless for deciding on how to invest resources in competing interventions in the health care sector. However, they are common because they are used by, for instance, the pharmaceutical industry, to draw attention to the costs of a disease. CS are used for marketing by the sponsoring company just about to launch a product. Such studies tell us that, for example, diabetes costs many billions and heart disease even more.

Such disease costings reveal nothing about how a disease can be treated efficiently with treatments that minimize costs and maximize benefits. They are discussed here to emphasize that they are not a form of economic evaluation as there is no comparison of alternative interventions, but are common elements of the marketing armoury of commercial companies seeking NHS funding.

Cost minimization analysis

Cost minimization analysis (CMA) involves the identification, measurement and valuation of the costs of the competing therapies. In such a study it is assumed that the outcome of the alternatives is identical. Thus the focus of the analysis is partial. It seeks to identify which of two alternatives is cheapest.

One of the early examples of the CMA approach was an analysis of alternative methods for treating varicose veins. Piachaud and Weddell (1972) identified two interventions: surgery and injection–compression therapy in an outpatient clinic. They measured the costs of health service resource use and the individual costs to patients in terms of time and costs of entering treatment. The authors also examined the wage cost losses of those treated but made no attempt to value unpaid activity such as the services of carers.

The study was based on a randomized clinical trial that showed that after three years of follow-up the results for patients under 60 were equally good. The authors concluded that as the cost of injection was less than a third of surgery, and the loss of earnings was much less than in the non-surgical arm of the trial, injection therapy was to be preferred as it was less costly.

However, subsequent follow-up of the patients in the trial showed that at five years the assumption of equivalence of outcome was valid only for patients aged less than 35 in whom there were no signs of venous insufficiency. For the majority of patients, the outcomes of surgery were superior and thus decision makers faced the choice of whether to fund an intervention that was more expensive but gave better results.

Cost-effectiveness analysis

Cost-effectiveness analysis (CEA) is an approach devised by the United States military during the Korean War. Their problem was to identify the cheapest way of killing enemy soldiers. For instance, what were the relative costs of bombing the enemy, napalming them, using tanks and using infantry, and how successful were these methods as measured by 'body count'?

This grim example demonstrates the essence of CEA. The method involves the costing of the alternatives and the use of an intervention specific measure of success. In health care where our interest is in improving the length and quality of patients' lives, the CEA approach involves costing the alternatives and using outcome measures such as reductions in blood pressure or lives saved.

It is obvious that CEA has a particular use. It can identify which alternative intervention in a particular clinical area is the best. However, CEA does not enable us to make evaluative comparisons across specialities. The measurement of reductions in blood pressure provides information about whether drugs, exercise and diet alone, or in combination, have a beneficial effect and hence reduce the risk of heart attack and stroke. Using dialysis or transplantation to treat chronic renal failure produces additional years of life. However, these two areas of study do not inform us as to which, treating renal failure or reducing blood pressure, is the better area for investment.

A good example of the use of CEA addresses the issue of treating chronic renal failure with hospital dialysis, or transplantation (Klarman et al. 1968). This study was incomplete in some aspects. In analyzing the mix of treatments, such as dialysis before transplant (which is usual) and hospital dialysis before home dialysis (which is community based and used to train recipients for home treatment), the study showed that transplantation is the cheapest way of producing additional years of life for such patients. This option also produces the best quality of life for survivors. The great problem is insufficient supply of spare parts available to meet patient demand.

Cost utility analysis

The absence of a generic benefit measure that informs choices between interventions between therapeutic areas in CEA has led to the development of cost utility analysis (CUA). Initially devised by the United States Office of Technology Assessment in the late 1970s, it was developed in the United Kingdom by Williams (1985) and now is a core element in the appraisal process for new technologies used by NICE. The goal of CUA is to identify the cost of producing an additional unit of benefit, the QALY. A QALY combines estimated increases in survival with health status valuations using quality of life measures such as EQ5D. One QALY is one year of perfect health and because it is measured on an interval scale, two half QALYs can be summed to one QALY.

Thus, if treatment A for hypertension is valued at 0.85 QALYs and treatment B is valued at 0.60 QALYs, the incremental difference in utility is 0.25 QALYs or 250 QALYs per 1,000 patients per year.

In using QALYs a major issue is whose valuation of quality of life should be used? Doctors and nurses are better informed about health states and interventions. However, patients are informed about the health states they experience, but not about those that they have not experienced. Typically patients rate health states higher than health care professionals. An alternative source of evaluation is the wider society, which mixes informed and uninformed views, and typically gives values lower than patients.

There continues to be considerable argument about the validity of QALY estimates. Typical challenges include: Do they really measure what they claim to measure? Are they reliable (that is, reproducible and consistent)? Are they sensitive to small health state changes? Are they stable over time and independent of the duration of time in a health state? One pragmatic response of QALY adherents is that they may be imperfect, but they are the best approach available.

Cost benefit analysis

Cost benefit analysis (CBA) involves the identification, measurement and valuing of both the monetary costs of each alternative treatment considered in an evaluation and the monetary value of the benefits. This is an ambitious enterprise requiring the analyst to elicit values as regards how much is given up (the opportunity cost) and how much is gained (that is, the value of reduced pain and increased length and quality of life).

Translating the stream of benefits from any intervention into monetary equivalents is done by contingent valuation (CV) or willingness to pay (WTP) studies whose purpose is to elicit a monetary valuation for common or societal goods, such as pollution and services, for example control by the patient over their symptoms. These goods are not traded in markets. CV seeks measures to value all health factors such as the length and quality of life outcomes, and non-health factors such as privacy and politeness in the treatment process.

This type of study involves investigating how much individuals are willing to pay to avoid ill-health or to improve their health. For instance, let us assume that you are in pain. There are two treatments: drug X and drug Y. You are informed that drugs X and Y are equally effective in controlling your pain. However, drug X gives 1 patient in 100 stomach bleeds, while drug Y gives bleeds to 3 in 100 patients. How much would you be willing to pay, to get drug X? How much will you pay to reduce the risk of a stomach bleed from 3 to 1 per cent?

This approach is burgeoning in both health economics and environmental economics. However, it poses some difficulties. For instance, there is evidence that the method used to elicit valuations affects the values given. There is also a risk that respondents may state high values for their preferred alternative as in the NHS they do not actually have to pay. The principal concern about this method is that the values are hypothetical. Despite these concerns, work in this field progresses with practitioners seeking to devise methods to test for bias.

Case study: Coronary artery bypass grafting: overview of types of economic evaluation

Conjoint analysis (willingness to pay) studies, cost-effectiveness work and cost utility analyses increasingly fill not only the pages of specialist health economics journals (such as *Health Economics*), but also medical journals. Clinicians increasingly recognize that the development and use of new technologies is not now determined on the basis of clinical effectiveness alone, but also on economic efficiency. In reviewing data or carrying out your own studies, it is important to adopt the appropriate approach for the task in hand and to use a checklist to ensure that the design of the study is robust and comprehensive. This will now be explored through questions raised about coronary artery bypass grafting, as set out in Box 14.3.

Box 14.3 *Coronary artery bypass grafting*

Questions relating to coronary artery bypass grafting

Should the number of coronary artery bypass grafting interventions be increased, decreased or maintained at the current level?
Elaborating on this:

- Which groups gain least and most per unit of cost from this procedure?
- Which groups gain more per unit cost from related cardiac procedures such as pacemaker insertion, transplantation, angioplasty and valve insertion?
- Which groups gain more per unit of cost from other procedures outside heart disease (for instance, renal dialysis and transplantation)?

Source: Williams (1985)

(Continued)

CASE STUDY

(Continued)

In this respect, the following comments may be made:

The author, Williams (1985), took the Rosser matrix valuations of different combinations of health state, in particular disability and distress, where 1 was healthy and 0 was dead (Rosser et al. 1982). At the time there was no clinical data that gave information on quality of life, so Williams used (only) three cardiologists to give him their judgements on the health profiles of patients with angina who had or did not have coronary artery bypass grafting (CABG). With this information the author derived Figure 14.1, which gives the expected length and quality of life gained for patients with severe angina and left main vessel disease. The judgement was that, for 67 per cent of patients with CABG, it would give considerable health gains, whilst 30 per cent would get no advantage and 3 per cent would die. The author derived different results for patients with differing levels of angina and disease spread and location. The benefits were discounted at 5 per cent.

The author also used available cost data from the Department of Health and international data to adjust the figures. Costs were also discounted at 5 per cent. A range of results was computed. For instance, the cost per QALY from treating a patient with severe angina and left main vessel disease was just over £1,000 in 1985 prices, whereas a pacemaker for atrioventricular heart cost produced a QALY for £700. A heart transplant and a kidney transplant were estimated as producing a QALY for £5,000 and £3,000 respectively.

This is shown in Figure 14.1 where quality of life based on the Rosser values is indicated on the vertical axis and the duration of survival is shown on the horizontal axis. Three curves on this quality–duration of life space depict three outcomes: the outcome with CABG, the outcome with medical management of angina, and the operative mortality rate. The gain from the CABG is the difference between the first and second curves, minus the area under the curve reflecting the mortality outcome.

The valuation of benefits has developed substantially since this study with the development of generic quality of life measures such as EQ5D. It is instruments such as this that are now required in technology appraisals by regulatory agencies such as NICE. The study was a major development as it switched attention away from benefit measurement merely in terms of survival, and towards quality of survival, which is a major attribute of CABG. The valuation of costs has improved, but further development is needed. NHS data are improving but remain crude and the creation of private cost data remains challenging.

The use of ranked cost–QALY data in 'league tables' that rank technologies has been criticized because, *inter alia*, such estimates have

(Continued)

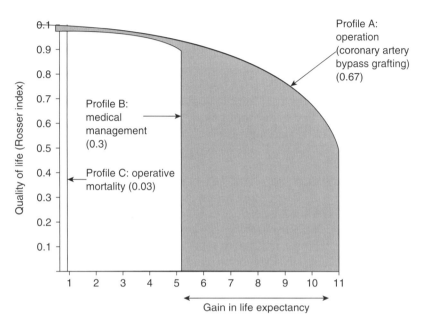

Figure 14.1 *Severe angina and left main vessel disease*

Source: Williams (1985) Reproduced with permission from BMJ
Publishing Group

been developed using differing methods (Maynard 1991). This approach
illustrates how increasingly the relative ranking of technologies can
determine regulatory sanction or rejection (see Maynard et al. 2004).

Typically, the system of ranking reflects the CUA characteristics of the
technology — that is, their costs and benefits in terms of QALYs. Some argue
that the value of a QALY for different groups might be weighted to reflect
equity concerns: for example, whether an additional QALY for a poor recip-
ient as opposed to a rich one is of greater value to a society interested in
decreasing health inequalities. Williams (1997) proposed the concept of a
'fair innings' whereby elderly citizens could give up use of efficient interventions to fund the inefficient treatment of young people who would
otherwise die prematurely after a short life span. Technology assessments
typically do not use weights based on social class or age, but there
continues to be a vigorous academic debate about such issues.

CONCLUSION

The influence of economic evaluations has grown considerably in recent decades due to the influence of Alan Williams and his students such as Michael Drummond. This has been the product of increasing recognition that the rationing of health care should not be based on the advocacy of those who shout loudest, but on the evidence base about clinical and cost effectiveness. The battle continues with patients often urgently seeking potentially life-saving care and their clinicians anxious to provide such care, but with the NHS having to assign priority between competing medical interventions and patients.

Economic evaluation techniques offer an explicit framework into which evidence of cost and effect can be inserted, often as probabilistic statements. This facilitates the critical analysis of data and helps to inform those charged with making the difficult rationing choices facing society. The chapter has made a distinction between different types of economic evalvation and what they aim to do. It has also drawn attention to the weaknesses of many studies. The reader should look for rigour and objectivity in the research that underpins economic assessments. An exercise now follows in which the reader can apply some of the principles covered in this chapter.

Exercise: Which treatment alternative in implant surgery should be funded?

Implant A has the lowest rate of complications. Implant B produces a quality adjusted life year at least cost. Implant C is the least expensive, and therefore its adoption facilitates the treatment of the largest number of patients from a given budget. Answer the following questions:

1
- Which of the following choices might be regarded as 'equitable'?
- Which of these choices is most clinically effective?
- Which of these choices is efficient?

Choices and consequences: There are 500 patients requiring treatment and the Primary Care Trust (PCT) has a budget of £500,000 for implants. Implant A costs £2,500 per patient and produces a QALY at a cost of £425. Implant B costs £1,500 and produces a QALY at a cost of £415. Implant C costs £1,000 and produces a QALY at a cost of £700.

(Continued)

2

- With implant A, how many patients can be treated and what is the total number of QALYs produced?
- With implant B, how many patients can be treated and what is the total number of QALYs produced?
- With implant C, how many patients can be treated and what is the total number of QALYs produced?

3

- If this PCT is maximizing improvements in health (as proxied by the level of QALY production) as it should in the NHS, how many patients will be left untreated?
- What information would you seek as the chief executive of the PCT to provide a case for increasing the budget allocation for these implants?
- What are the costs and benefits of adopting implants?

RECOMMENDED FURTHER READING

Drummond, M., Sculpher, M.J., Torrance, G.W., O'Brien, B. and Stoddart, G.L. (2005) *Methods of Economic Evaluation of Health Care Programmes*, 3rd edition. Oxford: Oxford University Press.
This book is an essential guidebook for practitioners on the issues raised in this chapter.

Jefferson, T., Demicheli, V. and Mugford, A. (2000) *Elementary Evaluation in Health Care*. Oxford: Oxford University Press.
This is more of an elementary and introductory guide to the use of economics in health research.

REFERENCES

Drummond, M. and the British Medical Journal Economic Evaluation Working Party (1996) 'Guidelines for authors and peer reviewers of economic submissions to the BMJ', *British Medical Journal*, 313: 275–83.
Drummond, M., Sculpher, M.J., Torrance, G.W., O'Brien, B. and Stoddart, G.L. (2005) *Methods of Economic Evaluation of Health Care Programmes*, 3rd edition. Oxford: Oxford University Press.

EuroQol Group (1991) 'Euroqol: a new facility for the measurement of health related quality of life', Health Policy, 16: 199–208.

Freemantle, N. and Maynard, A. (1994) 'Something rotten in the state of clinical and economic evaluations?', *Health Economics*, 3 (2): 63–67.

Jefferson, T., Demicheli, V. and Mugford, A. (2000) *Elementary Evaluation in Health Care*. Oxford: Oxford University Press.

Klarman, H.E, Frances, J.O. and Rosenthal, G.D (1968) 'Cost effectiveness analysis applied to the treatment of chronic renal failure', *Medical Care*, 6: 48–54.

Maynard, A. (1990) 'The design of future cost-benefit studies', *American Heart Journal*, 119 (3): 761–65.

Maynard, A. (1991) 'Developing the health care market', *Economic Journal*, 101: 1277–86.

Maynard, A. (1997) 'Evidence based medicine: an incomplete method for informing treatment choices', *Lancet*, 349: 126–28.

Maynard, A., Bloor, K. and Freemantle, N. (2004) 'Challenges for the National Institute for Clinical Excellence', *British Medical Journal*, 329: 227–29.

NHS Centre for Reviews and Dissemination (CRD) (2001) *Undertaking Systematic Reviews*. Report No. 4.

Philips, Z., Ginnelly, L., Sculpher, M., Claxton, K., Golder, S., Riemsma, R., Woolacoot, N. and Glanville, J. (2004) 'A review of guidelines for good practice in decision analytic modelling in health technology assessment', *Health Technology Assessment*, 8 (36): 1–158.

Piachaud, D. and Weddell, J.M. (1972) 'The economics of treating varicose veins', *International Journal of Epidemiology*, 1: 287–94.

Rosser, R., Kind, P. and Williams, A. (1982) 'Valuation of quality of life: some psychometric evidence', in M. Jones-Lee (ed.), *The Value of Life and Society*. Amsterdam: Elsevier.

Williams, A. (1976) 'The cost benefit approach', *British Medical Bulletin*, 30 (3): 252–56.

Williams, A. (1985) 'Economics of coronary artery by-pass grafting', *British Medical Journal*, 291: 326–29.

Williams, A. (1997) 'The rationing debate: rationing health care by age. The case for', *British Medical Journal*, 314: 820–5.

PART IV
Contemporary Issues in Researching Health

15

Governance and Ethics in Health Research

PRISCILLA ALDERSON

INTRODUCTION

This chapter considers formal and informal approaches to ethics review and governance and how issues of ethics can best be addressed in health research. The final part of the chapter discusses more explicitly the politics of research ethics and governance. To begin with some definitions, 'participants' is the current term used for people taking part in research. This implies an active involvement and a shared control of the research process between researchers and participants. In practice, this does not always occur as people may have little or no awareness about why they are being researched and what the process involves. In such cases, people are being treated as the subjects, or even the objects, of the research rather than as participants so the term 'subjects/participants' is used here. The term 'medical' is used to refer to clinical scientific research on the body and body parts, and the term 'social' includes all the disciplines that research people's views and experiences of health and illness.

At present, a spectrum of views about research ethics and governance is found among researchers. This ranges from active interest and support to resignation and resentful compliance; from a lack of awareness of ethical matters to a hostile impatience with the process. Researchers may also hold mixed views. They may accept the value of some governance, but feel confused by the rapid burgeoning of guidance documents. They may feel irritated by having to complete the time-consuming application forms now necessary for ethics approval, and may also see a rejection as unfair and a hindrance to research.

THE CHANGING CONTEXT OF HEALTH AND MEDICAL RESEARCH ETHICS

The history of research ethics

The history of medical ethics records doctors' gradual movement from rejection, for example see Tobias and Souhami (1993), to general support for research ethics and governance. In the first half of the twentieth century, there were few formal ethics guidelines and committees. For instance, during the 1930s to 1940s the guidance in Germany did little to prevent harmful research, which was also widely conducted in the United States, Europe and the Far East (Proctor 1988; McNeill 1993), and has continued into this century. Sharav (2003) reports contemporary unethical psycho-pharmaceutical trials on children in the United States. Even a leading British paediatric journal has published a report of unethical research without comment. For example, 'non-therapeutic' research on newborn babies with severe cardiac defects included 60–90 minutes of extra anaesthesia with administration of carbon dioxide before surgery (Hoehn et al. 2005).

From the 1970s and 1980s, research ethics committees and, in the United States, institutional review boards for medical research began to be introduced widely. In the 1980s and 1990s, philosophy departments at risk of closing set up flourishing medical ethics centres and courses, and there are now numerous medical ethics journals and well-attended conferences. However, as the neonatal cardiac example illustrates, research ethics committees still allow high-risk research that contravenes the guidelines set by the World Medical Association (1964/2000) and the Royal College of Paediatrics and Child Health (2000).

Research ethics and methodology

Research ethics and methodology are closely connected. Burgess and Bulmer (1981: 478) described methodology as 'the systematic and logical study of the principles governing enquiry'. Burgess (1989) identified three main areas for ethical attention: sponsorship in terms of how sponsors may assist with, or impede, research; research relations that may raise issues of access, power, deception, harm and secrecy; and the dissemination of research findings. Gouldner (1971: 50–1) also pointed out the inescapably ethical or value-laden nature of research when he wrote that research methodology is 'infused with ideologically resonant assumptions about what the social world is, and what the nature of the relation between them is'. According to this view, ethics is not a matter of adding a paragraph or veneer of respect for rules, but involves thinking about ethics in every aspect of the research project. In a more recent study, Alderson and Morrow (2004) have divided projects into 10 stages and reviewed the ethical questions that arise at each stage.

Sociologists generally have tended only recently to consider formal ethics governance seriously within their own discipline. The influences that stimulated interest in research governance include factors such as:

- The risk, cost and litigation, and the increase in the formal management of mistrust (Beck 1992).
- The institutionalized increase and formal management of mistrust.
- A few highly publicized cases of the death of a research subject.
- The exponential growth of governance and legalistic bureaucracy in institutions that sponsor and house research.
- The desire for standards to promote and protect profits from research and development.
- The many recent acts and conventions on human and children's rights and on data protection.

As a consequence, in the past five years various funding bodies, research agencies and professional academic associations have revised their ethics guidelines, and most universities in Britain now have research ethics committee to safeguard research subjects/participants, researchers themselves and the standards and reputation of research. Reputation matters when institutions undertaking research depend heavily on public funding and the willingness of people to take part. Their involvement in projects depends upon their interest and trust in research findings. So the context of this chapter is rapid change and considerable debate on the pros and cons of health research ethics and governance; whether the relevant disciplines require different forms of ethics governance; and how various disciplines can work together.

DEVELOPING A FRAMEWORK FOR MEDICAL ETHICS

I first joined a medical ethics committee in 1981 and over three years we met monthly as a group and published a book on ethics and medical research with children (Nicholson 1985). The group, modelled on the United States National

Commission for the Protection of Human Subjects in Medical and Behavioral Research (1977; 1978), included doctors, lawyers, a nurse, lay people, philosophers and psychologists. In the light of the history of unregulated medical research on children, our debates were critical and challenging. We worked to identify and agree on principled but flexible standards and examined how these could protect both child research subjects and also the interests of all future patients who might benefit from research findings. We were influenced by three main frameworks for medical ethics relating to the principles, rights and outcomes set out in Box 15.1.

Box 15.1   *Frameworks for medical ethics*

Principles, rights and outcomes

1   *Principles* of ethics that centre on a respect for autonomy, justice, doing no harm and using resources fairly and efficiently.
2   *Rights* that provide for basic needs with the best available health care; protect people from harm, abuse, neglect and discrimination; respect their freedoms, of information. expression, thought and conscience; and promote social inclusion and self-determination
3   *Outcomes* that aim to avoid or reduce harm and costs and to promote benefits.

Sources: United Nations (1989); Beauchamp and Childress (2000); United States National Commission for the Protection of Human Subjects in Medical and Behavioral Research (1978).

These principles, rights and outcomes, alongside other ethical frameworks such as virtue ethics, all have strengths but leave gaps, which are widely analyzed and debated (Gillon 2003). Moral questions about power, honesty and respecting or abusing people arise throughout the research process and, formally or less consciously, researchers tend to resolve questions by thinking about principles such as what is the right thing to do? They think about rights: how can we best respect and protect people's rights? And about outcomes: what might be the benefits to promote and the harms to avoid? Many researchers combine these approaches. Although the frameworks do not provide easy answers to ethical problems, they can help to identify and clarify problems and possible ways to solve them.

KEY ISSUES IN HEALTH RESEARCH ETHICS AND GOVERNANCE

The key questions for those concerned with research ethics and governance are:

- How can we prevent poor standards and promote high standards of research?
- How can ethics and governance be efficient and effective?

- What ethical questions arise throughout research projects?
- How can the many relevant disciplines and lay people involved in governance avoid conflicts with researchers that have a negative impact and how can they best work together?

In the United Kingdom, the *Research Governance Framework for Health and Social Care* (Department of Health 2004) defines governance as setting standards, defining ways to deliver standards, monitoring and assessing the arrangements, improving research quality, safeguarding the public by promoting good practice, reducing and preventing poor practice and misconduct, and ensuring that lessons are learnt from adverse incidents. These standards apply to all research conducted on health or social services in the United Kingdom and are likely to extend to other areas of research. Increasingly, funding bodies require the same standards too, irrespective of the disciplinary background of the researcher as inequities can occur when some subjects/participants are protected by formal ethics procedures, and others are not. The boundaries in health research may be drawn far more definitely by the methods used, or the participants involved, than by the researchers' particular discipline.

ISSUES OF CONCERN IN ETHICS GUIDELINES

A central question is whether guidelines are useful and effective. Some common confusions arise in the guidance, particularly on covert research, therapeutic research and harm–benefit equations.

Consent and covert research

In 1947, the first international guidance on research ethics, the *Nuremberg Code* (1947), said in Article One that the voluntary consent of the human subject is 'absolutely essential'. The code assumed that people could base their consent or refusal on an 'enlightened' decision. This emphasis on voluntary consent was lost later in the far more widely used *Declaration of Helsinki* (World Medical Association 1964) which emphasized the doctor's duty to relieve suffering, advance progress through research and to protect human beings' 'health and rights' (World Medical Association 2000). Consent is not mentioned until point 9. Although later points stress consent, power has shifted from the voluntary subject to the responsible medical researcher. The *Declaration of Helsinki* also does not mention covert research – that is, research carried out without the subject/participant's knowledge and consent – but appears to veto it by repeatedly stating that consent must always be sought.

Within social science, the British Psychological Society (2004) aims to 'protect the dignity of participants' but, like the British Sociological Association (2003), covert research, without people's knowledge or consent, is allowed. The code of the British Psychological Society (2004) says that the central principle to be determined is 'the reaction of participants when deception was revealed. If this led to [their] discomfort, anger or objections ... then the deception was inappropriate.' Yet an accurate prediction of people's later reactions is often not possible, particularly, perhaps, when the judgement is being made by researchers who have decided to deceive them.

Therapeutic research

Until 2000, the *Declaration of Helsinki* used the somewhat misleading phrase 'therapeutic research', which implies directly beneficial research, and required lower ethical standards for this than for 'non-therapeutic research', which was seen to be of no direct benefit to patients. However, all research concerns collecting data, but not providing care or directly benefiting people. Researchers might do so coincidentally, if they provide care/treatment that they are also researching or evaluating, but the main purpose of research is systematic enquiry. The term 'therapeutic' implies benefits that the researcher cannot ensure. Indeed, many people have been classed as being in 'therapeutic research' when the treatment was later shown to be useless or harmful. If they were in a placebo control group they would, by definition, be receiving a non-treatment. Research ethics committees still sometimes evaluate potentially dangerous drug trials as 'therapeutic' and therefore permissible, while criticizing 'non-therapeutic' collection of data, which might later prove to be far more useful, such as in understanding the aetiology or process of disease, or the experiences and needs of patients.

For decades the care-based concept of 'therapeutic research' has tended to confuse medical ethics discussions as it is used to excuse risks that might be accepted in treatment giving, but not in research. This confusion is also found in social research, when researchers justify intrusive interviews by claiming that people like to talk or find relief in relating their experiences. They may do, but that is not the aim or purpose of the encounter, and cannot be guaranteed. The claim blurs the reality that subjects/participants are helping the researcher by providing data. To recognize that the research encounter is essentially a meeting between strangers can help to promote protection and respect. However, existing guidelines for social workers, for example, including those involved in health research, may blur the roles of researcher and service provider. Butler (2002: 245) comments:

> Both the process of social work/care research, including the choice of methodology, and the use to which any findings might be put, should be congruent with the aims and values of social work practice and, where possible, seek to empower service users, promote their welfare and improve their access to economic and social capital on equal terms with other citizens.

The statement does not explain how the process of collecting and reporting data can either meet the aims of social work/care to provide a service, or directly benefit and empower a client. Promises directly to help participants can undermine the key principle of respect for consent or refusal that is freely given. Such promises have the potential to mislead researchers, participants and gatekeepers into believing that the supposed direct benefit of taking part in research should not be refused.

Turning to other research areas, some clinical trialists claim that patients do better simply by being in a trial, although the evidence for this is inconclusive (Vist et al. 2005). Feminist research ethics also tends to emphasize the ethic of care in research (Edwards and Mauthner 2001). This can imply a direct benefit of care from the researcher or from being in a research project. It risks over-conceptualizing the subject/participant as dependent and needy. In contrast, codes of medical ethics have placed emphasis on respect for the person's independence from the researcher as being crucial to the research process. In sum, there are vital distinctions between treatment and research, and between both the relationship of practitioner–patient/client and of researcher–subject/participant. As Cooter (1992) records, well-meant 'caring' intentions have on occasion cloaked and excused extremely harmful 'welfare', dietary and medical practices in research.

The harm–benefit analysis

Another longstanding confusion in the guidelines relates to the harm–benefit analysis. Too often, likely risks, harms, costs and inconvenience to subjects/participants were weighed against the supposed direct benefits to them of taking part in research and/or of receiving the treatment being tested. Participants might also have received the treatment outside the research. Alternatively, if a treatment were only available within trials then its efficacy would be likely to be too questionable to count as a definite assured benefit. *The Declaration of Helsinki* (World Medical Association 2000: 16) still makes this error in mentioning 'the foreseeable benefits to the subject' but does add 'or to others'. The real balance is between possible harm to subjects versus possible benefit to future people, and this should be explained to each potential participant so that they can make a decision on the basis of a personal harm–benefit assessment.

Ethics guidelines can be vague, confusing and contradictory and it has been argued that practice cannot be made to fit written codes, however well they are devised. For instance, two or more factors can have 'different, even conflicting implications' (Lindsay 2000: 18). However, ethics guidelines do address complex questions of justice, respect, harm and benefit that have been debated without clear resolutions for many centuries. Moreover, they raise vital questions that science and research methods do not deal with directly, and also help to promote a gradual rise in ethical standards in research.

GOVERNANCE THROUGH RESEARCH ETHICS COMMITTEES

The role of research ethics committees

The uncertainty about interpreting ethical guidelines is arguably one reason for having formal reviews and independent discussion to decide on the complex arguments, instead of leaving decisions to individual researchers alone. Research ethics committees serve several vital purposes. They can:

- Act as a protective barrier between researchers and potential participants.
- Raise awareness about ethics within the research community.
- Check whether a project is worth doing and if the anticipated benefits are likely to justify any risks to participants.
- Veto unethical research early and warn and advise about potential ethical problems that might be avoided or prevented.
- Check that potential participants receive clear written information and have an opportunity for discussion so that they can give informed consent or refusal.
- Check that certain groups are not over-researched, that particular needs are met, such as the need for interpreters, and that the protocol is not too onerous.
- Collect data on best practice and disseminate ideas.

A particularly crucial aspect of ethics review is to ensure that subjects/participants have clear written information for their own records. Furthermore, consent must be informed and not made under pressure so that people can freely refuse to take part. The review of basic science is also important and raises questions such as: Is the research worth doing? Do the hoped-for benefits justify the risks and costs? Will the research duplicate previous work? Are the methods likely to answer the research questions? Is the sample size large enough? How original and useful might the research findings be?

It may be claimed that only specialists in the particular research discipline can be competent reviewers and are sufficiently expert to examine these matters. However, the research can only be ethical if it is explained and justified clearly enough to enable people to give informed consent or refuse to take part. Research ethics committees are made up of people with a range of knowledge, expertise and experience who try to look at proposals from the point of view of the ordinary person and what they may wish to know about the purpose of the research, what will be required of them as participants, and what possible misunderstandings and anxieties about risk they might have. Lay members are better able to raise and debate such questions than a group of experts sharing similar assumptions (West and Butler 2003).

Guidance on ethics committees on the website www.corec.org.uk and in the monthly *Bulletin of Medical Ethics* contributes to training. These sources could be more widely used by social science health researchers as they offer information on asking and analyzing ethical questions; updates on new guidelines and laws about privacy, data protection and consent; ethical methods for selecting, accessing and involving participants and advisers in research; and standards for drafting patient/participant information sheets.

COMMON CRITICISMS OF RESEARCH ETHICS COMMITTEES

One criticism of research ethics committees is that the lay members are not 'representative'. Yet professional members are not 'representative' either as they are also appointed on the grounds of their personal qualities and expertise. A principle of research ethics is to transfer as much information and control as possible from researchers to participants. Lay members can encourage this when they ask seemingly naive questions on behalf of potential participants, so that the committees' discussions can involve both a practical and symbolic transfer.

Research ethics committees are biased against social science methods

Some social scientists have criticized medically based research ethics committees for dismissing social research questions, theories and methods (see Lewis 2002; Christensen and Prout 2002; Glendenning and McKie 2003; Iphofen 2004; Brindle 2005). However, if social scientists cannot convince ethics committee members of the worth of their research, are they likely to be able to convince potential participants? And if they cannot achieve this, how can they gain the informed consent from participants necessary for conducting ethical research? Current practice in ethics governance challenges researchers to refine their skills, for example in explaining appropriate qualitative methods and writing clear protocols, which helps to increase public understanding of research.

Increasingly, medically based research ethics committees are supporting social research.

Social research cannot harm people, as medical research risks doing

Medical research can cause harm and distress, and so can social research, and social aspects of medical research. For example, the parents who protested after their deceased children's organs were removed for research at Alder Hey Hospital said that they were not against scientific/medical research on the children's organs. Their main objection was a social concern that they were not informed or asked for their consent. In the 1980s, women enrolled into covert breast cancer trials expressed similar views and said that they felt wronged, and deeply distressed. Even the seemingly innocuous social research question 'Tell me about who you live with at home' can distress people who may be going through domestic turmoil.

Research ethics committees prevent ethnography, developing new questions during a project, and opportunistic and informal research

Research that is funded usually requires detailed planning, justification and safeguards for participants to satisfy funding requirements as well as research ethics committees. In practice, ethnographic and other social research methodologies are frequently approved by health care ethics committees if the objectives and methods are clearly described and feasible. If questions and methods alter during a project in a major way, then research ethics committees and participants can be informed. Indeed, in some projects participants may share in planning the initial project and any changes (see Chapters 8 and 18).

Research ethics is said to be based on widely held principles, but there are no such principles

The argument that there are no agreed principles in research ethics is amply challenged by the long history that shows how highly principles of respect for autonomy and consent are valued. The argument may be being used to defend researchers' own autonomy and to ward off interference from research ethics committees. Ironically, this defence invokes the very Kantian principles that such speakers deny – that is, treat others as you, or an average person, would wish to be treated in a similar situation. It is likely that critics would want to apply such principles not only to their own work, but also to any medical research in which they might become subjects. While the critical analysis of ethics and principles, their complex meanings, and their use and misuse, can be an extremely valuable activity, there are problems when this moves from being the *topic* of research into being the research *method*, as it can lead to the potential abuse of subjects/participants.

Research ethics committee forms are complicated and take weeks to complete

As mentioned earlier, this problem also applies to funding applications and information leaflets for participants. Filling in forms correctly is an inevitable part of efficient research. Sylvester and Green (2003) expressed concern that the lengthy process of ethics review delayed their students' research with people having palliative (terminal) care. The ethics review process does take time to complete as there will be a cycle of meetings, which needs to be anticipated. Delays can occur, although there is now guidance on time limits. Sylvester and Green also warned that students taking Masters degrees may have to undertake literature reviews instead of research with people because of the barrier of getting through the ethics review process. Yet it can be argued that a literature review may be preferable to exposing very ill, vulnerable 'participants' to hurried and therefore potentially unethical research by Masters students.

Research ethics committees lack competence

It has been alleged that research ethics committees approve poor and harmful protocols, reject good ones and nit-pick over trivial points. Without investigation, it is impossible to substantiate these points. It may be the case that ethics committee members have too little time and training to do their (unpaid) work properly, and certainly they need training and support. It is also possible that some committees may be dominated, and possibly misled, by an assertive minority. However, there are ways in which the researcher can seek a dialogue with a research ethics committee. For example, they may make a request to present their research to a committee in person.

THE POLITICS OF RESEARCH ETHICS AND GOVERNANCE

Research ethics governance is a contentious area, with researchers from different disciplines having to protect their own interests while they compete for research opportunities and for funds. There is a struggle for power and influence. Medical research has always dominated health research in terms of methods of bioscience and resources, and also through its strongly established institutions. Medical research ethics and guidelines have been well developed and medical researchers tend to belong to extensive social, collective and international networks that support dissemination. In addition, as Chapter 19 demonstrates, lay people have been highly involved in medical ethics for some time, and indeed often chair the research ethics committees.

It can be argued that, paradoxically, social science research ethics is less socially and collectively developed. Many social researchers still believe in the efficacy of the private ethics of 'self-regulation' and personal conscience (Economic and Social Research Council 2001; British Sociological Association 2003; Lewis 2002). The involvement of lay people in social science ethics committees is unusual even though social issues are likely to be easier for lay people to understand than, say, biochemical research. It may also be that, as a research community, social scientists are less aware of ethical issues in research. For example, in reporting on their research, Lewis et al. (2003: 4) state that: 'It was unexpected to find that a considerable number [of researchers] reported the absence of [consent] procedures.' Nevertheless, a subsequent project (Webster et al. 2004; Boulton et al. 2004) reported more support among social researchers for research ethics committees and for ethics training.

Some authors criticize ethics rules and formal review as: too inflexible; unable to deal with unforeseen situations; too easily becoming a routine or a fig leaf; and no substitute for the active engagement of the individual researchers and the social science community as a whole with ethical issues (Christensen and Prout 2002). Others have said that formal guidelines and research ethics committees can unethically 'invite the individual to surrender the moral conscience to a professional consensus' (Homan 1992: 331) and that there are dangers in bureaucratic ethics (Bauman 1993). Lewis et al. (2003: 1–4) warn that there is a danger of 'ethical inflation' and imposed 'external drivers' that could 'restrict the conduct of important, high quality, social science research'. They warn that overly prescriptive, imposed, 'highly formalised or bureaucratic ways of securing consent' could undermine the desirable ethics that is 'embedded' in everyday research. They consider that formal review is 'marginal to fostering relationships in which a process of *ongoing* ethical regard for participants could be sustained', and that it conflicts with what 'constitutes good (necessary, relevant) practice'. They add that 'ethical vigilance' should be 'proportionate to the risks borne by research participants'.

To dismiss ethics as yet another discourse of power ignores how researchers themselves have a vested interest in maximizing their autonomy as researchers, itself a form of power. Some researchers who oppose ethics governance seem to assume that it will either induce researchers to observe higher standards, or force researchers to lower their standards. Yet surely researchers would accept that the first point is reasonable and the second is unlikely. Opposition to ethics governance also denies the value of formalized ways of criticizing unethical research. Furthermore, in practice, morality in research is not exclusively either a private or a collective concern, but rather a complicated combination of the two. Social researchers' reservations about ethics governance suggest that, as with medical ethics education, 'ethical literacy' courses will have to involve them in academic debate beyond brief superficial training sessions.

LEARNING FROM SOCIAL RESEARCH ETHICS

While medical ethics has tended to dominate and inform policies on research ethics generally, there is also a value in a transfer in the opposite direction. Social research ethics can indeed contribute to medical ethics, which has been seen as too abstract and impersonal. To illustrate, one philosopher claimed that it was necessary to clear away the contingent 'rubbish' of social experiences in order to see the ethical issues and dilemmas clearly (Raphael 1976), to which a feminist philosopher replied that ethical issues are constituted from this everyday 'rubbish' (Grimshaw 1986). Grounded in practical everyday experiences, social research ethics can introduce the practical, realistic insights that tend to be ignored in abstract ethics. Social scientists may contribute to the development of a practical research ethics in three ways by:

- Allowing for feelings in the research process.
- Acknowledging practical problems.
- Acknowledging explicitly the social and political context of research.

Feelings and emotions in the research process

Researchers have feelings and emotions and can better handle the challenges of research by looking inwards to their hopes and fears about their work; their anxiety about mistakes; stress from lack of time and resources. Researchers gain from sharing satisfaction about new data and theories, as well as responding to the hopes and fears of the participants. Although emotions can mislead and cloud judgement, there are grave dangers if researchers lose empathy and pity. MacIntyre (1966) has analyzed how overly rational Kantian ethics validated Nazi research. This allowed researchers to become detached from their 'moral self constituted by responsibility' and blindly obedient to rules, instead of also carefully negotiating a way forward through unpredictable and ambiguous interactions (Bauman 1993: 11). During stressful and often sensitive research in the health field, it is important, and ethical, to support and debrief researchers and reflexive sessions can inform the research analysis.

Dealing with practical problems in research

Numerous practical and unpredictable problems arise during research projects, when solutions must be found. Hallowell et al. (2005: 142) review these rarely reported problems and contend that social research 'is first and foremost a moral activity'. It is about negotiating human relationships and achieving a complicated balance between many opposing options. They conclude that at every stage ethical research relies on codes, research ethics committees and researchers' good intentions. Ethics connects with researchers' skills when they respect participants' views, reflect on their own work and try to raise practical standards in an open and transparent way. Researchers consider ethics when they try to avoid misusing power differences between researchers and participants and within research teams. Forms of power within research methods and relationships can have greater force the less visible or acknowledged they are (Lukes 2005). Hence, it is important to be explicit in the consent process and watch for cues that participants might feel too intimidated to refuse to take part or withdraw.

The wider social and political research context

Research takes place within a broad social and political context. This influences the types of research that can, or cannot, attract funds and the support of policy makers. Research may challenge or complement the aims and interests of powerful groups. The political dimension raises questions about the contribution that social research does, might or should make to society. Medical ethics has tended to concentrate on standards during the central research stage of collecting data when there is contact with participants. It tends to ignore the initial selection of topics and the later stages of analyzing, reporting and disseminating the findings. A social science research ethics could contribute by increasing attention to ethical questions at every stage of each research project (Alderson and Morrow 2004).

Research reports can affect research participants/subjects and also, potentially, everyone associated with the group that is being researched, for instance people affected by HIV/AIDS. To take the example of children, for the last hundred years research has been driven largely by medico-psychological research. Public opinion and policy now treat childhood as a socially excluded state to the great disadvantage of children (Mayall 2002). Ethical analysis should involve examining how the eventual research reports raise, or lower, participants' social status and public perceptions of them as victims, offenders or resilient contributors. For example, researchers and reviewers could assess both the accuracy and ethics of final reports, their processes and possible effects.

At the time of writing, social research ethics is under review and there are some weaknesses in the current research ethics committee system (Wald 2004; Ward et al. 2004). There would be advantages and opportunities in social and medical researchers working jointly with other concerned people to achieve greater transparency and accountability within a national research ethics forum. They could debate problems, develop consensus and promote higher standards of research ethics 'literacy' and governance as well as set standards to protect researchers and participants. If this develops, social research ethics will have to be recognized as public, social, negotiated and political, as well as personal and private. There are many urgent questions to be addressed such as: When can researchers rely on children's consent without needing their parents' permission? How can personal privacy be respected in national surveys of disease or in family genome research?

Health care research ethics committees recognize that ethics is not only the private concern of researchers but must be fair to participants and accountable socially and politically to society. Currently, guidance in health research, laid down centrally by the Department of Health, relates to cross-disciplinary research ethics committees usually housed within health institutions. There is some guarantee of independence. In contrast, single-discipline research ethics committees within educational or other institutions may deal with applications from close colleagues within a single discipline. Critical independence is harder to achieve.

CONCLUSION

During debates about research ethics, opinions are sharply divided between regarding formal regulations and reviews as inhibiting research, or as essential to protect research subjects/participants and high standards in research. The chapter has aimed to highlight the nature of these arguments. The practical implication for researchers is that care must be taken at every stage of the research process, from initial plans to final dissemination, to ensure high ethical standards throughout.

Finally, key aspects of ethical research practice include working with participants as far as possible, from the initial planning and selection of topics, questions, methods and samples. Participants or their representatives can advise and encourage respectful approaches, and a deeper understanding of research subjects' motives and values, during data collection and analysis, report writing and dissemination. Further discussion on these matters may be found in Chapter 19, but the exercise below should also sensitize the readers to some of the issues involved.

Exercise: Writing a leaflet for participants in health research

Medically based research ethics committees require researchers to write a leaflet for potential participants to accompany the project application form. The leaflet must include the following:

A short project title

Researcher's name, institution and contact details

Information on:

- the nature, timing and purpose of the research
- the key questions and methods
- the potential harms/risks
- the benefits that any findings might yield
- participants' rights:

    - to withdraw from the project, or to refuse to take part
    - to have their data protected
    - to anonymity in reports.

Write a clear and respectful leaflet up to two A4 sides about one of your own projects. Assume that the people reading it will have a reading age of about 10 years, and use short words and sentences. See www.corec.org.uk for further details.

RECOMMENDED FURTHER READING

Alderson, P. and Morrow, V. (2004) *Ethics, Social Research and Consulting with Children and Young People*. Barkingside: Barnardo's.
This book breaks research projects into 10 stages and discusses the many ethical questions that can arise for researchers at each stage.

Hallowell, N., Lawton, J. and Gregory, S. (2005) *Reflections on Research: The Realities of Doing Research in the Social Sciences*. Buckingham: Open University Press.
This is an unusually honest book in which social researchers discuss ethical and other difficulties that occurred during their research projects and how they tried to resolve these.

World Medical Association (2000) *Declaration of Helsinki*. Fernay-Voltaire: WMA.
This is the basic international guide to medical research ethics, which has been regularly updated since it was originally agreed in 1964 and is relevant to all health researchers.

REFERENCES

Alderson, P. and Morrow, V. (2004) *Ethics, Social Research and Consulting with Children and Young People*. Barkingside: Barnardo's.

Bauman, Z. (1993) *Postmodern Ethics*. Oxford: Blackman.

Beauchamp, T. and Childress, J. (2000) *Principles of Biomedical Ethics*. New York: Oxford University Press.

Beck, U. (1992) *Risk Society*. London: Sage.

Boulton, M., Brown, N., Lewis, G. and Webster, A. (2004) *Implementing the ESRC Research Ethics Framework: The Case for Research Ethics Committees*. York: SATSU, University of York and School of Social Sciences and Law, Oxford Brookes University.

Brindle, D. (2005) 'Getting permission for social research is now a nightmare', *Guardian*, 5 February: 5.

British Psychological Society (2004) *A Code of Conduct for Psychologists*. Leicester: BPS.

British Sociological Association (2003) *Guidelines for Good Professional Conduct and Statement of Ethical Practice; Statement of Ethical Practice*. Durham: BSA.

Burgess, R. (1989) *The Ethics of Social Research*. London: Falmer.

Burgess, R. and Bulmer, M. (1981) 'Research methodology teaching', *Sociology*, 15: 447–89.

Butler, I. (2002) 'Critical commentary: a code of ethics for social work and social care research', *British Journal of Social Work*, 32: 239–48.

Christensen, P. and Prout, A. (2002) 'Working with ethical symmetry in social research with children', *Childhood*, 9 (4): 477–97.

Cooter, R. (ed.) (1992) *In the Name of the Child: Health and Welfare 1880–1940*. London: Routledge.

Department of Health (2004) *Research Governance Framework for Health and Social Care; Implementation Plan for Social Care*. London: HMSO.

Economic and Social Research Council (2001) *Research Ethics and Confidentiality*. Swindon: ESRC.

Edwards, R. and Mauthner, M. (2001) 'Ethics and feminist research: theory and practice', in M. Mauthner, M. Birch, J. Jessop, and T. Miller (eds), *Ethics in Qualitative Research*. London: Sage.

Gillon, R. (ed.) (2003) *Principles of Health Care Ethics*. Chichester: Wiley.

Glendenning, C. and McKie, L. (2003) 'BSA working in partnership with SPA: ethics in social research', *BSA Network*, Summer: 15–16.

Gouldner, A. (1971) *The Coming Crisis of Western Sociology*. London: Routledge.

Grimshaw, J. (1986) *Feminism and Philosophy*. Brighton: Wheatsheaf.

Hallowell, N., Lawton, J. and Gregory, S. (2005) *Reflections on Research: The Realities of Doing Research in the Social Sciences*. Buckingham: Open University Press.

Hoehn, K., Wernovsky, G., Rychik, J., Gaynor, J., Spray, T., Feudtner, C. and Nelson, R. (2005) 'What factors are important to parents making decisions about neonatal research?', *Archives of Disease in Childhood*, 90: 267–69.

Homan, R. (1992) 'The ethics of open methods', *British Journal of Sociology*, 42 (3): 321–32.

Iphofen, R. (2004) 'A code to keep away judges, juries and MPs', *The Times Higher Education Supplement*, 16 January: 24.

Lewis, J. (2002) 'Research and development in social care: governance and good practice', *Research Policy and Planning*, 20 (1): 3–9.

Lewis, G., Brown, N., Holland, S. and Webster, A. (2003) *A Review of Ethics and Social Science Research for the Strategic Forum for the Social Sciences, Commissioned by the ESRC. Summary.* York: SATSU, University of York.

Lindsay, G. (2000) 'Researching children's perspectives: ethical issues', in A. Lewis and G. Lindsay (eds), *Researching Children's Perspectives.* Buckingham: Open University Press.

Lukes, S. (2005) *Power: A Radical View.* Basingstoke: Palgrave Macmillan.

MacIntyre, A. (1966) *A Short History of Ethics.* New York: Macmillan.

McNeill, P. (1993) *The Ethics and Politics of Human Experimentation.* Cambridge: Cambridge University Press.

Mayall, B. (2002) *Towards a Sociology for Childhood.* London: Routledge/Falmer.

Nicholson, R. (1985) *Medical Research with Children: Ethics, Law and Practice.* Oxford: Oxford University Press.

Nuremberg Code (1947). Available at: ohsr.od.nih.gov/guidelines/nuremberg.html

Proctor, R. (1988) *Racial Hygiene: Medicine under the Nazis.* Cambridge, MA: Harvard University Press.

Raphael, D. (1976) *Problems of Politics and Philosophy.* London: Macmillan.

Royal College of Paediatrics and Child Health (2000) 'Ethics Advisory Committee: guidelines on the ethical conduct of medical research involving children', *Archives of Disease in Childhood*, 82: 177–82.

Sharav, V. (2003) 'Children in clinical research: a conflict of moral values', *American Journal of Bioethics*, 3 (1): 1–99.

Sylvester, S. and Green, J. (2003) 'An excess of governance? Social research and Local Research Ethics Committees', *Medical Sociology News*, 29 (3): 39–44.

Tobias, J. and Souhami, R. (1993) 'Fully informed consent can be needlessly cruel', *British Medical Journal*, 307: 1199–2001.

United Nations (1989) *Convention on the Rights of the Child.* New York: UN.

United States National Commission for the Protection of Human Subjects in Medical and Behavioral Research (1977) *Research Involving Children: Report and Recommendations.* Washington, DC: DHEW.

United States National Commission for the Protection of Human Subjects in Medical and Behavioral Research (1978) *The Belmont Report: Ethical Principles and Guidelines for the Protection of Human Subjects of Research.* Washington, DC: DHEW.

Vist, E.G., Hagen, K., Devereaux, P., Bryant, D., Kristoffersen, D. and Oxman, A. (2005) 'Systematic review to determine whether participation in a trial influences outcome', *British Medical Journal*, 330: 1175.

Wald, D. (2004) 'Bureaucracy of ethics applications', *British Medical Journal*, 329: 282–85.

Ward, H., Cousens, N., Smith-Bathgate, B., Leitch, M., Everington, D., Will, R. and Smith, P. (2004) 'Obstacles to conducting epidemiological research in the UK general population', *British Medical Journal*, 329: 277–79.

Webster, A., Lewis, G., Brown, N. and Boulton, M. (2004) *Developing a Framework for Social Science Research Ethics: Project Update for ESRC.* York: SATSU, University of York and School of Social Sciences and Law, Oxford Brookes University.

West, E. and Butler, J. (2003) 'An applied and qualitative LREC reflects on its practice', *Bulletin of Medical Ethics*, 185: 13–20.

World Medical Association (1964/2000) *Declaration of Helsinki.* Fernay-Voltaire: WMA.

16

Mixed Methods and Multidisciplinary Research in Health Care

JONATHAN TRITTER

INTRODUCTION

The key aim of this chapter is to examine the benefits and limitation of mixed methods and multidisciplinary research in health care and the implications these have for project management. This will include describing mixed methods and multidisciplinary research; outlining the strengths and weakness of mixed methods and multidisciplinary research; considering the implications for research design and project management; and providing an illustrative example and a problem-solving exercise.

Increasingly, those who fund research and publishers of professional journals require health research that is based on data collected through different methods and draws on expertise from both the biomedical and social sciences. A project may draw on physiological measurement, epidemiological data as well as data that explore people's understanding of their illness collected, for example from illness diaries or narratives. As researchers, one of the initial questions we face in designing a study is the nature and type of data we wish to collect and the methods we use to do so, and frequently projects use a range of different methods and types of data. These data often require analysis using a range of disciplinary frames of reference and knowledge. This chapter explores some of the reasons for adopting mixed methods in research and illustrates a number of typical research designs. It identifies some of the difficulties that can arise in multidisciplinary research and suggests ways of meeting the challenge. Fundamental to this is careful forethought and a strategic approach to research.

MIXING METHODS: SOME TYPICAL APPROACHES

Beginning with qualitative enquiries

As earlier chapters have discussed, different research methods are associated with different kinds of research question. However, the same method may serve different purposes depending on the order in which it is applied within a research project. Often research in an area about which little is known begins with an open approach that seeks to identify relevant issues or topics. Exploratory research rarely has explicit questions or a hypothesis to be tested. Instead, these are developed in the initial phase using a qualitative method such as observation, in-depth interviews or focus group discussions. This should yield the key dimensions that can then be used to frame a later stage of the project that will adopt other methods.

For example, we know from epidemiological studies that asthma has become more prevalent, and the incidence is increasing among children. In order to understand the experience of children with asthma of different ages, say in secondary schools, initially research might begin with observing playground activities or physical education lessons. Another approach might be to convene a number of focus groups to include children of the same age for a discussion of how they think asthma affects their life in school. Each strategy would yield different information, but both provide a way of identifying key issues for research participants. Other methods could be used to measure these more precisely.

Interviews or focus group discussions can also help to develop and refine research instruments. For example, the focus group discussion could be used to identify five key areas where children felt their school experience was affected by asthma. These could provide a basis for an unstructured interview topic guide or be used to design a questionnaire.

This type of approach can ensure that research is grounded in the experience of those who are the object of study. Research that builds on the health needs expressed by a population group being studied is especially relevant when the objective is to evaluate or develop a health service. It has been argued that the increased policy emphasis on user involvement in research (Lowes and Hulatt 2005) and on patient and public participation in health policy (Tritter and McCallum 2006) may privilege studies that adopt such approaches.

Laying the groundwork with quantitative methods

A different approach is to undertake a survey of a sample population to establish the frequency of a certain phenomenon. Using the example of asthma from above, a survey could be used initially to identify the number of children with asthma in secondary schools in a given area. These data could then be used to provide a sampling frame to identify a sample for further investigation. We might be interested in how children of different ages in different schools experienced and managed their illness. We could use the survey data to identify a sample of children that was stratified according to age, school and gender and use this to invite children to a focus group or interview. The second qualitative phase of the research would explore the meaning of illness for these children – a very different type of research question than prevalence.

The ethnography and case study approach

Some research approaches such as ethnography and case studies are dependent on using mixed methods. Ethnography relies on observation as an essential aspect of its methods toolkit, but this is typically augmented by interviews, focus groups and sometimes surveys. Similarly, case study research is premised on collecting multiple forms of data. This may include a critical review of organizational literature, observation and interviews. For both of these instances, the convergence of multiple sources of evidence is the key to obtaining more rounded and, arguably, more valid findings.

Research design and mixed methods

The various ways that different kinds of research methods can be combined have been outlined. The order and combination of methods must be planned carefully to accrue maximum benefit. Simply applying a range of methods to a research problem – a shotgun approach – is likely to yield little additional benefit. The particular research problem or question must be determined first. It is only after such decisions are made that actual methods and research instruments can be defined, evaluated and adopted.

   An important consideration in a mixed-method research design is the intended relationship between the types of data to be collected. Most designs rely on data collected in an early research phase to influence later phases, through the definition of a sample or the development of a research instrument. A further vital issue is how different kinds of data collected from different sources can be integrated analytically. Furthermore, it is important to consider at an early stage how research findings that draw on different forms of data will be presented in a final report.

Triangulation

The use of multiple sources of data is one of the principles behind the notion of triangulation. Triangulation, a navigational term based on using two bearings to locate an object, has been used in two ways in the social sciences. In the first, the term has been used to imply that the aggregation of data from different sources can validate a particular truth, account or finding (see Denzin 1970). In the second, multiple methods can be used in order to gain a greater understanding of a particular phenomenon – it can be seen from a number of different perspectives. Triangulation is used in the latter sense here. Collecting different kinds of data (for example, first-person accounts of an experience, observational video, survey data from participants and focus groups with participants) provides the opportunity to build a holistic understanding of the object of study. It does not attempt to privilege one account over another. The account given of a phenomenon through different methods will be based on a particular theory and the structure and meaning provided by that perspective (see Silverman 1993).

The application of an independent but coordinated analysis of the same data from a range of different perspectives is another aspect of triangulation. By using a mixture of methods in a research project, a number of researchers, often with diverse disciplinary backgrounds, may independently analyze and interpret the different types of data collected (Patton 2002; Yin 1994). Such an approach seeks to understand the phenomena being studied from multiple perspectives. Similarly, using a number of analysts who agree a common coding framework and then independently apply this to all of the data before meeting to reach a consensus on interpretation and findings can also lead to far more robust results.

THE VALUE OF MULTIDISCIPLINARY RESEARCH IN HEALTH CARE

Towards a more holistic approach to health

The impact of lifestyle and the importance of patient participation in decisions about health care are now recognized as key aspects in ensuring good health. It is also acknowledged that chronic conditions and recovery from trauma or illness can be managed more successfully with patient and carer participation. No longer can health outcomes be simply understood as the product of medical intervention or pharmaceutical treatment alone. How patients access services, the ways they participate in decisions about treatment and the social context in which they are treated, live and work are all important to health outcomes. The implication of this 'holistic' model of health for research is that a number of different disciplines and research methods are required to study the impact of health and illness in the round.

For instance, smoking is associated with many millions of deaths worldwide annually. Smoking changes the metabolism and retards healing. Therefore, smoking cessation is important from a public health perspective, and is also recommended as part of the 'treatment' for many medical conditions from asthma to coronary heart disease (Mackay and Eriksen 2002). But there is no way to 'prescribe' smoking cessation, or to understand the meaning of smoking, without considering the social context and the lifestyle of the patient (Copeland 2003).

Another factor leading to a more holistic view of health and, *inter alia*, the importance of research using mixed methods and a multidisciplinary approach, is the recognition of the impact of long-term, chronic conditions on health expenditure. This has placed greater emphasis on the possibilities for professional/patient partnership and on day-to-day self-management. The adoption of the Expert Patient Programme by the NHS is one example of this (Department of Health 2001). The programme is a development from an earlier initiative developed at Stanford University in the United States and now covers an estimated 13,000 patients, providing support and training for patients to manage their own condition.

This broader view of heath has in turn contributed to an interest in, and acceptance of, patient narratives as an important method and type of data in designing health services. Patient narratives take many forms, but in general they provide a temporal framework for the patient experience and help people to explore the impact, meaning and understanding of their illness experience and how this affects broader social networks and lived experience (Kleinman 1988; Frid et al. 2000; Bury 2001). The use of patient narratives and the study of patient pathways or journeys through the illness and treatment process put further pressure on health care to be more human and holistic (Carlick and Biley 2004). Furthermore, acknowledging the value of qualitative research in health in terms of providing access to the patient experience is potentially an effective mechanism for increasing patient satisfaction and their willingness to follow medical advice. This may be one factor behind the increasing acceptance of qualitative methods among physicians.

At a more macro policy level, the recent report by Wanless (2004) on future health strategy in the United Kingdom urges the government and the NHS to pursue a 'fully engaged scenario' in order to mitigate the impact of chronic illness, and to ensure that all members of the public feel responsible for their health and are encouraged to act in ways that work with, rather than against, clinicians. This is a challenge for the researcher as it implies a reconceptualization of 'health work' as an activity that takes place both outside and inside clinical settings.

The consequences for researchers of a holistic approach

The implication for researchers is that research methods suited to exploring lifestyle and the experiential aspects of health care as well as classic epidemiological data about incidence, morbidity and mortality are required. Researchers must also consider various types of theoretical and conceptual frameworks to explain their findings. Clinical knowledge must be integrated with social science expertise as well as other disciplines, such as history and statistics, in order to explore and understand contemporary health care. Multidisciplinary research in health care is challenging as it goes against the historical hierarchies of knowledge in medical care. Researchers must now attempt to draw in the range of health professionals who are concerned with diagnosing, treating and caring for people. These factors indicate increased complexity in the research process and underline the importance of good research management.

Research credibility

For research to have an impact on policy, on practice and on the thinking of professionals and academics, the findings must be credible. Many factors affect credibility, such as the research methods used; the findings and outcomes from research; the reputation of researchers; the status of the funding body; and the peer review process. The most fundamental factor is the first: the logic of the design, the management and process of the research, the methods used to collect data and their link to research questions, and the acceptance of the analytical framework adopted. These will all affect the perceived validity of the findings. The degree of fit or triangulation between the findings when using different methods is an important mechanism for ensuring acceptance of research findings.

Multiple forms of data derived from different methods, but analyzed and interpreted in an integrated fashion, are now seen to yield greater validity. However, in biomedical circles, as noted elsewhere in this volume, the randomized controlled trial (RCT) is still seen as representing the most powerful form of research evidence. The RCT yields quantitative, statistically validated results but, as suggested in Chapter 2, constructs physiological and social factors in a very particular way. The lack of recognition of epistemological differences is at the heart of some of the difficulties in integrating qualitative and quantitative data.

The credibility accorded different kinds of data is a reflection of different disciplinary cultures. The dominance of quantitative data and the RCT is in part a consequence of their centrality to epidemiology and medical training that draws on bioscience. This creates a culture in which issues of sampling, the representativeness of a sample and generalization are central to the evaluation of research findings. These criteria are antithetical to qualitative methods and interpretive data analysis. It is worth noting that in health care many of the decisions are made by a managerial or policy elite who may not be clinically trained. In the past, the longstanding bias of decision makers for 'hard' quantitative data with numerical measures of outcomes and effects is well known (Bowling 2002). This has undermined the opportunity for qualitative and mixed-method research to make a significant impact on health planning and policy, although it is worth noting that there were significant exceptions – for example, the work of Stacey on the care of children in hospitals (Stacey et al. 1970; Hall and Stacey 1979).

Despite this dominant tradition, there is growing appreciation of the value of other methods and multiple-methods research. Dixon-Woods et al. (2001) and Donovan et al. (2002) argue that qualitative, and quality of life, measures should be integrated into RCTs. It is also apparent that an increasing number of published articles in health journals adopt a mix of methods. Similarly, it has also been recognized that multiple methods employed by a multidisciplinary research team are likely to maximize the opportunities to present a study and research findings as legitimate and valid. One of the values of a multidisciplinary research team is their familiarity with a range of audiences and dissemination routes. This will enable a tailoring of the findings and a presentation of the research design that is more appropriate and acceptable to different kinds of research consumers.

Case study: Mixed methods and multidisciplinary research in practice

An example of a project highlighting the benefits of mixed methods and multidisciplinary research is *Developing and Evaluating Best Practice In User Involvement in Cancer Services*, which was part of the United Kingdom Health in Partnership initiative that the author led between 2000 and 2003. It provides a good example of a collaborative project that used a variety of methods and relied on the participation of a range of organizations as well as managers, health professionals, service users

(Continued)

(Continued)

and academic researchers from a number of disciplinary backgrounds. The project was funded by the Department of Health over a three-year period, and was based at Avon, Somerset and Wiltshire Cancer Services. Two universities, the West of England and Warwick, and two voluntary organizations, the Bristol Cancer Help Centre and Cancerlink Macmillan, collaborated in the project as did a number of NHS Trusts. Drawing on the different expertise of the academic, voluntary sector and health service partners, the project aimed to identify how user involvement was understood and practised within one cancer network. Specifically, it aimed to:

- Identify the variety of definitions of user involvement and methods that had been used by different health organizations and multidisciplinary cancer teams.
- Develop a consensus statement on user involvement in cancer services that could be supported by a range of stakeholders.
- Explore the impact of user involvement on both providers and users.
- Document the influence of user involvement in training and support programmes.
- Identify facilitators and barriers to success in user involvement activities and find examples of good practice.

The research team adopted different research methods to fulfil these aims and research tasks were disaggregated into five phases that are described below.

Mapping user involvement activities across the network

The first task was to undertake a mapping exercise of existing mechanisms for user involvement in cancer services in the region. We focused on activity in the health service and the cancer voluntary sector, but also collected data from hospices and local government. Focus group discussions were used to construct two questionnaires: one for the voluntary and one for the statutory sector. These were then piloted extensively. In late 2000, the statutory questionnaire was administered to 65 individuals with a 68 per cent response rate. In early 2001, 70 local voluntary organizations providing support services were sampled from a database and the questionnaire administered in January 2001. The response rate was 57 per cent. From the data, a range of different definitions of

(Continued)

user involvement was identified. The analysis also showed the scope of user involvement and provided examples of implementation across the cancer network.

Consensus development around user involvement

In the second phase, we undertook a formal consensus development exercise applying both a two-stage Delphi exercise and the Nominal Group Technique to obtain information. Bowling (2002) describes these techniques (see also Daykin et al. 2002). She sees the Delphi technique as an efficient way of getting information from a large number of people. A postal questionnaire asking open-ended questions is sent to a range of experts on a topic who give answers anonymously. Their responses are recycled into a questionnaire and participants are asked to rank their level of agreement with the ranking. In the nominal group, or expert panel, process a small number of experts (around 12) decide their individual views on a topic or health intervention by ranking factors on a Likert scale from 0 (never use) to 9 (always use). At a subsequent meeting and sometimes after reading additional literature, the results are summarized, discussion takes place and panel members re-rank their views. In the cancer project, the techniques were used to agree a consensus statement on best practice in user involvement in cancer care. We drew on the expertise of 367 individuals from key stakeholder groups such as cancer doctors, managers, general practitioners, cancer nurses, users, cancer voluntary organizations and academic researchers. Our final statement identified nine key aspects that all participants agreed were central to user involvement.

Interviews with users about their experience of involvement

In the third phase, we undertook interviews with users about their understanding, experience and satisfaction with user involvement. Our sample of 37 users of cancer services included three groups: those with experience of user involvement; those who had taken part in a training programme alongside health professionals; and those with no experience. The interviews allowed us to explore factors that contributed to users' conceptions of what it meant to be involved and their level of satisfaction.

(Continued)

(Continued)

A survey of users' willingness to be involved

In the fourth phase based on the above interviews, a questionnaire was developed to survey users' attitudes towards involvement and their willingness to contribute to the evaluation and development of cancer services in the future. A random sample of 700 users that met particular inclusion/exclusion criteria was extracted from cancer registry data. The accuracy of the data was checked against patient records and, with approval from clinicians, 388 users were surveyed in the summer of 2002. The response rate was 67 per cent. The survey was the first to give an indication of the proportion of cancer patients who were willing to be involved in service development, and the factors that affect willingness to participate, such as demographic characteristics, cancer type and the level of satisfaction with care received. Based on a verified random sample of 388 surviving cancer patients drawn from the Regional Cancer Registry database in January 2002, 19 per cent had some experience of contributing to service development. Of these, 71 per cent said they would be willing to be involved again. Almost half (49 per cent) of those who had no experience said they would be willing to participate in the future (Evans et al. 2003).

Selected case studies of a cancer multidisciplinary team in three Trusts

The fifth phase of the study aimed to understand the differences in the interpretation, attitude and experience of user involvement within different trusts, and within the multidisciplinary teams responsible for treating different types of cancer. We conducted case studies in three trusts, one in each of the health authorities covered by the cancer network and with varying levels of user involvement. In each setting, we looked at the multidisciplinary teams delivering services to people with the same range of cancers – breast, colorectal, lung and prostate cancer – as well as palliative care. Key providers and managers were interviewed to establish policy, rationale and practice and those data were used to evaluate the user involvement system against criteria developed in the earlier stages of the project and from the literature.

Project management

This project also highlights the importance of project management in mixed methods and multidisciplinary research. Members of the team

(Continued)

came from different disciplines and were employed by different organizations outside of the project. Specific roles were established within the team to ensure appropriate management and support for researchers and administrative staff associated with the project. We set up a steering group to include service users. Following advertisements in local media and surgeries and clinics, two users agreed to serve although only one stayed throughout the project. We paid a monthly fee to users to cover reading, preparation and an additional fee for attending the steering group and associated travel costs. Time was allowed for discussion with cancer service users before and after meetings to keep them well briefed.

Much of the research in health necessarily involves working in a clinical context and with clinical colleagues. A major benefit from working in a clinical setting with a multidisciplinary team is the virtually open access it brings to health care professionals and to patients and patient data that would otherwise require lengthy negotiation. In particular, access to medical staff and medical networks can bring great benefits to the research process. From negotiating research ethics committees to gaining agreement from staff to participate in interviews or identify potential respondents, medical personnel add legitimacy to a research team. These benefits are often directly related to the seniority as well as the discipline of the staff member. In health care settings, status differentiation still runs along professional lines. For example, having the senior cancer consultant and ex-director of the Oncology Centre working in one of our projects helped to identify the names and location of key clinical managers within the eight area hospitals in the study. His experience of working in the local area for 20 years and his high profile in cancer care nationally helped to ensure that the team were well prepared when seeking access as well as providing credibility to the project.

THE CHALLENGES OF, AND STRATEGIES FOR, MULTIDISCIPLINARY WORKING

The experience of working on a multidisciplinary project suggests that a number of common difficulties and challenges arise when working across different institutional and disciplinary cultures.

Workplace style and culture

A culture may be so embedded in a workplace that members of a work team may be unaware that their working lives are governed by particular norms until these norms are breached. There were a number of occasions when this occurred on the cancer project. For example, the research team were based in local health authority accommodation provided for cancer network adminis- trative staff. Researchers had access to a 'hot-desk' in a large room shared by the administrative staff. Local researchers spent considerable time out of the office collecting data or attending meetings. The administrative staff kept to health service working hours arriving at 8.30 a.m. and leaving at 5.00 p.m. Researchers were accustomed to looser academic timetables. One team mem- ber, anxious to meet a writing deadline, completed a report at 8.00 p.m. only to find all the lights turned off in the building and the main entrance locked. They were only released after contacting the off-site security company.

Differences in the work cultures of academe and the public sector were evi- dent in differences in the requirements on employees for a visible physical presence at the workplace. For example, in the health service, people were only deemed to be working if they were visibly present at the desk or clinic. In acad- eme more emphasis is placed on work outputs and there is a greater degree of flexibility on where and when work is done. Management styles between the health service and academe also differed. Initially on the project, there was pressure for a directive and bureaucratic form of project management, in which critical dialogue about the direction and progress of the research was seen as rebellion. It was also expected that reports and potential publications would be vetted – possibly because there was fear of repercussions from above in response to negative comments on findings or process. Conversely, the acade- mic culture tends to be based on a higher degree of autonomy and flatter col- league relationships and puts a high value on critical comment.

Over time, team members became aware of different expectations and sensi- tivities and sufficient trust was built to reach accommodation on the require- ments of the various cultures of employment. However, multidisciplinary projects need to anticipate and allow for such learning.

Balancing the research team

In developing a research proposal, balancing the composition of the project team with the requirements of the research design is one of the primary objec- tives. Projects that adopt mixed methods are also likely to incorporate researchers from a range of disciplines. The specialization of individuals in particular methods may be a key justification for their inclusion in a research team. However, this can lead to a series of separate mini-research projects each of which has been conducted independently. Such an approach may serve as a barrier to a common conceptualization of the research problem and the opportunity to adopt an integrated approach to the analysis and the interpretation of data. The benefits of using different methods and data through triangulation may be lost and this in turn may undermine the validity of the research findings.

The challenge for research management

The difficulties of research management are likely to be increased when research teams come from different institutions and/or there is a separation of research responsibilities. Inevitably members of research teams who have had little history of working together and are drawn from different disciplinary backgrounds and work contexts will have different experiences and expectations of how to conduct research. Furthermore, applied research may be based on collaboration with staff who have little experience of research. Their expectations may be very different from those of the project team and funders. Lack of knowledge about work cultures, responsibilities and styles of working can lead to confusion, disagreements and inefficiency. Good project management, regular team meetings and investment of time in creating a common conceptualization of the whole project, the contribution of each objective to the project as a whole and their relationship to each other are the best way to avoid fragmentation.

Many projects establish an advisory group as an aid to project management. Typically such groups include representatives of stakeholders such as user groups, funding bodies, statutory authorities or independent experts with particular skills. These can be useful sources of advice and data for a project but can also add layers of communication that increase the administrative workload and may slow down decision making. It is important to establish roles and responsibilities at the start. Furthermore, the research team should be clear on what they want from an advisory group and prepare well for meetings.

Writing up results in multidisciplinary teams

The process of writing up and the attribution of authorship vary significantly between disciplines. For example, it is common in scientific disciplines for authorship to include the entire research team, while in the social sciences team members are credited in the text but do not necessarily appear as authors. As other chapters in this book point out, issues of authorship can cause unhappiness and conflict, so they are best tackled early. For a long-term project, items written late in the life of a project may cause particular difficulties. Junior members of the team may have left to take up other posts. Certain kinds of funding may not include time to write up findings for publication. Wherever possible, this should be costed and written into research proposals. These matters are discussed further in Chapter 21.

Moving from multidisciplinary to interdisciplinary research

The issues raised above highlight the different forms of collaboration in research and also suggest the distinction between multidisciplinary and interdisciplinary projects. The latter is premised on working through the differences in perspective and arriving at a consensus on an approach that is acceptable methodologically to all team members. The resulting research will be far more integrated and coherent and has greater potential to yield methodologically interesting results. However, interdisciplinary research requires a great deal of time and contact early in the project, in order to learn about and from the different member of the research team. Multidisciplinary research will yield important results but they will be different from those emerging from interdisciplinary work.

Box 16.1 *Example: globalization and citizens in health care*

Exploring the role of users, choice and markets in European health systems

This project aimed to explore the impact of the health care reforms in Finland, Britain and Sweden focusing on competition, marketization, patient choice and user involvement within the context of European Union and international legal regulation as reflected in the policies promoted by the Organization for Economic and Cooperation Development, the World Health Organization and the World Trade Organization. The project was funded by the Academy of Finland.

The majority of the research team were fluent in three languages: Finnish, Swedish and English. The language used within the team was English, but reports to the funder needed to be made in Finnish. The Advisory Group included Finnish, Swedish and British experts. The approach to policy making differed between the three countries and so did the scope of publicly available documentation. Furthermore, the same pieces of European Union legislation had been implemented at different rates as well, with different effects.

Cultural differences added to the complexity. For example, August tends to be a public sector holiday month in Britain. In Finland and other Nordic countries, however, this is considered early autumn and July is the main summer holiday month. The scheduling of interviews at the same time over the summer period is therefore difficult.

International research

Research that has an international aspect, because the study either draws data from different countries or involves researchers from different national backgrounds, presents particular challenges. Language differences themselves may make communication or comprehension difficult. If data are sourced in different languages the costs of translation must be taken into account. Translation may hide rather than reveal different underlying cultural assumptions. The example in Box 16.1 describes an international project and provides an illustration of some of the cross-cultural and cross-national issues that arise.

CONCLUSION

The use of a range of methods in a single research project is becoming commoner, as indeed is the multidisciplinary and international research explored in this chapter. Indeed, many of the chapters in this book illustrate these themes and Chapter 20 is devoted to the challenge of comparative research. Using mixed methods and working with colleagues both nationally and internationally can be achieved in small-scale as well as larger projects. There are both benefits and pitfalls and, as the research process becomes more complex, managing and planning the process becomes a major task.

In terms of using a number of methods in a single project, as argued in the chapter, it is extremely important to consider the purpose and value of using a particular method when planning a project. The epistemological status of the data collected, that is the nature of data and the kind of knowledge produced, should also be considered. Where different methods are being used the purpose and added value to understanding should be examined carefully. A crucial decision to be made is the order of data collection using different methods. As has been demonstrated here and in other chapters, there may be an argument for first using a qualitative method such as a focus group or in-depth interviews, to explore concepts and understandings of the research participants. The insights gained may then be incorporated into a questionnaire to test the generalizability of a hypothesis or for frequency of occurrence. However, there may also be an argument for an initial questionnaire to explore the frequency of a particular phenomenon, followed by, for example, in-depth interviews to investigate a different aspect of the phenomenon. A variety of combinations is possible, but it is vital that the reason for using a particular combination of methods and the associated value added are clear and that they fall within the available budget. An exercise follows to facilitate further understanding of some of the issues raised in this chapter.

Exercise: Mixed methods and multidisciplinary research application to develop support for people with coronary heart disease

You want to apply to a regional government office to consider how the experience of carers could be used to develop support for people who have coronary heart disease.

The exercise is designed to make you think about how to design research using mixed methods and drawing on multidisciplinary expertise. While the material contained in this chapter may help you consider many of the issues, you may wish to access additional material from a library or the Internet. If you want to prepare a formal answer, then write a research proposal or protocol.

1
- What sort of methods will you use?
- Consider the range of possible respondents and sources of information (this will include patients, carers, voluntary organizations, health professionals and information leaflets).
- Consider the patient pathway and how you will ensure that your data reflect the needs of people at different points in their journey through the illness and care process.

2
- How will you select the sources of data that are relevant?
- Consider what sort of methods you want to use.
- How will you manage generalizability?

3
- How will you bring together the analysis of different kinds of data?
- What forms of coding and analysis will be appropriate for each?
- What mechanisms will you use to create a common analytical framework and the opportunity for joint interpretation of the findings?

(Continued)

4
- What sort of resources will you need?
- Can you plot the different activities over time and in relation to resources?
- How do various types of project meetings fit into this timetable?

5
- How will you present your findings and to whom?
- What would be your plan for dissemination?
- What are the implications for authorship?
- How would you begin to cost your proposal?

RECOMMENDED FURTHER READING

Dixon-Woods, M., Fitzpatrick, R. and Roberts, K. (2001) 'Including qualitative research in systematic reviews: opportunities and problems', *Journal of Evaluation in Clinical Practice*, 7: 125–33.
This is an interesting consideration of how qualitative and quantitative evidence can be synthesized together and influence clinical practice.

Strauss, A. and Corbin, J. (eds) (1997) *Grounded Theory in Practice*. London: Sage.
This book engages explicitly with the issues of integrating the analysis of different kinds of data – exemplified by different research projects with diverse designs and objects of study.

Yin, R. and Campbell, D. (2003) *Case Study Research: Design and Methods*, 3rd edition. London: Sage.
This definitive book on the case study as a form of research usefully illustrates how to bring together a range of methods to generate a holistic understanding of specific areas.

REFERENCES

Bowling, A. (2002) *Research Methods in Health: Investigating Health and Health Services*, 2nd edition. Buckingham: Open University Press.
Bury, M. (2001) 'Illness narratives: fact or fiction?', *Sociology of Health and Illness*, 23: 263–85.

Carlick, A. and Biley, F.C. (2004) 'Thoughts on the therapeutic use of narrative in the promotion of coping in cancer care', *European Journal of Cancer Care*, 13 (4): 308–17.

Copeland, L. (2003) 'An exploration of the problems faced by young women living in disadvantaged circumstances if they want to give up smoking: can more be done at general practice level?', *Family Practice*, 20 (4): 393–400.

Daykin, N., Sanidas, M., Barley, V., Evans, S., McNeill, J., Palmer, N., Rimmer, J., Tritter, J. and Turton, P. (2002) 'Developing consensus and interprofessional working in cancer services: the case of user involvement', *Journal of Interprofessional Care*, 16 (4): 405–406.

Denzin, N. (1970) *The Research Act*. Chicago: Aldine.

Department of Health (2001) *The Expert Patient: A New Approach to Chronic Disease Management in the Twenty-first Century*. London: HMSO. Progress updates available at: http://www.expertpatients .nhs.uk/ about_progress.shtml

Dixon-Woods, M., Fitzpatrick, R. and Roberts, K. (2001) 'Including qualitative research in systematic reviews: opportunities and problems', *Journal of Evaluation in Clinical Practice*, 7: 125–33.

Donovan, J., Brindle, L. and Mills, N. (2002) 'Capturing users' experiences of participating in cancer trials', *European Journal of Cancer Care*, 11 (3): 210–14.

Evans, S., Tritter, J., Barley, V., Daykin, N., Sanidas, M., McNeill, J., Palmer, N., Rimmer, J. and Turton, P. (2003) 'User involvement in UK Cancer Services: bridging the policy gap', *European Journal of Cancer Care*, 12 (4): 331–8.

Frid, I., Ohlen, J. and Bergbom, I. (2000) 'On the use of narrative in nursing research', *Journal of Advanced Nursing*, 32: 695–703.

Hall, D. and Stacey, M. (eds) (1979) *Beyond Separation: Further Studies of Children in Hospital*. London: Routledge & Kegan Paul.

Kleinman, A. (1988) *The Illness Narratives*. New York: Basic Books.

Lowes, L. and Hulatt, I. (eds) (2005) *Involving Service Users in Health and Social Care Research*. London: Routledge.

Mackay, J. and Eriksen, M. (2002) *The Tobacco Atlas*. Geneva: World Health Organization.

Patton, M. (2002) *Qualitative Research and Evaluation Methods*, 3rd edition. London: Sage.

Silverman, D. (1993) *Interpreting Qualitative Data: Methods for Analysing Talk, Text and Interaction*. London: Sage.

Stacey, M., Dearden, R., Pill, R. and Robinson, S. (1970) *Hospitals, Children and their Families*. London: Routledge & Kegan Paul.

Tritter, J. and McCallum, A. (2006) 'The snakes and ladders of user involvement: moving beyond Arnstein', *Health Policy*, 76 (2): 156–68.

Wanless, D. (2004) *Securing Good Health for the Whole Population*. London: HMSO.

Yin, R. (1994) *Case Study Research: Design and Methods*, 2nd edition. London: Sage.

17

Researching Orthodox and Complementary and Alternative Medicine

JANET RICHARDSON AND MIKE SAKS

INTRODUCTION

This chapter addresses the challenges in researching health across the boundaries of orthodox medicine and complementary and alternative medicine (CAM), arguing that there is a strong case for adopting a more eclectic approach centred on both quantitative and qualitative approaches. It includes a discussion of the evidence base in orthodox medicine and CAM, as well as some of the specific challenges to research-ing the latter, linked to the politics of health – with suggestions as to how these may be overcome. The key themes of the chapter are illustrated by a case study involving the Lewisham Complementary Therapy Centre, in which one of the authors was centrally involved.

In this context, orthodox medicine and CAM are both defined politically in terms of how far at any point in time they are formally underwritten by the state – as regards, for example, the level of research funding and their inclusion in the undergraduate medical curriculum (Saks 2003). The heavily state-supported current Western medical orthodoxy is usually seen as being based on the biomedical model outlined in Chapter 2. This tends to place emphasis on objective indicators of health and to focus on specialized surgical and other procedures involving specific areas of the body in cases of disease pathology (Stacey 1988). In this biomedical approach the randomized controlled trial (RCT) described in Chapter 12 has been proclaimed as the definitive standard in research evaluations. However, this chapter highlights the difficulties inherent in applying this model to health care interventions other than those involving drug trials – even within orthodox biomedicine.

Outside the bounds of biomedicine, such difficulties are most strongly exemplified in the case of CAM, on which this chapter is centred. CAM consists of a diverse range of therapies outside the political mainstream, from aromatherapy and crystal therapy to acupuncture and homoeopathy. These do not share a common philosophy, but tend to be ideologically positioned more towards the holistic end of the spectrum – in which the subjective views of clients and mind–body links are usually regarded by their proponents as more central than in orthodox medicine (Saks 2000). This can be illustrated with reference to classical acupuncture where clients are treated holistically according to their individual characteristics through the insertion and manipulation of complexes of needles in prescribed points to adjust the energy flow along a system of channels called meridians that are held to run through the body (Saks 2005b). The key question, however, is whether the RCT is applicable to this area and, if not, how such therapies are to be assessed. A number of possible solutions to this research dilemma will be set out in this chapter using examples from research practice. Ultimately, it will be proposed that health care research in CAM and orthodox medicine requires a multidisciplinary approach and the use of diverse research methods to address the wide range of issues that arise.

THE DEVELOPMENT OF EVIDENCE-BASED ORTHODOX MEDICINE

Historically, the purpose of orthodox medical research has been to understand the mechanisms of disease, produce new treatments and use them pragmatically, not to test for effectiveness using a rigorous scientific method (Smith 1995). Despite their introduction in the mid-twentieth century, many conventional treatments have not been subjected to RCTs and as a result new interventions have been introduced on a wide scale on the basis of opinion rather than evidence (Smith and Rennie 1995). Many have also been employed widely before being shown to be harmful and of little benefit – as, for example, in the use of insulin coma therapy, leucotomy and regressive electro-convulsive therapy (ECT) for the treatment of schizophrenia (Andrews 1989). Innovations in health service delivery have also been unregulated and unevaluated, and few decisions have been made on the basis of sound evidence regarding their efficiency and safety in pragmatic settings (Fitzpatrick 1994).

Lack of evidence has therefore inhibited the effective use of resources and led to wide variations in clinical practice in diagnostic procedures and health care interventions in orthodox biomedicine, centred largely on drugs and surgery (see, for instance, Bloor et al. 1976). However, this is not to deny some of the dramatic advances in medicine from the use of antibiotics to hip surgery which have been evidence based and brought about substantial patient benefit (Le Fanu 1999). The very thin and patchy application of rigorous evaluative approaches in orthodox medicine in the United Kingdom eventually gave rise to a systematic NHS research and development programme to create an NHS where decisions are evidence based (Department of Health 1993), the basic principles of which have since been restated and embellished (see, for example, Department of Health 2006). This has placed the RCT even more centrally at the heart of the NHS. Nevertheless, some clinicians fear that 'scientific' evidence-based medicine threatens the 'art' of patient care, and will lead to the neglect of good clinical skills and experience (see, for example, Grahame-Smith 1995).

DEBATES ABOUT 'EVIDENCE' IN ORTHODOX AND COMPLEMENTARY AND ALTERNATIVE MEDICINE

The question as to what constitutes 'evidence' in orthodox medicine remains. The strongest type of evidence in biomedicine is thought to be provided by systematic reviews of well-designed RCTs as outlined in Chapter 12. Here the overall approach is 'reductionist' – as opposed to the more individualistically tailored approach in CAM – emphasizing the generation of objective 'hard data' to establish particular cause–effect relationships for generically defined diseases (Brown et al. 2003). The experimental methodology in RCTs, where strenuous efforts are made to isolate independent and dependent variables and eliminate 'non-specific' variables, has fitted closely with the theoretical assumptions contained in the orthodox biomedical model (Pocock 1983). This approach, however, can exclude the role of social, psychological and cultural factors in the development and resolution of health problems, and the experiences of health problems of different individuals – issues which have been central to CAM.

CAM has seen a dramatic recent rise in popularity with the public in the United Kingdom and most of the developed world (Saks 2003). However, there remains a lack of credible evidence for the effectiveness of CAM therapies. Despite queries raised about the efficacy and safety of some CAM therapies

(Ernst 2006), the main problem has been, with a few notable exceptions, the lack of methodologically rigorous studies that might convince the sceptics (Saks 2006). The debate on the most relevant methodological approaches to evaluating alternative therapies pivots on the apparent contrast and conflict of two different and diverse world views or paradigms (Vickers 1996), as discussed in Chapter 2. It is frequently asserted by practitioners of CAM that research methods developed in the orthodox biomedical frame of reference are not transferable to the evaluation of more holistic CAM therapies – particularly in relation to the application of RCTs (see, for instance, the debate over their appropriateness in cancer care in Block et al. 2004).

This is in part because those practising CAM therapies typically claim to treat the individual client specifically rather than providing a standard treatment for a given condition, as in orthodox biomedicine. This makes organizing subjects into control and experimental groups in a randomized trial – with the administration of placebo treatment alongside the therapy being evaluated – more problematic in the case of CAM than in drug assessment (Saks 2006). In this regard, blinding procedures also raise considerable difficulties in the evaluation of CAM as compared with trials of pharmaceuticals. The purpose of blinding is to exclude non-specific factors or placebo effects which may produce a desirable outcome, but which are not due directly to the active intervention. Yet even for many orthodox health care interventions it may be extremely difficult to arrange a double-blind trial with a credible placebo (Pocock 1983). Anthony (1993) also suggests that blind designs may be impossible in CAM as the therapist is usually regarded as an integral part of the intervention.

This critique fails to acknowledge adequately that, despite the ideology of holism, some CAM therapies like osteopathy for bad backs can be as mechanistic and reductionist as many of those in orthodox biomedicine (Saks 1997). In the case of acupuncture, this is well illustrated by the formula, as opposed to the classical, variant which involves needling the same points for a given condition, irrespective of the individual patient (Saks 1992). Even in relation to more holistic therapies, moreover, RCTs may be conducted in which both patients and practitioners are not blind to the procedure, as has happened in evaluating the effects of psychotherapeutic techniques, healing and prayer (Vickers 1996). Nonetheless, Black (1996) has argued that in such instances, the artificiality of the trial may reduce the placebo element of any intervention. This may limit the extent to which the researcher can capitalize on the non-specific treatment effects, and as in the case of more mechanistic CAM therapies, the outcome of the trial may reflect the minimum rather than the maximum level of benefit that can be expected.

It can be argued therefore that it is important to evaluate care as it is normally delivered in clinical practice. Who then decides which evidence is important? Reilly and Taylor (1993) used a survey approach to produce a profile of evidence required by general practitioner trainees for CAM and orthodox medicine. The same profiles for both were demanded by 59 per cent of respondents. However, 44 per cent placed greater emphasis on the patient experience for CAM and clinical trials than for orthodox medicine. However, purchasers of health care are accountable and are driven by limited resources. They must therefore ensure the greatest cost–benefit and value for money. Although CAM is increasingly provided in the NHS, especially in primary care through either direct provision or subcontracting relationships (Thomas et al. 2003), such parameters have undoubtedly led to short-term 'quick-fix' planning. This may have worked to the prejudice of CAM, especially as there is relatively little state funding for research as compared with orthodox medicine (Saks 2005a). This is despite recent government capacity-building initiatives following the field-breaking report on CAM by the House of Lords Select Committee on Science and Technology (2000) which favoured greater investment in research into CAM.

Patients, however, may be looking for different health benefits than those indicated by the results of conventional RCTs based on a biomedical model, particularly when they have long-term chronic disease. Increasingly, lay people place importance on such factors as how far treatment enhances or sustains emotional well-being, a healthier lifestyle and more satisfying relationships. This may lead to very different perceptions by patients of what constitutes relevant evidence in evaluating the efficacy of CAM and other therapies as compared with orthodox practitioners and researchers (Mercer et al. 1995). Furthermore, studies suggest that patients frequently choose CAM due to the adverse effects of conventional treatments and have low-risk perceptions of its use (Vincent and Furnham 1996). Although this may be regarded as a rather blunt instrument for gauging the efficacy of therapeutic interventions in clinical circles, subjective levels of consumer satisfaction with CAM have been consistently high whatever their objective deficiencies or merits (Saks 2003). In this sense, patients may have been disempowered by RCTs with their emphasis on objective rather than subjective outcome measures (Brown et al. 2003).

ORTHODOX MEDICINE AND THE POLITICS OF RESEARCH IN COMPLEMENTARY AND ALTERNATIVE MEDICINE

In terms of the 'politics' of research, it is important to note that doctors who are the prime beneficiaries of state research funding in health care in the United Kingdom have an interest in restricting their research to areas where they are recognized as competent, which may operate to the detriment of CAM research. This may explain, for example, the long history of the rejection of acupuncture as a therapy in modern times. It may also explain why, following public pressure in the 1960s and 1970s, doctors have been keener to examine acupuncture from a neurophysiological perspective with reference to the production of endorphins, rather than the traditional focus on balancing *yin* and *yang* along meridians (Saks 1992). The effect of this has been to limit research in acupuncture to pain and the treatment of addictions, rather than a wider application based on classical Oriental theories. These tend to lie outside the knowledge and experience of Western medical researchers. Nevertheless, from the viewpoint of medical interests, acupuncture has opened up new areas for doctors to colonize while at the same time avoiding legitimating the growing numbers of traditional acupuncturists operating in private practice. In turn, this has helped to maintain the status, income and power of the medical profession (Saks 2005b).

From this standpoint, it can be seen that research into health care, and the choice of research methodologies, is not simply a technical operation, but is also related to maintaining dominant medical interests (Mulkay 1991). The influence of such interests may also extend to the powerful multinational pharmaceutical companies which have generally seen CAM as a threat (Walker 1994), even if it could be argued that they themselves are now being colonized through the range of CAM preparations for standard conditions now available in chemists' shops and supermarkets. This raises serious questions about the main drivers for state and privately funded research in CAM and other areas of health care – and the extent of toleration of more eclectic approaches to research and how far the policies adopted are synonymous with the wider public interest (Saks 2006).

A good example of research into CAM that showed that the medical establishment does not always live up to high 'scientific' standards was a study based on a trial by Bagenal and colleagues (1990) that led to an attack on the Bristol Cancer Help Centre. This study suggested that women with breast cancer attending the centre – which offered a range of alternative health provision – were more likely to die earlier than those receiving orthodox medical treatment. Unfortunately, though, there were a variety of flaws in this study, such as poorly matched subjects in the trial and the control group (Stacey 1991). This meant that the research findings were not supported by the data. The effects of their publication nonetheless were devastating for the women concerned, which led to suggestions that the study was part of a politically inspired medical campaign to demonize CAM.

CHALLENGES TO RESEARCH IN ORTHODOX AND COMPLEMENTARY AND ALTERNATIVE MEDICINE

The example of the Bristol Cancer Help Centre highlights that the RCT is itself socially constructed and is not a neutral approach, as it inevitably rests on certain paradigmatic assumptions (see, for instance, Richardson 2003). As ever, the decision to use RCTs depends on the nature of the research question being asked (Dyson and Brown 2006). There are also further criticisms of the RCT when used in either CAM or orthodox medicine (Kelner et al. 2003). One key instance of these is the contentious methodological assumption underlying the use of the RCT that patients have no treatment preferences (Fitter and Thomas 1997). Whilst the issues that this raises can be overcome by using patient selection criteria (Brewin and Bradley 1989), critics like Heron and Reason (1984) go further in seeing clinical trials as a source of alienation as they separate the individual from what is going on in their body and decisions about treatment. In order to help to resolve such dilemmas about assessing efficacy, a number of alternative and complementary approaches to health research are now considered in turn.

The role of pragmatic and explanatory studies

One approach that addresses some of the problems concerned with RCTs is to make a distinction between pragmatic trials and explanatory trials. In a pragmatic trial, the intention is to study the policy context in which a therapy will be used and ask whether the therapy will work in everyday practice. The explanatory trial, on the other hand, tries to separate the policy into its constituent parts – for example, time, active intervention and therapeutic setting – to discover which specific component of an intervention produces the outcome (Schwartz and Lellouch 1967).

The main difference between pragmatic and explanatory studies is the extent to which protocol violations, such as patient non-compliance, are considered in the interpretation of the results. The explanatory approach confines the analysis to only those patients who receive therapy according to the protocol. Pocock (1983), however, suggests that all eligible patients, regardless of compliance, should be included in the analysis where possible. In the pragmatic trial all patients, including those who withdraw from therapy, need to be accounted for, and all protocol violations and major deviations should be recorded. Withdrawals and deviations are considered in the analysis to avoid distorting treatment comparisons. This is particularly important if patients are withdrawn because of side effects as they will otherwise not be reported and may therefore create uncertainty about the results of the trial, even if a lack of response data from those who withdraw may sometimes mean that they have to be excluded from the analysis (Pocock and Abdalla 1998). In relation to assessing the efficacy of CAM in particular, the term 'pragmatic' refers to a research design that allows practitioners to treat patients individually in clinical practice, in a manner that capitalizes on, rather than restricts, non-specific placebo effects. Meade and Frank (1993) illustrate how such a pragmatic approach using individualized treatments compared the policies of outpatient management and chiropractic for the treatment of low-back pain. Knipschild (1993) also advocates the use of pragmatic trials in comparing the best orthodox and CAM therapy for patients.

Two major problems exist for patient selection to CAM research trials. The first problem also relates to trials in orthodox medicine and originates from the premise that patients play an active part in the outcome of their treatment. In this model, the patient's motivation to follow treatment regimens is held to be influenced by preferences before treatment is started. In general, the greater the need for participation (for example, by following a special diet), the greater motivation is likely to influence outcome. In pragmatic trials the objective is to discover the effect and outcome of 'packages' of management, even though most treatments are complex, mixing supposedly active components with contextual factors – including the way treatment is given. In explanatory, as opposed to pragmatic, trials the contextual factors are 'equalized' by randomization and artificial constraints which do not allow the role of expectations in treatment outcome to be evaluated. Brewin and Bradley (1989) therefore suggest that the alternative is to optimize motivation by ascertaining patients' preferences prior to randomization to a treatment or control group by allocating them to their preferred treatment choice.

The second problem relates to patient selection that can be based on diagnosis by orthodox medical or CAM system criteria. Wiegant et al. (1991) propose that there are four possible ways of dealing with this dilemma:

- To follow selection criteria based on orthodox diagnosis.
- To base selection on orthodox criteria, but allow the practitioner to treat the patient on an individual basis according to the therapy they are practising.
- To conduct an initial trawl based on orthodox diagnosis, then create subdivisions according to the appropriate CAM diagnosis.
- To define selection criteria by following the CAM diagnosis alone.

Whatever means is chosen, it should be consistently employed. Combining this precept with a pragmatic trial that accounts in some way for patient preference and allows practitioners to treat patients on an individual basis goes some way to addressing the criticisms of using RCTs in CAM. In this frame of reference, blinding should be included in the design where possible, and every effort made to identify and control for potential bias in order to ensure that the outcome is due to the intervention.

The use of appropriate outcome measures

Health care intervention is intended to maintain or improve functioning and well-being, and subsequently to improve the quality of life. It is therefore very important to measure patients' subjective experiences of illness and the care that they receive in CAM research if trials are to be employed, especially given the significance that is accorded to this in the CAM field (Kelner et al. 2003). Yet the biomedical model of disease is rooted in a belief that this is an objective and measurable state – a philosophy that has often been enshrined in RCTs. Moreover, attempts to evaluate interventions purely in terms of this model have been contested due to limited success in producing objective standards of assessment and different perceptions of health and illness (Turner 2003). One of the anomalies in contemporary practice is that patients' subjective perception of personal well-being may be discordant with their 'objective' health status – for example, a person can feel ill without medical science being able to detect disease and many people live with pathologies of which they are unaware (Bowling 2004).

It is therefore important to employ appropriate outcome measures. Dixon and colleagues (1994) found that most health outcome assessments in use were multidimensional, the main indices being included in the Short Form 36 (SF-36). This has the merit of being well validated and used frequently as a generic quality of life measure in outcome assessment, as well as having been employed to evaluate CAM therapies (see, for instance, Fitter and MacPherson 1995). Outcome measures such as the SF-36 ask specific questions about physical, social and emotional functioning. However, it is also important to define and measure what is significant to the patient. In this respect, the Measure Yourself Medical Outcome Profile (MYMOP) is a very helpful patient-generated, individualized, outcome questionnaire (Paterson 1996). It is problem specific, but includes general well-being. It is suitable for a range of symptoms, which can be physical, emotional or social. It is brief, with only seven items, simple to administer and sensitive to change. Prior to commencing a clinical research trial or outcome assessment the nature of the research questions about CAM need to be clearly defined, and the selected outcome measures should be appropriate, valid and reliable.

Qualitative approaches

It is also vital to note that using such quality of life measures and trials in orthodox medicine or in CAM studies does not facilitate a deeper understanding of the experience of health and illness. In order to address this question, qualitative research methods can usefully be deployed. They are particularly appropriate to new fields of study where the experiences of individuals are of concern – providing rich descriptions of what it is like to experience illness or suffering. Pope and Mays (1995) suggest that qualitative approaches should be an essential component of health service research as they allow access to areas not amenable to quantitative research, such as by providing a fuller understanding of lay and professional beliefs. Various dimensions of such research methods and the specific balance of benefits and costs are explored in the chapters contained in Part III of this volume. These are reinforced by the general criteria for the evaluation of qualitative research set out in Box 17.1.

Box 17.1 *Criteria for the evaluation of qualitative research*

Four general criteria can be given for the evaluation of qualitative research:

- *Truth value*: This is subject oriented and not defined by the researcher in advance. Here the researcher recognizes there are multiple realities and attempts to report the perspectives of the informants as clearly as possible
- *Applicability*: This is the criterion used to determine whether the findings can be applied in other contexts or settings
- *Consistency*: This is whether the findings would be consistent if the enquiry were replicated without the same subjects or in a similar context
- *Neutrality*: This is freedom from bias in the research procedure and results

---

Source: Lincoln and Guba (1985)

Such approaches to ensuring validity and reliability are fundamental to challenging the criticisms of qualitative methods as 'quick', 'dirty' and 'at the bottom of the hierarchy of evidence' (Greenhalgh 1998). This is particularly the case when they are used in the CAM area that is already marginalized compared with orthodox medicine.

A recent systematic review and thematic analysis of qualitative studies in CAM specifically found that qualitative methods enabled an assessment of the integrity and feasibility of interventions and study design prior to large-scale clinical trials (Richardson et al. 2004). Qualitative studies provide an understanding of the complexity of the patient experience, including how the experience of the intervention impacts on the patients' self-knowledge, and important self-directed changes in behaviour and lifestyle. The extent to which experiencing an intervention also clarified for patients issues of meaning – or allowed them to explore meaning – and brought about a desire for inner change was a common finding in a number of studies.

Whilst strenuous efforts to control 'extraneous variables' are desirable in controlled clinical trials, it should also be recognized that in reality the world is not best conceptualized by being polarized into 'objective' quantitative and 'subjective' qualitative studies. This is highlighted by the fact that the therapeutic effect of any intervention will be at least partly due to the way that intervention is delivered (Helman 2001). Researchers have therefore attempted in various ways to evaluate the benefits of CAM therapies from chiropractic to homoeopathy using pragmatic trials that assess therapies in the context in which they are practised in individualized treatments (Meade et al. 1990; De Lange de Klerk et al. 1994). In such trials, the intervention is often compared with an alternative or standard treatment or the use of a waiting list control group. This chapter concludes by indicating how the challenges that this poses can be addressed using a case study from the field – drawing heavily on the recent practical experience of one of the authors, Janet Richardson, in a CAM therapy centre in Lewisham.

Case study: The Lewisham Complementary Therapy Centre

The Lewisham Complementary Therapy Centre, on which this case study focuses, was recognized as a 'good model' of service delivery and evaluation that maintained the integrity of CAM therapies by basing its evaluation of effectiveness on pragmatic trials using sensitive approaches (Fulder 1996). It originated in June 1994 when an innovative new project was launched in Lewisham Hospital NHS Trust in South East London. The project introduced a number of CAM therapies into the NHS — acupuncture, homoeopathy and osteopathy — alongside an evaluation programme (Richardson 1995). The launch followed approximately four years of working towards raising the profile of CAM therapies within the hospital through study days, workshops, and establishing a massage and osteopathic service for staff within the hospital.

Janet Richardson established a steering group to draw together a proposal for funding the service. This was followed by setting up, organizing and managing the service once it was funded, and evaluating the outcome of the care it provided (Richardson 1996). The development of the service was based on a survey of local general practitioners to assess the level of support, followed by the generation of referral guidelines using a modified Delphi technique. The initial intention to conduct randomized controlled trials was hampered by lack of funding from medical research charities who considered funding the researcher but not the practitioners. A contract to provide the service was therefore sought and awarded by the relevant health authority. As agreed with the health authority, the evaluation took the form of an outcome assessment based on the SF-36 together with open-ended questions about expectations and experience, using the waiting list as a control group.

(Continued)

(Continued)

Patients attending the clinic for acupuncture, osteopathy and homoeopathy over a nine-month period were evaluated and their SF-36 scores, measuring eight dimensions of health, were compared with the waiting list controls. There were statistically significant differences in outcome between the treatment group (N = 179) and the control group (N = 151) on all dimensions of the SF-36 questionnaire with the exception of 'physical functioning'. Here the treatment group still had higher health status than the controls. As a result of a large non-response rate in the control group, sensitivity analysis was carried out in line with an 'intention to treat' approach. Based on the assumption that non-responders in the control group experienced a moderate clinical/social improvement, this demonstrated that the differences at outcome between the treatment and control group remained significant, except for mental health (Richardson 2004).

The evaluation of patient expectations prior to the intervention found that there was anticipation of relief of symptoms; a therapeutic/holistic approach; improvement in quality of life; provision of information; reduction of the risks of allopathic treatments; the need for self-help advice; and greater accessibility of such treatments on the NHS (Richardson 2004). Qualitative evaluation of the patient experience showed that patients experienced additional positive benefits such as relaxation and feelings of increased well-being; a therapeutic and 'holistic' approach; help to develop coping strategies; and being listened to by practitioners.

This service evaluation illustrates how a pragmatic approach can maximize the therapeutic effect, maintain the integrity of the intervention and benefit from both quantitative and qualitative research. It also provides an example of a systematic approach to service development. Fulder (1996) suggests that the Lewisham complementary therapy project was successful as a result of the specific referral guidelines that were established through intensive dialogue between doctors and the CAM therapists. The issue of dialogue was extremely important as the service was based on three 'complete' systems of treatment, two of which were grounded in world views very different from conventional medical science. Crucially, the focus of the dialogue was not inhibited by the different paradigms within which the CAM practitioners were working. For the local general practitioners, the issues were not about developing an understanding of health according to meridians in the case of traditional acupuncture, or the application of massively diluted substances containing no scientifically detectable active ingredient in the case of homoeopathy. They were about moving towards a collective

(Continued)

agreement about the kind of patients who might be helped by these treatments. This was achieved by the CAM practitioners translating their respective paradigms into a conventional diagnostic system.

Unfortunately, the Lewisham Complementary Therapy Centre had its funding withdrawn in spite of achieving positive therapeutic outcomes. This is a clear example of 'moving goal posts', and reinforces again how 'evidence' cannot be divorced from the politics of health care (Richardson 2003) – a theme which is very apparent in historical and contemporary debates over orthodox medicine and CAM in Britain and other societies (see, for instance, Saks 2003).

CONCLUSION

In summary, then, there are many questions to ask in research, and diverse questions require a range of approaches in researching CAM and more orthodox forms of medicine. Even very sophisticated RCTs can fail to detect the complexity that lies beneath the swampy lowlands in research linked to therapeutic outcomes (Richardson 2002). Researchers should therefore think very carefully about the nature of their questions, as well as their own motivation, and consider the possibility of a more eclectic approach to research methods in general and RCTs in particular, in line with the support given for mixed methods and multidisciplinary research in Chapter 16 of this book. The chapter has, therefore, suggested how research can be moved forward in relation to both orthodox medicine and CAM by going beyond the straightforward application of an RCT. It now winds up with an exercise for the reader that brings some of the themes the chapter has covered more sharply into focus.

Exercise: Researching the effects of massage on patients with cancer

With the question in mind of what is to count as evidence, and in light of the issues raised in this chapter about research questions and methodologies, consider the example below.

(Continued)

(Continued)

You are asked to design a study to evaluate the effects of massage on patients with cancer who are receiving supportive (palliative) care. Address the following questions:

1 What kind of study would you design and what method(s) would you use?
2 How would you recruit study participants and how many would you require?
3 What would you measure?
4 Who would you involve in the study — in terms of both researchers and practitioners?
5 Where would you apply for funding?

Finally, you may wish to consider what political issues may arise from the study.

RECOMMENDED FURTHER READING

Ernst, E. (ed.) (2006) *The Desktop Guide to Complementary and Alternative Medicine: An Evidence-based Approach*, 2nd edition. London: Mosby.
This is a good general overview which draws together some of the current international research evidence for CAM.

Richardson, J. (2004) 'Developing complementary therapy services: a systematic approach', *Health Psychology Update*, 13 (3): 23–33.
This article discusses further the establishment and evaluation of the CAM service established within an NHS setting in Britain, that is considered as a case study in this chapter.

Saks, M. (2003) *Orthodox and Alternative Medicine: Politics, Professionalization and Health Care*. London: Sage.
This is an important book for understanding the context within which orthodox and alternative medicine have developed in Britain and the United States and the significance of politics in the struggle for legitimacy in research and other areas.

REFERENCES

Andrews, G. (1989) 'Evaluating treatment effectiveness', *Australian and New Zealand Journal of Psychiatry*, 23: 181–86.

Anthony, H.M. (1993) 'Clinical research: questions to ask and the benefits of asking them', in G.T. Lewith and D. Aldridge (eds), *Clinical Research Methodology for Complementary Therapies*. London: Hodder & Stoughton.

Bagenal, F.S., Easton, D.F, Harris, E., Chilvers, C.E.D. and McElwain, T.J. (1990) 'Survival of patients with breast cancer attending the Bristol Cancer Help Centre', *Lancet*, 336: 606–10.

Black, N. (1996) 'Why we need observational studies to evaluate the effectiveness of health care', *British Medical Journal*, 312: 1215–18.

Block, K.I., Cohen, A.J., Dobs, A.S., Ornish, D. and Tripathy, D. (2004) 'The challenges of randomized trials in integrative cancer care', *Integrative Cancer Therapies*, 3 (2): 112–27.

Bloor, M.J., Venters, G.A. and Samphier, M.L. (1976) 'Geographical variations in the incidence of operations on the tonsils and adenoids: an epidemiological and sociological investigation', *Journal of Laryngology and Otology*, 92: 791–801.

Bowling, A. (2004) *Measuring Health: A Review of Quality of Life Measurement Scales*, 3rd edition. Buckingham: Open University Press.

Brewin, C.R. and Bradley, C. (1989) 'Patient preferences and randomised clinical trials', *British Medical Journal*, 299: 313–15.

Brown, B., Crawford, P. and Hicks, C. (2003) *Evidence-based Research: Dilemmas and Debates in Health Care*. Maidenhead: Open University Press.

De Lange de Klerk, E.S.M., Blommers, J., Kuik, D.J., Bezemer, P.D. and Feenstra, L. (1994) 'Effect of homoeopathic medicines on daily burden of symptoms in children with recurrent upper respiratory tract infections', *British Medical Journal*, 309: 1329–32.

Department of Health (1993) *Research for Health*. London: Department of Health.

Department of Health (2006) *Better Research for Better Health*. London: Department of Health.

Dixon, P., Heaton, J., Long, A. and Warburton, A. (1994) 'Reviewing and applying the SF-36', in *Outcomes Briefing*. Leeds: UK Clearing House on Health Outcomes – Nuffield Institute for Health, 4: 3–25.

Dyson, S. and Brown, B. (2006) *Social Theory and Applied Health Research*. Maidenhead: Open University Press.

Ernst, E. (ed.) (2006) *The Desktop Guide to Complementary and Alternative Medicine: An Evidence-based Approach*, 2nd edition. London: Mosby.

Fitter, M. and MacPherson, H. (1995) 'An audit of case studies of low back pain: a feasibility study for a controlled trial', *European Journal of Oriental Medicine*, 1 (5): 46–51.

Fitter, M.J. and Thomas, K.J. (1997) 'Evaluating complementary therapies for use in the National Health Service: "Horses for Courses". Part 1: The design challenge', *Complementary Therapies in Medicine*, 5: 90–93.

Fitzpatrick, R. (1994) 'Applications of health status measures', in C. Jenkinson (ed.), *Measuring Heath and Medical Outcomes*. London: UCL Press.

Fulder, S. (1996) *The Handbook of Alternative and Complementary Medicine*. Oxford: Oxford University Press.

Grahame-Smith, D. (1995) 'Evidence based medicine: Socratic dissent', *British Medical Journal*, 310: 1126–27.

Greenhalgh, T. (1998) 'Qualitative research', *British Journal of General Practice*, September: 1626–27.

Helman, C. (2001) *Culture, Health and Illness*, 4th edition. London: Arnold.

Heron, J. and Reason, P. (1984) 'New paradigm research and holistic medicine', *British Journal of Holistic Medicine*, 1: 86–91.

House of Lords Select Committee on Science and Technology (2000) *Report on Complementary and Alternative Medicine*. London: The Stationery Office.

Kelner, M., Wellman, B., Pescosolido, B. and Saks, M. (eds) (2003) *Complementary and Alternative Medicine: Challenge and Change*. London: Routledge.

Knipschild, P. (1993) 'Trials and errors', *British Medical Journal*, 309: 1706–1707.

Le Fanu, J. (1999) *The Rise and Fall of Modern Medicine*. London: Abacus.

Lincoln, Y.S. and Guba, E. (1985) *Naturalistic Inquiry*, Beverly Hills, CA: Sage.

Meade, T.W., Dyer, S., Browne, W., Townsend, J. and Frank, A.O. (1990) 'Low back pain of mechanical origin: randomised comparison of chiropractic and hospital outpatient treatment', *British Medical Journal*, 300: 1431–37.

Meade, T.W. and Frank, A.O. (1993) 'Manipulation and low back pain: an example of principles and practice', in G.T. Lewith and D. Aldridge (eds), *Clinical Research Methodology for Complementary Therapies*. London: Hodder & Stoughton.

Mercer, G., Long, A.F. and Smith, I.J. (1995) *Researching and Evaluating Complementary Therapies: The State of the Debate*. Leeds: Collaborating Centre for Health Service Research, Nuffield Institute for Health.

Mulkay, M. (1991) *Sociology of Science: A Sociological Pilgrimage*. Milton Keynes: Open University Press.

Paterson, C. (1996) 'Measuring outcomes in primary care: a patient generated measure, MYMOP, compared with the SF-36 health survey', *British Medical Journal*, 312: 1016–20.

Pocock, S.J. (1983) *Clinical Trials: A Practical Approach*. Chichester: Wiley.

Pocock, S.J. and Abdalla, M. (1998) 'The hope and the hazard of using compliance data in randomized controlled trials', *Statistics in Medicine*, 17: 303–17.

Pope, C. and Mays, N. (1995) 'Reaching the parts other methodologies cannot reach: an introduction to qualitative methods in health and health services research', *British Medical Journal*, 311: 42–45.

Reilly, D. and Taylor, M. (1993) 'Developing integrated medicine: Report of the RCCM Research Fellowship in Complementary Medicine, The University of Glasgow 1987–1990', *Complementary Therapies in Medicine*, 1 (Suppl. 1): 1–50.

Richardson, J. (1995) 'Complementary therapies on the NHS: the experience of a new service', *Complementary Therapies in Medicine*, 3: 153–57.

Richardson, J. (1996) 'Non-conventional therapy in the NHS: can it work?', *International Journal of Alternative and Complementary Medicine*, July: 20–21.

Richardson, J. (2002) 'Evidence-based complementary medicine: rigour, relevance and the swampy lowlands', Editorial, *Journal of Alternative and Complementary Medicine*, 8 (3): 221–23.

Richardson, J. (2003) 'Complementary and alternative medicine: socially constructed or evidence-based?', *Healthcare Papers*, 3 (5): 30–36.

Richardson, J. (2004) 'Developing complementary therapy services: a systematic approach', *Health Psychology Update*, 13 (3): 23–33.

Richardson, J., Smith, J. and Pilkington, K. (2004) 'Qualitative research in complementary therapies: is it of any value?', *FACT (Focus on Alternative and Complementary Therapies)*, 9 (1): 43.

Saks, M. (1992) 'The paradox of incorporation: Acupuncture and the medical profession in modern Britain', in M. Saks (ed.), *Alternative Medicine in Britain*. Oxford: Clarendon Press.

Saks, M. (1997) 'Alternative therapies: are they holistic?', *Complementary Therapies in Nursing and Midwifery*, 3: 4–8.

Saks, M. (2000) 'Medicine and the counter culture', in R. Cooter and J. Pickstone (eds), *Medicine in the Twentieth Century*. Amsterdam: Harwood Academic.

Saks, M. (2003) *Orthodox and Alternative Medicine: Politics, Professionalization and Health Care*. London: Sage.

Saks, M. (2005a) 'Improving the research base of complementary and alternative medicine', Editorial, *Complementary Therapies in Clinical Practice*, 11: 1–3.

Saks, M. (2005b) 'Regulating complementary and alternative medicine: The case of acupuncture', in G. Lee-Treweek, T. Heller, S. Spurr, H. MacQueen and J. Katz (eds), *Perspectives on Complementary and Alternative Medicine: A Reader*. London: Routledge/Open University.

Saks, M. (2006) 'The alternatives to medicine', in J. Gabe., D. Kelleher and G. Williams (eds), *Challenging Medicine*, 2nd edition. London: Routledge.

Schwartz, D. and Lellouch, J. (1967) 'Explanatory and pragmatic attitudes in therapeutic trials', *Journal of Chronic Disease*, 20: 637–48.

Smith, R. (1995) 'The scientific basis of health services', *British Medical Journal*, 311: 961–62.

Smith, R. and Rennie, D. (1995) 'And now, evidence based editing', *British Medical Journal*, 311: 826.

Stacey, M. (1988) *The Sociology of Health and Healing*. London: Unwin Hyman.

Stacey, M. (1991) 'The potential of social science for complementary medicine', *Complementary Medical Research*, 5 (3): 183–86.

Thomas, K.J., Coleman, P. and Nicholl, J.P. (2003) 'Trends in access to complementary or alternative medicines via primary care in England: 1995–2001', *Family Practice*, 20: 5.

Turner, B.S. (2003) 'The history of the changing concepts of health and illness: outline of a general model of illness categories', in G.L. Albrecht., R. Fitzpatrick and S.C. Scrimshaw (eds), *The Handbook of Social Studies in Health and Medicine*. London: Sage.

Vickers, A.J. (1996) 'Research paradigms in mainstream and complementary medicine', in E. Ernst (ed.), *Complementary Medicine: An Objective Appraisal*. Oxford: Butterworth–Heinemann.

Vincent, C. and Furnham, A. (1996) 'Why do patients turn to complementary medicine? An empirical study', *British Journal of Clinical Psychology*, 35: 37–48.

Walker, M. (1994) *Dirty Medicine: Science, Big Business and the Assault on Natural Health Care*. London: Slingshot.

Wiegant, F.A.C., Kramers, C.W. and van Wijik, R. (1991) 'Clinical research in complementary medicine: the importance of patient selection', *Complementary Medical Research*, 5 (2): 110–15.

18

Researching the Health of Ethnic Minority Groups

MARK R.D. JOHNSON

INTRODUCTION

It is now widely recognized that the United Kingdom is a multicultural society. In consequence, there is interest in, and a need for, research into the health of ethnic minority groups. Minority populations are growing in both size and complexity and new groups of migrant origin continue to be added to the national community. In the 2001 decennial census of the population, in England nearly 1 in 10 of the population gave their ethnic origin as being from one of the 'black and minority ethnic groups' (www.statistics.gov.uk/census2001/profiles/commentaries/ethnicity.asp). However, these figures may not include members of some white ethnic minorities, who may have found the new census categories inappropriate to their circumstances. The form only offered 'British, Irish and Other White' as sub-categories of the White group.

Particularly since the report of an official Commission of Inquiry in 1999, following the death of a young black man, Stephen Lawrence, both politicians and policy makers have given increasing attention to the needs of minorities. The Macpherson Report (1999) led to official recognition that many procedures and organizations were 'institutionally racist', as they did not take differences in ethnicity or culture into account. Subsequent legislation including the Race Relations (Amendment) Act 2000 and the European Human Rights Act has placed the rights of minorities on a stronger base. Consequently, increasing attention has been focused on the health and social care needs of minority groups. Both Labour governments and senior health officials have stated that identifying and meeting needs of these communities is a priority for the NHS (Crisp 2004).

This chapter argues that ethnicity is a key variable in explaining inequalities in health and therefore an important area of study. However, there are major challenges in identifying ethnic origin. Both narrow and broad definitions are considered together with some of the approaches commonly used by social researchers. Some useful national sources of baseline data on ethnic minorities are given and the chapter concludes with a case study of an action research project where members of the community helped to develop research questions and carry forward the research process. Some general principles for conducting action research are suggested.

KEY VARIABLES IN THE PATTERNS OF HEALTH AND DISEASE

Over recent decades, a consistent finding of research into health inequalities among ethnic minority groups has identified inequalities in access to care and in the outcomes of many health care interventions with ethnic minority groups having less good access and poorer health outcomes (Johnson 2003). It has also been established that for certain conditions and diseases there are distinctive patterns of prevalence; the prognosis for the course of the disease may differ; and so may treatment needs between ethnic minority communities and from other groups (Gill et al. 2002). In consequence, ethnic differences have attracted the attention of scientists seeking to understand diseases as ethnic variation provides the basis for a form of natural experiment: that is, cultural and genetic differences may explain variation in patterns of health and disease between groups within a population. There is a considerable literature that describes the patterns of health and disease associated with 'race' and 'ethnicity'.

'Race', culture and ethnicity are not the only factors that influence patterns of health and disease across groups. Social status or class factors have long been shown to affect health. However, there are difficulties in making a link between the class group to which people belong by virtue of their occupation, and the ill-health of particular individuals within that class. Social class is a crude label as class may be changed simply if occupation is changed. It does not reflect the lifetime experiences that contribute to health and ill-health. Gender also affects health in many and complex ways, and some social analysts will describe women as effectively a minority, at least in terms of their relationship to the main dimensions of power in society. Gendered inequalities in health – and also differences between gender groups in different ethnic or social communities – are very important, but cannot be fully explored in a short chapter. However, no research into ethnic minority groups should assume that the health needs of men and women are identical. Both gender and class factors within ethnic minority groups will have an effect on health status.

RESEARCHING ETHNIC MINORITY HEALTH: SOME CHALLENGES

A number of problems occur when starting to research 'ethnicity' in health. A first and critical problem is one of definition: what is meant by ethnicity and what is an ethnic group? Second, particularly if a quantitative method is being followed, there is the problem of sampling. In order to sample, the size of the population to be sampled from must be known. Such information may not be readily available and the population characteristics may not be known. These two issues complicate the questions of choosing the most appropriate research design, whether quantitative or qualitative, and developing the most appropriate instruments in a situation where language, access and accessibility will require careful and informed thought. The challenges are explored in the following sections of this chapter.

Problems of definition

Since the late 1970s following a world conference of social and physical scientists, the term 'ethnic' has almost entirely replaced the word 'race' in most scientific discussions of population migration and mixing. Here, it was agreed that 'race' as a concept had no essential scientific validity (Banton 1977). In common parlance, the term 'ethnic' is also used as a form of shorthand to describe people and groups of people who are 'different'. However, we must recognize that the terms 'race and racism' continue to be used in both popular and political discussion. The existence of racism, defined as a belief, or action based on a belief, that one's own group of origin is inherently superior to others, is a social reality. Indeed, many current tensions may be traced to the existence of racist ways of thinking and their consequences.

There is considerable uncertainty about the definition of ethnicity and the use of the term in scientific, medical or health and, social care research (LaVeist 1994). It is perhaps best to recognize, first, that 'ethnicity' is a complex, many-layered concept, and, second, that it is not fixed but dynamic. Culley (2000) observes that 'ethnicity' refers to a socially defined group of people who may be characterized by such factors as culture and language. However, ethnicity is also the ever-changing product of traditions and cultural practices. It is situational and contextual. Other key elements that mirror definitions in the legislation of the United Kingdom Race Relations Act include not only culture, language and religion, but also shared origins, or at least a shared 'myth of origin'. These myths may be passed from generation to generation. For example, Jews may trace their ancestry to Abraham and Isaac. However, myths of origin can also be relatively modern creations (Cashmore 1982).

In health-related research, the key elements of ethnic identity have been shown to have direct relevance to health care needs and outcomes (Johnson 2003). When used to describe groups of a particular migrant origin, ethnicity may be associated with cultural factors that may affect health status, with exposure to specific risk factors. Migration itself may also affect health, as well as the ability of migrants to access health services in their new country. Culture itself is a multilayered concept that includes many aspects of belief and behaviour, some learned and some linked to cherished aspects of identity. It might include language, religion and exposure to, or preferences for, certain types of music and art. History, including a sense of the history of a family, group or nation, may be a part of a culture as well as shared experiences of discrimination or exclusion.

Language is usually learned from the parent (hence the term 'mother tongue') and language may help to unite or divide. On the Indian subcontinent, the use of different scripts is the main marker between those described as speaking 'Punjabi' (used by Sikhs and Hindus in certain parts of India) and 'Urdu' (a language essentially similar in vocabulary to Punjabi when spoken, but using a written language derived from Arabic or the Persian Farsi). In the United Kingdom, many families of South Asian people who settled in British cities came from the Mirpur District of Kashmir. This is a region divided between the nation states of India and Pakistan, and there is a growing desire to describe their family language as 'Mirpuri'.

The politics of definition in researching ethnicity

The discussion above indicates that the choices of terms are themselves political matters. Categories and labels change over time and differ across countries. Many studies now include a short description of their use of terms. For example, a common justification of using the word 'black' is that it is a collective term used to indicate groups that share a common history of social exclusion and discrimination. In North America, the terms used to describe 'Native Americans' or 'Indians' have undergone a long process of evolution. Some authors use terms such as 'First

Nation' or 'Aboriginal'. The latter is also used in Australia, rather than the more pejorative term 'Aborigine'. The 'tribal' name of the group may also be used for the same reason. In North America, the label 'Asian' tends to refer to people whose origins are in 'South-East Asia', countries such as Vietnam, Cambodia/Khmer, Thailand or Korea. On the other hand, people from these countries may be grouped with those from the Pacific islands (Sadler et al. 2003).

In the absence of a scientific consensus, the most authoritative listing can be found in the National Institutes for Health (NIH) National Library of Medicine 'MeSH' (Medical Speciality Heading) catalogue used in PubMed and other databases. A recent revision states that the term 'Racial Stocks', pointing to categories of 'Australoid', 'Caucasoid', Mongoloid' and 'Negroid', has been abandoned because of the lack of scientific biological validity and its potentially offensive nature. Since 2004, 'Ethnic Groups' has been adopted as a term within the overall group heading of 'Continental Population Group origin'. This group includes an Oceanic Ancestry Group that refers to the Pacific islands and rim; European, African and Asian Ancestry Groups. The group formerly known as 'Black' in United States parlance is now recorded as African American, while Eskimos are generally known as Inuit (see www.ncbi.nlm.nih.gov/entrez).

In the United Kingdom, attempts have been made to break down the term Asian or South Asian (Bhopal et al. 1991). The exercise has been of some value in differentiating between the health experiences of some major groupings (Modood et al. 1997), although it could be criticized for being essentialist and/or creating adverse stereotypes. The majority of South Asian people living in the United Kingdom have fairly recent family connections to the larger states within the Indian subcontinent: notably India, Pakistan and Bangladesh. But many, including significant numbers of refugees and professionals, originally came from Sri Lanka, or were of 'Indian' origin when that was a single state under the English Raj. Some indeed had been settlers in various states in East Africa. Furthermore, India itself is one of the most populous and most diverse nations in the world, encompassing many distinctive languages and cultures, with significant numbers of followers for virtually every world religion.

The question of ethnic origin is important as United Kingdom data on health outcomes show that people of Muslim, particularly Bangladeshi and Pakistani, background have worse health and less satisfactory encounters with health services than those of other religions or national backgrounds (Acheson 1998). For this reason, it is necessary to consider precisely which system of ethnic categorization should be used in a particular health research project.

Self-identification and its limitations

One generally accepted approach among social scientists to the issue of 'ethnicity' is to insist that ethnic identity is a personal issue. The ascription of ethnic identity should therefore be made by the person being researched and not by the observer. For instance, an observer might easily ascribe a wrong label to a dark-skinned Devonian born in England or a light-skinned Pathan from Pakistan, if visual identification was used as a criterion, quite apart from any prejudices held by the observer. Guidance issued to the NHS and other bodies on 'ethnic monitoring' strongly supports the idea of self-identification. Public bodies are now required to collect data on ethnicity to overcome the disadvantages associated with racialized discrimination. However, a question such as 'To which ethnic group do you belong?' could create an almost infinite number of categories. It might also be impossible to compare any data collected with baseline data. This is a requirement for most scientific and health-care-related research.

There are also clinical reasons for wishing to identify members of certain ethnic groups who are at most risk of developing, or giving birth to children with, certain genetic conditions and a number of studies set out to test what category labels are most effective in identifying members of at-risk groups (Aspinall et al. 2003). Studies have found that it is possible to offer a selection of group labels which are meaningful to respondents and also have some predictive value for clinical purposes. Similarly, in epidemiological research it has been found possible to identify certain categorical labels that are recognized and accepted, and which also relate to clinical differences in health outcomes (Comstock et al. 2004). It is generally accepted that it is desirable when carrying out research to offer respondents a list of possible categories from which to choose, even if this restricts their choice. As in any social science research, the category 'other: please specify' provides a residual option.

The problem in data collection of shifting identities and social categories

National surveys and the decennial census are important sources of data on ethnic minority groups for researchers and, over the years, the Office of National Statistics (ONS) has devoted considerable effort to developing questions for these. The ONS notes that an individual's description of their ethnic group may change over time as, for quite legitimate reasons, a person may record themselves as belonging to one ethnic group at one time, and another when asked the same question on another occasion. Social and political attitudes change over time as noted above in relation to North American studies. In Britain, 'black' was at one time an unacceptable term, but it is now widely used as it stands for the groups concerned as a statement of political awareness and solidarity. In other words, any ethnic group label is only valid for the period and the context in which it is used. To overcome this problem, the ONS maintain a 'data-bridge' of categories to be used in surveys, including the census (National Statistics 2003). This provides a way of linking the terms used over time so that longitudinal work can be carried out.

In the United Kingdom, the decennial census is the major national set of data available to social science researchers which incorporates data on 'ethnicity' and it has become the accepted wisdom to use the so-called 'Census Ethnic Question' drawn from the 2001 Census for England and Wales, shown in Box 18.1. The question asked people to indicate 'which ethnic group' they felt best described their origins. The majority (over 85%) opted for 'White British' and thus, by definition, all other categories can be regarded as 'minority ethnic' groups. White British includes 'White Irish' and other white groups. The form makes it explicit that ethnicity is seen in terms of a 'cultural background' rather than seeking to identify place of birthplace, nationality or even descent. The higher level group headings, shown in bold below as 'Asian or Asian British', 'Black or Black British', make this point clearly. In Scotland and Northern Ireland, slightly different options were offered to take account of the much smaller numbers of people in the population from these minority groups.

Box 18.1   *'Minority Ethnic Group' categories in the 2001 Census*

What is your ethnic group? Tick the appropriate box to indicate your cultural background

White:
White — British
White — Irish
White — Any other White background (please write in)
Mixed:
Mixed — White/Black Caribbean
Mixed — White/Black African
Mixed — White/Asian
Any other mixed background (please write in)
Asian or Asian British:
Asian or Asian British: Indian
Asian or Asian British: Pakistani
Asian or Asian British: Bangladeshi
Asian or Asian British: Any other background (please write in)
Black or Black British:
Black or Black British: Caribbean
Black or Black British: African
Black or Black British: Any other background (please write in)
Chinese or other ethnic group:
Chinese or Other Ethnic group: Chinese
Chinese or Other Ethnic group: Any other (please write in)

Source: Adapted from ONS Census form (National Statistics 2003)

While this categorization has proved adequate for most national research and many local studies, it omits other identifiable groups such as Arab, Somali, Yemeni and Vietnamese. These population groups may be significant in particular localities or of interest for certain kinds of health care research. It has been recognized that such groups should be included in local listings, and guidance is available from the ONS on the best ways to incorporate these categories into data to make projections compatible with the census data (National Statistics 2003). This still does not take account of many groups, especially those who may be defined as 'new migrants', including refugees and asylum seekers. There is at present no solution to this – but, as there are no nationally available data on the ethnic or national background composition of refugees and asylum seekers in Britain, the requirement to collect data which can be used to compare with a baseline estimate does not apply.

In many health research studies designed to identify health needs and behaviours, a religion had been the label used to identify certain groups: for example, Jews or Sikhs (Johnson 2004; Bonney 2004). Consequently, it is advisable for the researcher to include a separate question on religious adherence or membership. The ONS has collected some national data using a well-tested question to cover this matter, as have the Fourth National Study of Minority Groups (Modood et al. 1997) and the Health Survey for England (Erens et al. 2001). In yet other studies, the ability to communicate in a particular oral or written form has been a marker for culture and ethnic identity. A question on language could be couched in terms of a 'preferred' language or communication, a 'mother tongue' or the language 'used at home' and used to explore the ways in which ethnic identity is constructed and expressed.

RESEARCHING ETHNIC MINORITY HEALTH IN PRACTICE

From a methodological perspective, it is clear that there is no single 'right answer' to the issue of researching the role and nature of ethnicity in health. The solution adopted by many researchers therefore is one of triangulation: that is, using a variety of approaches and perspectives to obtain a rounded picture (see also Chapter 16 for a discussion of triangulation). One particularly effective approach is the 'social action' research model. This combines elements of survey and ethnographic or qualitative methods, particularly through using focus groups or unstructured interviews with 'action research', where a process of capacity building and community or service development is incorporated into the research design (Fleming and Ward 1999; 2004). The advantages are that by working closely with members of the communities concerned many of the problems of being an outsider can be avoided. Working with a community can increase a researcher's understanding of the significance of what is observed by the researcher in terms of health behaviour and attitudes to health and illness. Questions may also be asked in a way that is relevant to the culture, as opposed to asking questions which have no relevance or cannot be answered within the terms of reference of the culture. The stages of the action research model developed by Morjaria-Keval and Johnson (2005) are shown in Box 18.2 – further discussion on experience and application can be found in Chapter 8.

Box 18.2 *Using a social action model in researching ethnic minority health*

The application of a social action model in researching ethnic minority health

Stage 1: Getting started
A health research study working with minority communities should be based on a sound review of needs. Data from national and local sources should be obtained and consultation undertaken with the 'expert' community. A literature review should be undertaken on scholarly sources and the 'grey' literature (see Chapter 2). Local reports often contain valuable information.

Stage 2: Recruit key worker(s)
Experience of working within minority cultural communities is necessary, as well as a commitment to change, and to the community. Once appointed, key workers need extensive training and briefing in all aspects of the project, including on health matters related to the project and the statutory and voluntary services provided locally.

Stage 3: Recruit and train community facilitators
The key element of the social action research model is the use of locally recruited community fieldworkers who are given basic training in research and substantive issues. If possible, this should be provided to a certificated level of competence. Our experience is that most local minority communities possess extraordinary reserves of well-qualified, highly committed and resourceful people. Some basic level of education and dual language ability is essential as well as personal qualities such as respect for community members and other groups.

Stage 4: Develop survey questions/topic guide for interviews
Expert advice should be sought from community facilitators to test the findings from the literature and the initial priorities of the project. During the training, community facilitators should be encouraged to comment on the research instruments and topic guides.

Stage 5: Conduct interviews
The agenda or topic guide may be used to establish the views and perceptions of communities, service users and providers against a common template. It is likely that facilitators will use their community's own language, and provide a translated report on the discussions or interviews.

Stage 6: Review, analyze and feed back
It is essential to confirm or validate the analysis of transcripts from interviews with the community facilitators and other informants. An opportunity to comment on the researchers' data analysis should be given prior to circulating reports to sponsors and service providers.

Stage 7: Take appropriate action – further intervention
It may be necessary to revise plans during the course of the project. The importance of assertive outreach and information giving is well established. Resources should be used flexibly to achieve this. It is essential to honour the pledge that the research will contribute positively to community development.

Stage 8: Evaluate and disseminate
The evaluation of outcomes and a dissemination strategy should be planned at the outset and modified as the project progresses. Key audiences include the communities that have taken part as well as practitioners and academic peers. Findings should become part of an official record in order for others to learn from the research.

Case study:	Ethnic minority health research using a social action approach

Background

In the 1990s, the NHS Executive Ethnic Health Unit was responsible for setting up a number of developmental projects, to bring about change in the way health care was provided and to promote improvements in the health status of minority groups across Britain (Chan 1997). One of the projects was the 'Sahara' project in Birmingham, designed to bring about change in the health behaviour of men in the Asian communities (Johnson and Verma 1998). In this case, 'Asian' was not defined. The project coordinators, including the author, interpreted their brief broadly. A central aim in the project was to explore existing perceptions of health and ill-health and to find out the priorities of males as previous studies had focused on women. The project also aimed to enable local community organizations to conduct the research through providing training and support. From a very early stage, project researchers worked closely with community organizations such as neighbourhood centres and religious groups who were responsible for finding community facilitators and recruiting the members of focus groups. Seven organizations were identified, who recruited 24 volunteers who were given training and paid as discussion group facilitators. The interviewers drawn from local groups were matched to the groups they were interviewing to ensure a better understanding of culturally specific concerns.

Refining the research questions

During the training, it became apparent that the men recruited represented, in their own terms, more than a dozen self-identified ethnic groups, so that the 'Pakistani' group contained representatives of people from the Kamalpuri/Campbellpur district; Pathans, Mirpuri or Kashmiri speakers; and people who described themselves as 'Pakistani Punjabi'. From the Indian side of the international border, there were also Hindu and Sikh Punjabis as well as Hindu Gujeratis.

Participants in the training were very vocal in discussing the appropriateness of certain questions, and suggested ways in which questions could be

(Continued)

(Continued)

phrased to ensure a worthwhile response. For instance, the normal practice in questionnaire design is to place the rather general question 'Are you happy with your health?' before a specific one: 'Are you happy with your level of energy?' We were advised by a representative that this would lead to the response for the second question: 'I have already said.' Placing the specific question first would allow the culturally appropriate response of 'no' while still expressing overall satisfaction with health. In other cases, we were advised to ask about 'some people' or 'others' in the community on the grounds that there were certain cultural taboos that community members would not breach. For example, it would be difficult for Muslims to admit to drinking alcohol, or Sikhs to say they used tobacco.

The social action research process

Following training, the community facilitators organized events and meetings in their community organizations, and obtained the agreement of groups of men to take part in focus group discussions that followed a predetermined topic guide. Discussions took place in a comfortable, familiar setting such as the community centre, or someone's home. Discussions were tape recorded, usually using the community language rather than English. The facilitators then wrote a report, transcribing relevant parts of the conversations, and added their comments on how these responses reflected community perceptions. During and after the discussion, facilitators also gave information about health, or offered help with specific queries. In this way, particular issues were raised and debated. In consequence, information began to reach those who had previously been outside existing systems of health promotion. Furthermore, we obtained extensive information on service use and, incidentally, the ease of access to, and use of, sport and exercise facilities that had not been included in the original survey design. It became clear that the different 'ethnic groups' had distinctive perspectives on their health needs and priorities. A major complaint was that 'Asian' services did not meet their needs, and, frequently, that one sub-group or another had managed to hijack the local agenda or facilities. This feedback was later used to develop facilities and health promotion locally.

This study demonstrated the potential for using locally recruited, community-based informants as research workers, as have other similar projects (Morjaria-Keval and Johnson 2005; Fleming and Ward 1999; Fleming and Ward 2004). Working with community members builds capacity, confidence

(Continued)

and a sense of ownership within communities that can be sustained after a project has finished. It also combats the accusation that needs are being ignored. Joint or collaborative studies can combine the rigour expected from scientific research with the virtues of insight from within the community. Box 18.2 illustrates the different stages of a social action research model, drawing on recent research in which the author was involved, supported by the Thomas Pocklington Trust and the Housing Corporation.

CONCLUSION

Research on health and access to health services is an important and relatively well-funded area of research, but full of pitfalls for the unwary. This chapter has looked at the problems of researching ethnicity, of which identifying the ethnic identity of research participants is a major issue. Various ways of thinking about, and determining, ethnicity have been discussed and key sources of baseline data identified.

Following up a theme addressed in Chapter 8 on action research, it is suggested that researchers in this area should aim to involve ethnic minority communities themselves in carrying out the various stages of research. Although this approach will require effective management of the research process, it has the advantage of working with, rather than on, communities as well as helping to improve the research from a technical perspective. Great care should be taken to honour any promises made to provide feedback to communities, or to seek service improvements as a consequence of the research.

Exercise: The take-up of services for the visually impaired from ethnic minority groups

The take-up of services for the visually impaired from ethnic minority groups is less than might be expected. Drawing on this chapter, consider from a health research perspective how you would address the following questions:

(Continued)

(Continued)

1 Why does it appear that people from ethnic minority groups are not taking up services for the visually impaired?
2 How would you raise awareness of and uptake of services currently being provided?
3 How far do we need to understand if 'needs' are the same or different from those of the majority community and whether different services or 'more of the same' are required?
4 Is the solution to work with communities to understand specific needs and generate materials to bring about change among service providers, as well as potential service users?

For more background information, see: http://www.pocklington-trust.org.uk/Templates/Internal. asp?Nodel D=89386

RECOMMENDED FURTHER READING

Johnson, M.R.D. (2006) 'Engaging communities and users: health and social care research with ethnic minority communities', in J. Nazroo (ed.), *Health and Social Research in Multiethnic Societies*. London: Routledge.
This chapter considers the merits and problems of engaging with communities in participatory action for empowerment through the social action research model, in a Department of Health commissioned handbook covering the major issues involved in research with ethnic minority groups.

Johnson, M.R.D. (2006) 'Ethnicity', in A. Killoran, C. Swann and M. Kelly (eds), *Public Health Evidence: Changing the Health of the Public*. Oxford: Oxford University Press.
This chapter discusses the nature of ethnicity and the problems in defining, measuring and using it as a research category, in a volume addressing a wide range of issues by leading experts in public health research.

Johnson, M.R.D. (2003) 'Research governance and diversity: quality standards for a multi-ethnic NHS', *Nursing Times Research*, 8 (1): 2–10.
This article discusses the ethical issues lying behind the design of health care research to meet the needs of the wider population and especially the inclusion of minority ethnic groups in that objective.

REFERENCES

Acheson, D. (1998) *Independent Inquiry into Inequalities in Health*. London: The Stationery Office.

Aspinall, P.J., Dyson, S.M. and Anionwu, E.N. (2003) 'The feasibility of using ethnicity as a primary tool for antenatal selective screening for sickle cell disorders: pointers from the research evidence', *Social Science and Medicine*, 56: 285–97.

Banton, M. (1977) *The Idea of Race*. London: Tavistock.

Bhopal, R.S., Phillimore, P. and Kohli, H.S. (1991) 'Inappropriate use of the term "Asian": an obstacle to ethnicity and health research', *Journal of Public Health Medicine*, 13 (4): 244–46.

Bonney, R. (2004) 'Reflections on the differences between religion and culture', *Clinical Cornerstone*, 6 (1): 25–33.

Cashmore, E.E. (1982) *Rastaman: The Rastafarian Movement in England*. London: George Allen & Unwin.

Chan, M. (1997) *Achievements of the NHS Ethnic Health Unit*. Leeds: NHS Ethnic Health Unit.

Comstock, R.D., Castillo, E.M. and Lindsay, S.P. (2004) 'Four year review of the use of race and ethnicity in epidemiologic and public health research', *American Journal of Epidemiology*, 159 (6): 611–19.

Crisp, N. (2004) *Race Equality Action Plan*. Available at Department of Health website: http://www.dh.gov.uk/PublicationsAndStatistics/Bulletins/BulletinArticle/fs/en?CONTENT_ID=4072494&chk=1e/oI7

Culley, L. (2000) 'Working with diversity: beyond the factfile', in C. Davies, L. Finlay and A. Bullman (eds), *Changing Practice in Health and Social Care*. London: Sage.

Erens, B., Primatesta, P. and Prior, G. (eds) (2001) *Health Survey for England 1999 Volume 1: Findings. Volume 2: Methodology and Documentation*. London: The Stationery Office.

Fleming, J. and Ward, D. (1999) 'Researcher as empowerment: the social action approach', in W. Shera and L. Wells (eds), *Empowerment Practice in Social Work*. Toronto: Canadian Scholars' Press.

Fleming, J. and Ward, D. (2004) 'Methodology and practical application of the social action research model', in F. Maggs-Rapport (ed.), *New Qualitative Research Methodologies in Health and Social Care: Putting Ideas into Practice*. London: Routledge.

Gill, P., Kai, J., Bhopal, R.S. and Wild, S. (2002) *Black and Minority Ethnic Groups in Healthcare Needs Assessment: Epidemiologically-based Needs Assessment Reviews, Third Series*. Oxford: Radcliffe Medical. Available at: http://hcna.radcliffe-oxford.com/bemgframe.htm

Johnson, M.R.D. (2003) 'Ethnic diversity in social context', in J. Kai (ed.), *Ethnicity, Health and Primary Care*. Oxford: Oxford University Press.

Johnson, M.R.D. (2004) *Towards An Epidemiology Of Ethnic Diversity*. Module in ENB/DH/Nursing & Midwifery Council Online Course for Cultural Competence. Available at: www.rcn.org.uk/Resources/Transcultural/Index.php

Johnson, M.R.D. and Verma, C. (1998) *It's Our Health Too: Asian Men's Health Perspectives*, CRER Research Paper 26, for Southern Birmingham Community Health NHS Trust and NHS Executive Ethnic Health Unit, Coventry: University of Warwick.

LaVeist, T.A. (1994) 'Beyond dummy variables and sample selection: what health services researchers ought to know about race as a variable', *Health Services Research*, 29: 1–16.

Macpherson, W. (1999) *The Stephen Lawrence Inquiry: Report of an Inquiry*. London: Home Office.

Modood, T., Berthoud, R., Lakey, J., Nazroo, J., Smith, P., Virdee, S. and Beishon, S. (1997) *Ethnic Minorities in Britain: Diversity and Disadvantage*, PSI Report 843. London: Policy Studies Institute.

Morjaria-Keval, A. and Johnson, M.R.D. (2005) *Our Vision Too: Improving the Access of Ethnic Minority Visually Impaired People to Appropriate Services*, Seacole Research Paper 4. Leicester: MSRC with Housing Corporation and Thomas Pocklington Trust.

National Statistics (2003) *Ethnic Group Statistics: A Guide for the Collection and Classification of Ethnicity Data.* London: Stationery Office/Office of National Statistics.

Sadler, G.R., Ryujin, L., Nguyen, T., Oh, G., Paik, G. and Kustin, B. (2003) 'Heterogeneity within the Asian American community', *International Journal for Equity in Health*, 2: 12. Available at: www.equityhealthj.com/content/2/1/12

19

Involving the Consumer in Health Research[1]

SOPHIE HILL

INTRODUCTION

Health consumers not only produce their health but now increasingly help produce health knowledge through participation in health research. At face value this represents a fundamental shift in social power. Is it a real phenomenon or is lip service paid to the participation by health consumers in health research? It may not be possible to answer this question conclusively but I address it by exploring the nature, features, advantages and disadvantages of consumer involvement in research, drawing on documents, mainly from the United Kingdom and Australia, concerned with promoting consumer participation.

The involvement of consumers in health research represents the intersection of two phenomena – on the one hand, the emergence of health social movements (Brown and Zavestoski 2004) and on the other, the development of theories, methods and knowledge in the clinical sciences. In this chapter, I first outline how this intersection is played out in myriad ways that often defy easy description, categorization and analysis. These tasks are made more difficult by the developmental, voluntary and political nature of consumer participation, which in many instances is not well documented or researched. Second, I assess the effect or impact of participation, outlining potential advantages and disadvantages from different perspectives. In the course of the chapter, I will present the views and experiences of consumers who have been involved in research in the Cochrane Collaboration, an international organization. This allows me to illustrate the ways in which consumer participation is happening in practice and to document some of the major barriers such as the impact of illness on the ability of individuals to participate; the knowledge and skills required by participating consumers; the language differences between experts and lay people; and the lack of resources to take part in activities. I will also explore how these may be overcome.

RESEARCH ISSUES: DEFINITIONS AND CATEGORIZATIONS

From patient to health consumer

Over recent decades across countries, many health consumer or patients' groups have not only raised awareness of problems with the outputs of health care in terms of services and policy, but also turned their attention to health and medical research: that is, to the knowledge inputs into health care. This shift in critical stance reflects a desire to influence health care, but also an increasingly sophisticated understanding of science and its methods by health consumer groups.

This shift is evident in language. In recent years, the patient is frequently called a 'consumer'. The use of the term 'consumer' is contested, reflecting various political, economic and social assumptions that have changed over time (Boote et al. 2002; Henderson and Petersen 2002; Herxheimer and Goodare 1999). In addition, the scope of health services has broadened, with greater attention to illness prevention and health promotion. This means that the consumer is commonly not a sick person: that is, not a patient in the traditional sense of the term. Internationally, a range of terms are used, including consumer, carer, lay person, volunteer, citizen, member of the public, in addition to patient. For this chapter, I will use the term that is most common in debates about people's involvement in health policy and research, namely the term health consumer. Drawing from United Kingdom and Australian definitions, the term consumer includes patients and potential patients; people who use health and social services; carers and parents; members of the public targeted by health promotion programmes; organizations that represent the interests of the public; communities that are affected by health, public health or social care issues; and groups asking for research because they believe they have been exposed to potentially harmful circumstances, products or services (INVOLVE UK 2006; National Health and Medical Research Council and Consumers' Health Forum of Australia 2001).

Participation or involvement, and by whom?

Australians use the term participation whereas the British literature favours involvement. The implied meaning is much the same. In the past, consumer involvement in research occurred through the participation by patients and members of the public as subjects in research carried out by professional or clinical researchers. Typically, they gave their informed consent to being a subject in a research project, but had no part in setting up the research or contributing to the design process. Nor were they necessarily informed of the outcomes.

The emphasis has now shifted to a more active involvement or 'partnership' in all stages of the research process from setting priorities to assessing outcomes (Consumers in NHS Research Support Unit 2000; Williamson 2001). According to an Australian joint consumer–researcher publication, this is 'where consumers and researchers work in partnership with one another to shape decisions about research priorities, polices and practices' (National Health and Medical Research Council and Consumers' Health Forum of Australia 2004a: 9). This implies that consumers have the right to be represented and some power to shape the decisions made.

This level of involvement cannot occur without some organization and structuring within the health sector to harness the contribution of increasingly active and informed citizens and the expansion and diversification of health consumer groups and associated organizations. Consumers of health care have been classified by Boote et al. (2002). This is shown in Box 19.1.

Box 19.1   *Classification of consumers*

Classification of consumers in health research

Individuals may participate as:

- Service users and carers
- Patient representatives
- Patient advocates
- Citizens
- Members of the public who are potential users of health services

Local groups may participate through:

- Population groups
- Support groups
- Groups convened to discuss health matters such as citizens' juries and health

(Inter)national consumer organizations

- Statutory bodies
- Charities
- (Inter)national support groups

Source: Boote et al. (2002)

In what kinds of research are health consumers involved?

In a guide for consumers who want to be involved, research has been defined as 'planned, cautious, systematic and reliable ... Good research addresses soluble problems, has realistic aims, adopts sound research methods and addresses important issues' (Consumers in NHS Research Support Unit 2004: 6). In Australia, the National Health and Medical Research Council and Consumers' Health Forum of Australia (2004b) have categorized health research into various health domains under the following headings:

- *Basic research*: Research that happens in the laboratory, using test tubes and micro-scopes and operating at the level of cells, not people. Consumer involvement could occur at a policy level, such as reviewing the ethics of specific tests and proce-dures. At the level of the research body, consumers could donate specimens such as blood, sperm or ova for study.
- *Clinical research*: Research that is seeking to understand the causes of, or treat-ments for, ill-health and that may happen in the laboratory or in other health set-tings in contact with people. At the macro level, consumers could be involved in identifying priorities for research. Within clinical research, they could be involved in identifying important outcomes or advising on how results should be dissemi-nated. This is the domain in which they are most commonly subjects.
- *Public health research*: Research involving the study of communities or popula-tions, which aims to identify factors that contribute to ill-health and how those fac-tors can be influenced to reduce ill-health, and which commonly happens outside health care settings. Consumers could be involved by helping to formulate research questions by raising questions about potential cause and effect relationships. At the other end of the spectrum, they could advise researchers and governments on how findings could be used to change practice and programmes, for instance providing advice on the implications of social diversity.
- *Health services and health systems research*: Research that aims to improve the delivery of health care, and which may focus on issues of access, equity, cost and effectiveness. Consumers could review recruitment strategies, such as how to recruit people from 'hard to reach' groups, or they could participate in the devel-opment of training programmes to be used for consumer advocates for reviewing the quality of care.

The National Health and Medical Research Council and Consumers' Health Forum of Australia (2004b) define the stages of research as deciding what to research; deciding how to do it; doing it; letting people know the results; and deciding what to research next. Recent attention to the science of implementa-tion would imply that we can add getting research into practice as another important phase. The list emphasizes that consumers may be involved at all stages and that research is an ongoing or cyclical process. Furthermore, the role of consumers, who is involved and the methods used will depend on the stage and activity.

What are the different models and methods of involvement?

Oliver and colleagues (2004) have developed a comprehensive framework for categorizing consumer involvement in research. It has eight key features that explore a range of roles, functions and methods, and has wide applicability (see Nilsen et al. 2006; Paterson 2004). The framework can assist in analyzing the dimensions of consumer involvement in a particular project by using a checklist that covers a number of characteristics. These are as follows:

- Who are involved: individuals or people representing a consumer organization?
- Who initiated the involvement: consumers or researchers?
- What was the degree of involvement? This can be disaggregated by consultation, collaboration or consumer-controlled research.
- What are the forums for exchanging ideas? For example, this can be through citizens' juries or focus groups.
- What are the methods used for collective decision making? As an example, this can be through developing a method for ranking research priorities.
- What are the practicalities for involvement? For instance, this may be achieved through resources for training or other forms of skill development.
- What is the context for agenda setting? The setting may be described according to such factors as institutional type, geographical coverage, or the background of participants in terms of consumer activism.
- What particular theory underpins the strategy for consumer involvement? For example, there may be an implicit belief that involvement should be researcher led, consumer led or even professionally led.

The framework provides a structure for analyzing consumer involvement that makes explicit reference to the power relationships in health research, and the potentially dynamic nature of participation. Thus, for example, the third item above suggests a power continuum from 'consultation', a process for seeking or inviting views, through 'collaboration', an active and ongoing relationship, to 'consumer-controlled research', where the process is led by consumers.

The National Health and Medical Research Council and Consumers' Health Forum of Australia (2004a) have placed an emphasis on developing the conditions for effective consumer participation. These include developing organizational leadership and capacity; integrating participation into the structure of organizations; earmarking resources for participation; and recognizing that time is needed to change attitudes. However, while there has been some recognition by governments and research bodies of the need for consumer participation in research policy, this has not always been the case for semi-autonomous research institutes and the universities (Dickersin and Schnaper 1996; National Health and Medical Research Council and Consumers' Health Forum of Australia 2004a).

THE CONSUMER CHALLENGE: WHAT DO CONSUMERS HOPE TO ACHIEVE AND WHY?

There are several intertwined strands in what consumers hope to achieve through participation. First, the challenge to medical authority and autonomy from social movements in general (such as women, people with HIV/AIDS, indigenous people), and health social movements in particular, has laid the ground for extending that challenge to health and medical researchers (Brown and Zavestoski 2004; Dickersin and Schnaper 1996; Sepkowitz 2001). The need for a more 'patient-centred care' has been embraced by politicians for some decades.

A second and related point is that it cannot be assumed that health researchers understand or reflect the perspective of the people who ultimately 'consume' the research knowledge, in terms of ultimate treatments and services (Entwistle et al. 1998). Indeed, consumers have different priorities from those who research (Tallon et al. 2000). For this reason, consumers and their representatives have asked for a 'seat at the table' where decisions are made (see Breast Cancer Network Australia).

Third, it has been argued that better quality decisions will be made if consumers participate in research and the way findings are applied will also be more relevant and responsive to the actual needs of current and future patients and the public (O'Donnell and Entwistle 2004). Moreover, research where consumers take part in the formulation and conduct of the study is more likely to measure outcomes of importance to those who may be affected by the research results (Sakala et al. 2001).

Fourth, within a rights and ethical framework for consumer involvement, the rationale is that people have a right to influence the development of new knowledge, procedures or processes that affect what happens to their bodies or those of future patients (National Health and Medical Research Council and Consumers' Health Forum of Australia 2001; Williamson 2001). This argument is frequently strengthened with the disclosure of research that has seriously transgressed and harmed those who participated (Goodare and Smith 1995). In recent years, research malpractice as well as large-scale system failures have led to a climate with closer scrutiny of research practice and greater accountability of researchers both upwards to professional bodies and government departments as well as downwards to local communities (Cartwright Inquiry 1988; Bristol Inquiry 2001; National Health and Medical Research Council and Consumers' Health Forum of Australia 2001).

Finally, consumer groups and researchers have argued that society benefits from having a knowledgeable public, aware of research, how it is done and what it implies. Consumer participation is seen as a means for achieving informed consumers and consumer organizations that can disseminate information to the wider community (National Health and Medical Research Council and Consumers' Health Forum of Australia 2001). This argument has been developed particularly in relation to what the public should know about pharmaceutical companies, the research they conduct and how they promote the end products of their research (Moynihan 2005). However, it has been notable that pharmaceutical companies themselves have a commercial interest too in informing consumers about their products and involving them in research (Oliver et al. 2004). Market opportunities are expanded if products are tailored to the needs of consumers, especially with the development of designer drugs.

In this sense, the debate about consumer participation is dialectic and reflexive. As well as having a 'self-interest', citizens and groups have been drawn into the policy arena to serve governmental interests in developing a more responsive health policy. In consequence, other interests, professional, commercial and institutional, have seen consumer involvement in research as a 'policy requirement' and also an advantage in achieving their own particular policy aim (O'Donnell and Entwistle 2004).

In summary, a great deal rides on consumer involvement in research. It may produce research that reflects the health problems of the community, conducted with the community and not on the community, for improved health outcomes within the context of an accountable and ethical system.

THE ADVANTAGES OF CONSUMER PARTICIPATION: WHAT IMPACTS AND EFFECTS HAVE BEEN DEMONSTRATED?

A Cochrane systematic review of trials of methods of consumer participation across a broad range of domains including research shows that little research has been done to find the best ways of involving consumers in health care decisions at the population level. In the research domain, two studies, which compared using consumer interviewers with staff interviewers as data collectors for patient satisfaction surveys, found small differences in satisfaction survey results, with less favourable results obtained when consumers were the interviewers (Nilsen et al. 2006).

The review of consumer involvement in the process of agenda setting for research by Oliver and colleagues (2004) provides some evidence on impact, although their conclusions are tentative. They suggest that the extent of influence in terms of identifying and prioritizing research topics is related to the degree of consumer participation and control. Collaborative approaches where interaction is active and ongoing appear more effective in influencing the agenda than consultation alone. To be effective, consumer involvement requires an investment of time; training for skill development for consumers and researchers; establishing effective working practices for committees; involving consumers who are well networked; and providing them with information, resources and support for consulting with their peers. Dialogue, to be constructive, must be ongoing with frequent reflection and review.

There are also certain organizational requirements (Oliver et al. 2004). The activity should be endorsed by senior staff; staff should be experienced in consultation and collaboration techniques; there should be a commitment to building ongoing and constructive relationships with communities; the knowledge and experience of consumers should be valued; and whatever representative mechanisms that are put in place should recognize different groups within the communities.

WHAT ARE THE DISADVANTAGES OF CONSUMER PARTICIPATION?

The disadvantages of consumer involvement must be seen from the perspective of the various interests involved. For example, within medicine concerns have been expressed that consumers will be insufficiently knowledgeable; may be biased in their views; and would only 'represent' themselves and not others (Entwistle et al. 1998). Moreover, they might be simply troublesome, and hinder decision making. From the perspective of research funding bodies, given the lack of consensus and uncertainties about the benefits of the process, there have been concerns that consumers may dominate a project. This may occur, for example, in the context of public lobbying for new treatments in association with powerful pharmaceutical or manufacturing interests (O'Donnell and Entwistle 2004). In consequence, guides to consumer involvement have proliferated in recent years, such as those cited above.

From the point of view of consumers, a disadvantage may be token involvement. Consumers have identified the following problems: feeling outnumbered and isolated on committees full of professionals; of not being listened to; of being manipulated; or having no real opportunity to influence the research agenda, the research project itself and the research process (National Health and Medical Research Council and Consumers' Health Forum of Australia 2001). The review by Oliver et al. (2004) identified problems associated with poor-quality consumer representation, poor communication and dysfunctional relationships within committees, as well as serious time constraints. In a review of consumer involvement in research to promote best practice in the use of medicines in Australia, Kirkpatrick et al. (2005) showed that most research projects were dominated by health professionals despite a policy commitment to consumer involvement. The authors also highlight the importance of adequate resources and a robust infrastructure to support the development of initiatives from consumer groups.

It should also be stressed that most research has a long lead time. Oliver (1999) argues that a contribution to research is an evolutionary process. Knowledge of the consumer perspective is cumulative and must be created, shared and applied within a consultative framework that includes people's experiences (see DIPEx.org database of personal experiences of health and illness). Moreover, researchers may have to understand differences in experience in terms of culture, class and age, and gender differences in terms of life experience, as well as the differing perspectives of the ill person and the carer. Undoubtedly, there is a tension between the individual experience and the way that research questions are structured and addressed (Beard 2004; Ong and Hooper 2003).

There are also inherent inequalities in access to resources between research professionals and consumers. Participation by consumers is commonly on a voluntary basis. Many consumer groups are resource poor. They juggle with many competing objectives and must choose their policy priorities carefully. In this context, it is not surprising that the study by Baggott et al. (2005) of health consumer groups in the United Kingdom showed an increase in active relationships between consumer groups and pharmaceutical companies.

For groups, collaboration with a pharmaceutical company may provide additional funds for projects and activities and provide access to information on recent developments, research or products. Some groups, such as those representing people with a disease where management or cure is dependent on the company's products, may have a shared agenda with pharmaceutical interests. However, the dilemma is the potential for loss of integrity and independence in a relationship where there is inequality in terms of power and wealth and where profit is the overriding goal for companies. There have been concerns about the lack of transparency. In the United Kingdom, the Parliamentary Health Select Committee (2005) recommended that companies should disclose donations and funding to health consumer groups and this is also endorsed in guidelines by the Association of the British Pharmaceutical Industry (2002).

For their part, peak or national organizations in the United Kingdom have developed codes of practice for their members in relation to funds received from companies (Baggott et al. 2005; Herxheimer 2003). Similarly in Australia, the Consumers' Health Forum, together with the peak body for research-based pharmaceutical companies, have produced a guide, *Working Together*, to inform consumer groups about relationships they may form with pharmaceutical companies (Consumers' Health Forum of Australia and Medicines Australia 2005). The two organizations recognize the increasing number and complexity of these relationships and provide guidance through posing a series of questions such as: Will any funding arrangement be perceived as appropriate? Have the benefits and risks of funding or sponsorship been assessed? Interestingly, in this respect, the benefits are listed but not the risks.

Case study: The Cochrane Collaboration

Many of the advantages and disadvantages of consumer participation may be illustrated by reference to the international Cochrane Collaboration which is provided as a case study of consumers in research in practice.

The aim of the Cochrane Collaboration

Established in 1993, the Cochrane Collaboration (www.cochrane.org) is an international non-profit and independent organization set up to ensure that up-to-date, accurate information about the effects of health care interventions is readily available worldwide. This is achieved by coordinating and publishing systematic reviews of studies on the effects of interventions in an Internet-based library of specialized data-bases called *The Cochrane Library*. The Collaboration's 2003 Strategic Plan includes the principle 'Enabling wide participation in the work of The Cochrane Collaboration by reducing barriers to contributing and by encouraging diversity.' This principle is realized through various structures and processes. These include setting up a network so that consumers can participate; introducing consumer representation from the network at steering group level; the active encouragement of consumer involvement in organizations producing reviews; and support and funding for consumers to participate in annual scientific meetings and training programmes (Ghersi 2002). Table 19.1 lists the main functions carried out by consumers.

A recent survey identified that many consumers wanted to be more involved in the Cochrane Collaboration, yet faced a range of personal and structural barriers. Personal barriers included the financial costs of participation such as wages forgone, the cost of attending meetings, the health costs for those with chronic illness, language barriers, and the feeling of being isolated from other consumers (Horey 2002: 18–19).

Structural barriers included the lack of clarity within the Cochrane Collaboration of the roles of consumers and communication about changes; the lack of access to computers and other technology to enable

(Continued)

Table 19.1   *The functions carried out by consumers in the Cochrane Collaboration*

Different stages of research	The roles and tasks of consumers
Deciding what to research	Identifying review topics or priorities
Deciding how to do it	Identifying issues from a consumer's perspective and important outcomes Commenting on drafts of Cochrane reviews and protocols as referees
Doing it	Hand-searching journals for research missed by database searching Translating documents Researching and writing a review, as co-reviewers Working as editors and coordinators Running training courses
Letting people know the results	Writing lay versions of reviews for simultaneous publication with full reviews Disseminating the results, giving presentations, writing newsletters, linking to consumer groups
Deciding what to do next	Representing consumer members on the organization's management and working groups Encouraging others to participate

Source: Horey (2002)

some people to participate; the complexity of the scientific language and concepts; poor communication between the institutions contributing to the Cochrane Collaboration and consumers; the short time scale in which to complete complex tasks; and the patronizing or insensitive attitudes of professionals and researchers (Horey 2002).

Overcoming barriers to consumer participation

A small number of Cochrane groups have written up their experiences, documenting their strategies to establish consumer involvement in the research and the measures taken to overcome barriers to participation. The Cochrane Musculoskeletal Group, which coordinates the production of reviews of treatments for musculoskeletal conditions and is based in

(Continued)

(Continued)

Ottawa, Canada, provides dedicated resources to consumers in all stages of its work, with roles, functions and tasks similar to those listed above. Access to people who might be interested in volunteering was made easier by the Group's close relationship with the Arthritis Society of Canada, which itself had built a broad network of interested people with arthritis. Despite these advantages, the Group reported difficulties in maintaining its consumer membership as people faced health problems, competing priorities in their lives or both. People also complained about the costs for individuals of participation (Shea et al. 2005).

The Haematological Malignancies Group based in Cologne, Germany, faced similar difficulties that in its case were compounded by language barriers and serious illness. It was found that the appointment of a dedicated consumer coordinator, one-to-one support for consumer representatives, time spent on consulting and listening, and training programmes for consumers assisted the process (Skoetz et al. 2005). Most of the consumer participants came from a self-help group relevant for people with haematological malignancies. Individuals had an interest in research but also wanted to take back what they had learned to the consumer group.

Both of these groups had the benefit of significant support at a senior level for consumer participation and dedicated resources. They established or improved relationships to existing organizations which already had consumers involved. Both also emphasized the importance of intensive and ongoing interaction to sustain commitment. Once established, the relationship enables both consumers and researchers to report back to consumers more generally on the influence or impact of consumer participation in terms of ideas or actions taken, a process for improving transparency of research and accountability of researchers. The findings suggest, though, that whilst the Cochrane Collaboration is global in coverage, local or regional support is necessary to sustain activity.

Supporting consumer participation in health research

The Cochrane Collaboration has expected health researchers to support consumer participation and to respond to the issues raised by consumers. The intellectual dominance within the Cochrane Collaboration of questions on the effectiveness of clinical and pharmaceutical interventions itself suggests the question: is the impact of consumer participation important enough to warrant the investment in time and resources?

(Continued)

This attractive, but facile, question obscures other and broader challenges within health research. Brown and Zavestoski (2004: 680–1) write: 'Science and technocratic decision-making have become an increasingly dominant force in shaping social policy and regulation.' They suggest that one cost to society for the dominance of science is that: 'Scientists are asked to answer questions that are virtually impossible to answer scientifically due to data uncertainties or the infeasibility of carrying out a study.' A second cost is that: 'The scientization of decision-making delegitimizes the importance of those questions that may not be conducive to scientific analysis.' These processes, they argue, diminish the capacity of the public to participate as citizens in framing and contributing to policy debates.

I would argue that these processes in fact provide a compelling rationale and justification for seeking effective ways of enabling health consumers to participate in the production of knowledge. After all, it is their bodies and their lives that are affected by the uncertainties. Their participation may enable impossible questions to be reframed and to be addressed in meaningful ways.

CONCLUSION

This chapter has summarized briefly some of the ways that consumer involvement in research is happening. In conclusion, there are two important questions that will require further exploration. First, for researchers, the question is how to establish and sustain a meaningful relationship that accommodates epistemologically and practically the intersection of the experience of illness with producing new knowledge about illness and health (Hess 2004). Second, for consumers, the challenge is how one moves from critique to participation. Effective participation must balance a critical viewpoint and independence with understanding and involvement in the concerns of researchers. These are exciting questions to explore, but to be answered they require more than token commitment to consumer participation, and a greater awareness that consumer participation is more complex than has been assumed. Readers can test the latter point further by attempting the exercise below on developing a policy for consumer participation for a health research organization.

Exercise: Develop a policy for consumer participation in research for a health research institute

Imagine you are working in a health research institute and the board has decided that it needs a consumer participation policy. Further, all new projects are expected to involve consumers. The board asks you to develop a consumer participation policy, to identify where consumers could be 'found', their roles and some indication of achievements for the first 1–2 years.

1 *The evidence base and the social setting*: Identify sources of evidence that will assist you to develop a policy position paper. In addition to the sources in the references, you may wish to check the following:

- The Cochrane Library, including the databases of the Cochrane Database of Systematic Reviews and the Database of Reviews of Effectiveness, to identify recent reviews of evidence.
- Medical and health research databases, in addition to databases of activities and projects for consumer participation in research.
- The websites of local or national consumer groups who would have an interest in the research in your Institute.

2 *The development of a plan*: Consider using the framework for consumer involvement developed by Oliver and colleagues (2004), to form a plan for consumer participation in your institute. Against the eight main features, document your proposed strategies. Remember to identify what type of research is undertaken in your institute and for whom. Consider whether you would consult consumer groups and researchers to identify their interest in consumer participation, the prospect for ongoing relationships, and the skills that people may require. Build this into your plan. Identify realistic achievements for the first 1–2 years, using the available literature to substantiate your proposals where possible. Formulate a strategy for obtaining support for your plan and the outcomes from the board and chief executive officer.

3 *Evaluation*: The policy should have an evaluative component that establishes a process of reflexive practice involving consumers and researchers. Identify indicators of success or impact, and how these will be measured.

NOTE

1   My thanks to Dr Dell Horey for her thoughtful comments on the practicalities of consumer participation in research, and in particular for her insights into pharmaceutical
funding for consumer groups; and to Dr Sandy Oliver for showing me a connection
between research and change.

RECOMMENDED FURTHER READING

Brown, P. and Zavestoski, S. (2004) 'Social movements in health: an introduction',
Sociology of Health and Illness, 26 (6): 679–94.
This is good reading for those interested in acquiring a sociological understanding of
health social movements.

Nilsen, E.S., Myrhaug, H.T., Johansen, M., Oliver, S. and Oxman, A.D. (2006) 'Methods
of consumer involvement in developing healthcare policy and research, clinical practice guidelines and patient information material', *Cochrane Database of Systematic
Reviews*, Issue 3. Art. No.: CD004563. DOI: 10.1002/14651858.CD004563.pub2.
This key reference is a Cochrane systematic review of evaluation studies relevant to consumer participation in research, which is regularly updated.

Oliver, S., Clarke-Jones, L., Rees, R., Milne, R., Buchanan, P., Gabbay, J., Gyte, G., Oakley,
A. and Stein, K. (2004) 'Involving consumers in research and development agenda
setting for the NHS: an evidence-based approach', *Health Technology Assessment*,
8 (15). Available at: http://www.ncchta.org/fullmono/mon815.pdf
This provides the detailed background on the development of the framework for
analyzing consumer participation in research.

REFERENCES

Association of the British Pharmaceutical Industry (2002) *The Code of Practice for the
Industry*. London: ABPI.
Baggott, R., Allsop, J. and Jones, K. (2005) *Speaking for Patients and Carers: Health
Consumer Groups and the Policy Process*. Basingstoke: Palgrave Macmillan.
Beard, R.L. (2004) 'Advocating voice: organisational, historical and social milieux of the
Alzheimer's disease movement', *Sociology of Health and Illness*, 26 (6): 797–819.
Boote, J., Telford, R. and Cooper, C. (2002) 'Consumer involvement in health research: a
review and research agenda', *Health Policy*, 61: 213–36.
Breast Cancer Network Australia. *A Seat at the Table Program*. Available at: http://
www.bcna.org.au/cms/details.asp?NewsID=56
Bristol Inquiry (2001) *Learning from Bristol. The Report of the Public Inquiry into Children's
Heart Surgery at the Bristol Royal Infirmary 1984–1995*. Available at: http://www.bristol
inquiry.org.uk/final_report/index.htm

Brown, P. and Zavestoski, S. (2004) 'Social movements in health: an introduction', *Sociology of Health and Illness*, 26 (6): 679–94.

Cartwright Inquiry (1988) *The Report of the Committee of Inquiry into Allegations Concerning the Treatment of Cervical Cancer at National Women's Hospital.* Auckland: WHA.

Consumers' Health Forum of Australia and Medicines Australia (2005) *Working Together: A Guide for Relationships between Health Consumer Organisations and Pharmaceutical Companies.* Available at: www.chf.org.au/Docs/Downloads/361_manual_relationships.pdf

Consumers in NHS Research Support Unit (2000) *Involving Consumers in Research and Development in the NHS. Briefing Notes for Researchers.* Eastleigh: Consumers in NHS Research Support Unit.

Consumers in NHS Research Support Unit (2004) *Getting Involved in Research: A Guide for Consumers.* Available at: http://www.invo.org.uk

Dickersin, K. and Schnaper, L. (1996) 'Reinventing medical research', in K.L. Moss (ed.), *Man-made Medicine: Women's Health, Public Policy and Reform.* Durham, NC, and London: Duke University Press.

DIPEx.org database of personal experiences of health and illness. Available at: http://www.dipex.org

Entwistle, V.A., Renfrew, M.J., Yearley, S., Forrester, J. and Lamont, T. (1998) 'Lay perspectives: advantages for health research'. *British Medical Journal*, 316: 463–66.

Ghersi, D. (2002) 'Making it happen: approaches to involving consumers in Cochrane reviews', *Evaluation and the Health Professions*, 25 (3): 270–83.

Goodare, H. and Smith, R. (1995) 'The rights of patients in research', *British Medical Journal*, 310: 1277–78.

Henderson, S. and Petersen, A. (2002) 'Introduction: consumerism in health care', in S. Henderson and A. Petersen (eds), *Consuming Health: The Commodification of Health Care.* London: Routledge.

Herxheimer, A. (2003) 'Relationships between the pharmaceutical industry and patients' organizations', *British Medical Journal*, 326: 1208–10.

Herxheimer, A. and Goodare, H. (1999) 'Who are you and who are we? Looking through the eyes of some key words', *Health Expectations*, 2: 3–6.

Hess, D.J. (2004) 'Medical modernisation, scientific research fields and the epistemic politics of heath social movements', *Sociology of Health and Illness*, 26 (6): 695–709.

Horey, D. (2002) *'It takes time to find your role': A Survey of Consumers in the Cochrane Collaboration in 2002.* Email survey available at: http://www.cochrane.org/consumers/docs/reportcochraneconsumersurveyDH.doc

INVOLVE UK (2006) http://www.invo.org.uk

Kirkpatrick, C.M.J., Roughead, E.R., Monteith, G.R. and Tett, S.E. (2005) 'Consumer involvement in Quality Use of Medicines (QUM) projects – lessons from Australia', *BMC Health Services Research*, 5: 75. Available at: http://www.biomedcentral.com/1472-6963/5/75

Moynihan, R. (2005) 'The marketing of a disease: female sexual dysfunction', *British Medical Journal*, 330: 192–94.

National Health and Medical Research Council and Consumers' Health Forum of Australia (2001) *Statement on Consumer and Community Participation in Health and Medical Research.* Commonwealth of Australia, Canberra. Available at: http://www.nhmrc.gov.au/publications/synopses/r22syn.htm

National Health and Medical Research Council and Consumers' Health Forum of Australia (2004a) *A Model Framework for Consumer and Community Participation in Health and Medical Research. December 2004*. National Health and Medical Research Council, Commonwealth of Australia, Canberra. Available at: http://www.nhmrc.gov.au/publications/synopses/r22syn.htm

National Health and Medical Research Council and Consumers' Health Forum of Australia (2004b) *Resource Pack for Consumer and Community Participation in Health and Medical Research. December 2004*. National Health and Medical Research Council, Commonwealth of Australia, Canberra. Available at: http://www.nhmrc.gov.au/publications/synopses/r22syn.htm

Nilsen, E.S., Myrhaug, H.T., Johansen, M., Oliver, S. and Oxman, A.D. (2006) 'Methods of consumer involvement in developing healthcare policy and research, clinical practice guidelines and patient information material', *Cochrane Database of Systematic Reviews*, Issue 3. Art. No.: CD004563. DOI: 10.1002/14651858.CD004563.pub2.

O'Donnell, M. and Entwistle, V. (2004) 'Consumer involvement in research projects: the activities of research funders', *Health Policy*, 69: 229–38.

Oliver, S. (1999) 'Users of health services: following their agenda', in S. Hood, B. Mayall and S. Oliver (eds), *Critical Issues in Social Research*. Buckingham and Philadelphia: Open University Press.

Oliver, S., Clarke-Jones, L., Rees, R., Milne, R., Buchanan, P., Gabbay, J., Gyte, G., Oakley, A. and Stein, K. (2004) 'Involving consumers in research and development agenda setting for the NHS: an evidence-based approach', *Health Technology Assessment*, 8 (15): 1–148. Available at: http://www.ncchta.org/fullmono/mon815.pdf

Ong, B.N. and Hooper, H. (2003) 'Involving users in low back pain research', *Health Expectations*, 6 (4): 332–41.

Parliamentary Health Select Committee (2005) (HC 42–1) 4th Report 2004/5. *The Influence of the Pharmaceutical Industry*. London: TSO.

Paterson, C. (2004) '"Take small steps to go a long way": consumer involvement in research into complementary and alternative therapies', *Complementary Therapies in Nursing and Midwifery*, 10: 150–61.

Sakala, C., Gyte, G., Henderson, S., Neilson, J.P. and Horey, D. (2001) 'Consumer–professional partnership to improve research: the experience of the Cochrane Collaboration's Pregnancy and Childbirth Group', *Birth*, 28 (2): 133–37.

Sepkowitz, K.A. (2001) 'AIDS – the first 20 years', *New England Journal of Medicine*, 344 (23): 1764–72.

Shea, B., Santesso, N., Qualman, A., Heiberg, T., Leong, A., Judd, M., Robinson, V., Wells, G. and Tugwell, P. (Cochrane Musculoskeletal Consumer Group) (2005) 'Consumer-driven health care: building partnerships in research', *Health Expectations*, 8 (4): 352–59.

Skoetz, N., Weigart, O. and Engert, A. (2005) 'A consumer network for haematological malignancies', *Health Expectations*, 8 (1): 86–90.

Tallon, D., Chard, J. and Dieppe, P. (2000) 'Relation between agendas of the research community and the research consumer', *Lancet*, 355: 2037–40.

Williamson, C. (2001) 'What does involving consumers in research mean?', Editorial, *Quarterly Journal of Medicine*, 94 (12): 661–64. Available at: http://qjmed.oxfordjournals.org/cgi/reprint/94/12/661

20

Comparative Health Research

VIOLA BURAU

INTRODUCTION

Health, health care and policies have become more international over recent decades, reflecting a number of factors. The development of mass media and communication technologies means that information about health problems and health services in individual countries has become more readily and widely available. This trend is also supported by the work of international organizations such as the World Health Organization (WHO) and the Organization for Economic Cooperation and Development (OECD), which not only gather but also disseminate information about health care across a wide range of countries. Health policies are also increasingly made at the international level. For example, the European Union is now involved in a wide range of areas from public health to pharmaceutical policies. Finally, many health problems are shared across countries. HIV/AIDS affects countries across the world. Industrialized Western countries share a concern about how to respond to ageing populations and infectious diseases, such as the respiratory disease SARS, across country borders.

With the internationalization of health care, the cross-country, comparative perspective has become increasingly significant in understanding contemporary issues in health. Although there are methodological challenges, comparative health research allows the evidence from more than one country to be used in a systematic way. The notion of comparison may be incorporated into a flexible research design and draw on a range of different methods.

APPROACHES TO COMPARATIVE HEALTH RESEARCH

Comparative health research can deal with a wide range of substantive areas in health and take a range of perspectives. Researchers should be aware of different approaches prior to embarking on a study and Øvretveit (1998) and Clasen (2004) provide useful overviews. One area of study is to focus on the health needs of particular patients. For example, the needs of asthma patients could be approached in two ways: either through an analysis of how the organization of health services across different countries addresses the needs of asthma patients or, alternatively, through focusing on health professionals. How do doctors and nurses across different countries respond to asthma patients and what services do they provide?

Studies can also be undertaken at different organizational levels. First, a macro-level study may test a hypothesis and use statistical analysis. For instance, Huber (1999) examined how the public–private mix in the funding of health care shaped the impact of cost containment measures using OECD health figures to analyze health care expenditure in 29 countries. Second, meso-level studies focus on the organization of health services. There is a large literature on health policy and reform – for example, Blank and Burau (2004), Freeman (2000) and Moran (1999) use the categories of funding, provision and regulation of health care, to understand why policy responses to health problems vary across countries. Third, micro-level studies are concerned with specific aspects of health care behaviour and practice. In their analysis of care arrangements of older people in Britain and Germany, Chamberlayne and King (2000) use qualitative methods to study the biographies of individual carers and identify different 'cultures of care' within particular countries.

THE PURPOSE OF COMPARISON

Beyond the choice of substantive area and level of analysis, another important consideration is the purpose of comparison. Comparison may be about:

- Exploration
- Explanation
- Evaluation.

Exploratory studies

Exploratory comparative health research aims to investigate the same 'phenomenon' in different countries. This can be anything from the organization of palliative care and public health policies to cancer survival rates and public expenditure on hospital care. Here, the aim is to broaden the 'basis of evidence' by considering cases from very different contexts to get a better idea of the potential variation in service delivery.

Exploratory studies help to avoid both false particularism ('everywhere is unique') and false universalism ('everywhere is the same') as they aim to identify what is different and what is similar. In this respect, studies may adopt a static perspective and focus on the differences and similarities as such. For example, Raffel (1997) analyzes the differences and similarities in the organization of health services across 10 industrialized countries. A study may adopt a more dynamic perspective and analyze how countries are *becoming* more different, or similar. This approach is particularly dominant in studies that analyze processes of convergence, whereby health problems, services or policies tend to become more similar over time. Gibson and Means (2000) analyze recent reforms in long-term care in Britain and Australia and show how two initially very differently organized regimes have become more alike.

Explanatory studies

Explanatory studies investigate deeper questions, notably about why it is we find certain differences and similarities (Klein 1997). For example, a study by Haug (1995) of the division of labour between doctors and nurses in Britain and Germany starts with the observation (based on OECD health statistics) that the ratio between doctors and nurses in the two countries differs significantly. She uses the remainder of her study to examine various explanations for this difference. Although exploratory studies give an indication of findings, explanatory studies make better use of the analytical potential of the comparative research design. The particular explanations considered depend on the specific theories underlying the research questions. For example, theories of policy making are the basis for the central assumption of Haug (1995) that the influence nurses enjoy at both the macro and micro levels of organization explains the different ratio of doctors to nurses within different systems.

Evaluation studies

Finally, there are health studies using comparison as a method of evaluation. Here, the main aim is to assess the impact of health care and policies in different countries against specific criteria of relative success or failure. An important example is the 2000 World Health Report by the World Health Organization (2000). The report compares the performance of different health systems and makes recommendations about how the performance of health systems can be improved within available resources. Evaluative studies build on two more or less explicit assumptions. First, the evaluation of health involves making judgements, often by identifying exemplary cases or so-called 'best practice'. This implicitly suggests that there is a best way of doing things and the promotion of market-based mechanisms in health care is a prominent example. Second, evaluative studies assume that best practices can be transferred across countries and that in this way countries can learn from each other in very practical ways. However, both assumptions are problematic as the next section shows.

THE POLITICS OF COMPARATIVE HEALTH RESEARCH

The interest of both governments and international organizations in comparative health research has led to an increasing politicization of comparative studies. This is reflected particularly in more applied studies where the aim is explicitly to evaluate evidence from different countries in order to identify what works best in relation to, for example, organizational reform, the use of medical technologies or in particular care pathways. Governments identify existing problems and seek 'solutions' by looking at other health systems (Rose 2000). For instance, in the United Kingdom, the NHS has been seen as 'underfunded' when compared with other countries which spend higher levels of GDP on health care (Dunne 2002). For policy makers, the attraction of cross-country comparison lies in the fact that it resembles a kind of 'natural experiment', which allows 'testing' individual reform instruments and assessing their relative suitability and success.

   This is especially attractive in two respects. First, policy making informed by comparative research potentially allows learning from the mistakes of others, and thereby holds the implicit promise of avoiding policy failure altogether. This is an attractive promise in any policy area, not least health, which is high on the political agenda of many countries reflecting the importance of health services to the general public. Second, policy making informed by comparative research enjoys greater credibility, because it is informed by more than the personal judgement of policy makers. As such, comparison can be part and parcel of a more 'evidence-based' style of policy making. In the case of the increase in NHS funding referred to above, it was precisely the comparison with other countries that offered additional credibility to an otherwise controversial policy decision. This is also in line with the distinctively anti-ideological and pragmatic approach of the New Labour government in the United Kingdom (Rose 2000).

The process of 'comparing for policy making' is not a neutral, but a highly politicized, activity and the literature on policy learning and transfer refers to a number of constraints (Dolowitz and Marsh 1996; Klein 1997) as follows:

- The process of policy learning itself is selective and more often than not reflects the specific, domestic agendas of policy makers. For example, the internal market reforms of the British NHS in the early 1990s were influenced by health care practice and thinking in the United States, precisely because of the common neo-liberal market orientation of the two governments at the time. Policy learning from other countries therefore is often concerned with finding additional arguments for a political decision already made.
- Best practices are deeply embedded in highly specific national, social, economic and political contexts and therefore cannot be transferred easily. Indeed, the literature suggests that health policies follow country-specific paths and reflect existing institutional frameworks in health care and the broader political system (Freeman 1999) and past policy choices may constrain the scope for policy learning (Peterson 1997). This also means that the relative success of individual best practices is highly conditional and depends on specific organizational settings. Any transfer is likely to be partial and require some adaptation. For example, although market mechanisms were the central focus of health reforms in the 1990s across Europe, countries implemented market mechanisms in very different ways. This reflects differences in specific policy goals, in the political institutions and in the structure of health systems (Jacobs 1998).

What are the implications for the researcher undertaking comparative health research? The literature suggests that researchers must be aware of the limitations of research for policy. They should recognize that the most desirable comparative research design for policy makers may not necessarily be the most fruitful analytically. Researchers also need to be sensitive to the specific contexts and conditions under which best practices may be considered as 'best'.

THE METHODOLOGICAL CHALLENGES OF COMPARATIVE HEALTH RESEARCH

Sampling: Choosing cases

The first challenge is related to sampling. Sampling requires clarifying the rationale for comparison. What is it that comparison is supposed to explain? Individual studies should focus on either differences or similarities depending what it is they aim to analyze and/or explain. For example, a study looking at the effect of the introduction of market forces in health care cannot, in the same study, both analyze convergence towards market mechanisms in health care reforms and analyze differences in the implementation of health care markets.

Sampling is about choosing suitable countries or more generally 'cases' for comparison; that is, cases from which one can learn most in terms of what the study aims to analyze and explain. The choice of cases is closely tied to the underlying theoretical framework of a study. For example, the widespread reference to 'market forces' in health reforms may reflect processes of policy learning and transfer. Relevant theories suggest that such cross-country learning is more likely where there are similarities in the mode of health care delivery between countries. Thus, Britain and Sweden, with their tax-funded national health systems, can be used as comparators (Glennerster and Matsaganis 1994).

In contrast, if the focus of attention is on analyzing why markets in health care have been implemented in very different ways across European countries, it would be more appropriate to include countries with contrasting or dissimilar health systems (Ranade 1998). In terms of theory, neo-institutionalist theories suggest that differences in policy outcome reflect differences in the institutional setting. In the literature on comparative research methods, these two approaches to the choice of cases are also referred to as the 'most similar' and the 'most different' design (see Mackie and Marsh 1995). However, both research designs require that the cases chosen are comparable in the first place. Here, Lijphart (1975) defines comparability as a strategy, whereby the theoretically insignificant 'background variables' are held constant. This can be achieved by choosing countries with comparable levels of economic wealth, with stable democratic political systems and with developed welfare states.

Equivalence: Ensuring comparability

A second challenge relates to 'equivalence', which can be understood as identifying comparable units for cross-country comparison (see Øyen 2004). This question arises at the research design phase – however, comparing 'apples with apples' rather than 'pears' is less straightforward than it appears. The units of comparative health research can be anything from specific health workers to professional practices, disease patterns, health services, health policies or health outcomes.

Identifying such units of comparison across countries is complicated as it involves being aware of not only differences in the use of language, but also differences in the specific cultural meaning and the related function of such units. In the literature, this is referred to as the difference between 'formal' and 'functional' equivalence. For instance, units that have similar cultural meanings (and functions) may have different names; conversely, units with the same name may have very different cultural meanings (and functions). Health care is culturally embedded within society (Freeman 1999). The concept of the hospital is an example. Although the English term 'hospital' can be translated directly into other European languages (as *hôpital* in French, *Krankenhaus* in German or *sygehus* in Danish), this disguises differences in cultural meaning and function. For example, English hospital trusts are providers of specialist health care and cover both inpatient and outpatient services, whereas their German counterparts focus on inpatient specialist care only. This reflects the fact that the majority of outpatient specialist care is delivered by office-based specialists.

To secure the validity of a piece of comparative research, it is essential to identify similar units for comparison. It is, however, a complex process requiring translation of both words and meanings and an acknowledgement of the social construction of concepts (Eyraud 2001). One way of taking account of linguistic and cultural differences while ensuring comparability is to work with 'functional equivalents'. This means the researcher makes a choice of the unit of analysis on the basis that its substantive functions are comparable. For example, a British–German comparison of hospital care could use the unit 'inpatient specialist care' as a focus of study.

Managing complexity: Processing and interpreting data

A third challenge of comparative health research is to manage the quantity, diversity and complexity of the data collected in a systematic and theoretically meaningful way. This must be achieved through all the phases of the research from data collection to data processing and interpretation where more that two countries are included. It is especially important to process the material emerging from comparative health research in a systematic way by specifying clearly what material is relevant and in what way. This is about labelling and categorizing, but is more than a technical exercise. Instead, processing comparative research material is at the centre of the interpretation itself. To be done systematically, analysis must be theory led. Processing has to reflect the specific hypotheses that are expected to explain differences or similarities across countries.

The use of ideal types

One method used for data processing and interpretation is to cluster explanatory factors into 'ideal types'. These are constructs and can be understood as the basic variants of a particular phenomenon and have been a particularly important tool in meso-level comparative health research (Burau and Blank 2006). For example, a commonly used typology of health systems defines health systems as representing specific sets of macro-institutional characteristics and such a typology can be used to explain specific variations of health policies across different countries. In this case, the typology is based on variations in the funding of health care and corresponds to differences in the organization of health care provision (OECD 1987). It distinguishes three basic models of health systems: the national health service model with funding out of general taxation; the social insurance model with compulsory social insurance funded out of employer and employee contributions; and the private insurance model funded by individual and/or employer contributions.

The underlying assumption of this typology of health systems is that the public funding of health care, or lack of it, is the defining characteristic of the extent of state involvement in health care. Thus, Freeman (2000) uses the typology to explain specific variations in the politics and policies of health care across a number of European countries. The ideal type model of health systems helps not only to describe and categorize the organization of health care, but also to explain why countries respond to health problems in certain ways. In consequence, the analysis moves beyond the specificity of individual countries, towards more insight into the health system in general.

The limitations of typologies

Using typologies is not without its problems, many of which arise from the ambiguous relationship between ideal types and real systems. Ideal types of the health system are abstractions drawn from real health systems and are meant to help in understanding the organization of health care. Typologies aim to simplify reality but, in doing so, they may limit understanding of actual systems. In Singapore, for example, health care funding comes from private sources in the form of personal savings accounts, although payment into such accounts is mandatory. The health system of Singapore therefore fits poorly into the typology of health systems referred to above. In this case, the typology raises more questions than it answers (see Blank and Burau 2004).

Another danger is that analyses become divided by individual ideal types and do not effectively compare across different countries. An example is the international literature on health professions, which is often based, more or less explicitly, on a typology centred on the Anglo-American professions (Collins 1990). Its limited explanatory power has resulted in single-country case studies dominating the literature. Cross-country comparative studies have been few (see, for example, Hellberg et al. 1999).

In comparative health research, there is an underlying tension between uniqueness and generalization. As Mabbett and Bolderson (1999) point out, broad-brush characterizations often do not hold up when confronted with the complex detail of actual arrangements. Yet, the dilemma is that once one departs from such characterizations, research can become merely descriptive, which militates against identifying clear and all-encompassing contrasts.

CASE STUDY

Case study: Comparative health research in practice

The following discussion is based on a comparative study of nursing in Britain and Germany (Burau 1999a; Burau 1999b; Burau 2005). The initial interest in the study arose from the following puzzle. Although nursing is the single largest occupation in most health systems in Europe, relatively little is known about nursing across countries. The comparative literature on health care and policy is notable for its silence on nursing. The study addressed the following research questions: What are the different strategies used for governing nursing as an occupation? How can the differences between nursing in Britain and Germany be explained?

The study used two sets of theories. Theories of the professions were used to identify the main strategy for occupational governance and the substantive focus for occupational governance. Typically, the literature associates occupational governance with strategies for 'professional closure' through state-licensed self-regulation in relation to overseeing education and maintaining a register of the qualified. In addition, the strategies for occupational governance are used to explain intra-professional dynamics. However, as feminist writers have noted, the state often plays an influential role in the governance of women-dominated occupations such as nursing. The study therefore also used institutionalist theories to explain the specific strategies of occupational governance of nursing. These theories suggest that institutional rules backed by coercion as well as norms and values shape the interests and resources of actors involved in the governance of nursing. In this instance, actors included nurses themselves, both individually and collectively, health care providers as employers of nurses, and the state. The interplay of these various interests shaped the strategies for the occupational governance of nursing.

The research questions and the choice of theoretical framework had implications for the design of this cross-country comparative study. The effect of institutions is relatively easy to identify where institutions are different, and the study used a 'most different case' design as the independent, explanatory variable. The institutional arrangements for the occupational governance of nursing differ between Britain and Germany and so does the organization of health care and the role of the state. Britain has a tax-funded, publicly provided health service with the highly centralized political system providing important levers in relation to the occupational governance of nursing. In contrast, the health system

(Continued)

in Germany is funded by social insurance contributions and health service provision is a public/private mix. This provides the basis for extensive joint self-governance by providers and insurers. Moreover, the federal structure devolves governance to the more local level. In consequence, the role of the state in health care organization, and the occupational governance of nursing, is limited.

To examine how strategies for occupational governance had been shaped by different institutional arrangements required a two-part analysis: an analysis of the structures of occupational governance in the two countries on the one hand, and a case study of the strategies for occupational governance of nursing on the other. For the case study, comparable units of analysis had to be chosen to deal with issues of equivalence. This proved to be challenging. Although in both countries there is a policy emphasis on providing nursing care outside hospital, there was no equivalent to 'primary' or 'community care' in Germany. Nor was there a category of 'practice nurse'. Primary care remains highly medically oriented. However, in both countries home-based nursing services exist, albeit organized in different ways. In Britain, specialist 'district nurses', general nurses and health care assistants deliver care to patients in their homes. In Germany, general nurses, geriatric carers (*Altenpfleger*) and care assistants provide home-based care and there is no specific term for nurses delivering this type of care.

In this study to ensure functional equivalence, the research focused on the occupational field of home-based (nursing) care rather than on individual occupational groups. To allow for the different meanings of home-based (nursing) care, the study used the term 'district nurses' only in the British context. When referring to Germany or both countries, the more neutral term 'community nurses' or 'community nursing staff' was used.

As with most comparative research, complex data had to be gathered, managed and analyzed. The study used existing meso-level typologies of health systems and health care states to order the material on the structure of nursing occupational governance. The distinction between 'Anglo-American' and 'Continental' types of professions was less useful as this was developed on the basis of influential, male-dominated professions.

CONCLUSION

In attempting to carry out a piece of comparative research, a number of choices have to be made in terms of strategy, and this chapter has aimed to provide a structured approach to making those choices and negotiate the pitfalls of a complex field. First, a choice must be made about the unit for comparison across countries. It has been suggested that there should be formal or functional equivalence in what is being compared. Second, in choosing the countries in a study, the best strategy is to compare countries that are relatively similar. Here, typologies or ideal types are a useful device, although one that should be used cautiously as real systems rarely conform fully to a concept that is based on an abstraction. Third, the researcher should then decide whether in making comparisons their strategy is to look for lines of difference or lines of similarity. They should also decide whether the study they are undertaking is exploratory, explanatory or evaluative. Finally, any analysis of similarity or difference should be theory led: that is, the researcher should identify a general proposition or hypothesis about the way in which policies, organizations, groups or individuals function that they are seeking to explain. To conclude the chapter, a practical exercise for the reader follows.

Exercise: Comparing health care expenditure and cost containment policies

In principle, health policy in most developed capitalist democracies has been based on achieving three goals: the provision of high-quality services; equal access for all citizens to health care; and cost-efficient provision (Blank and Burau 2004). In the first two decades following the Second World War, health policy initiatives were particularly concerned with the first two goals. Since the 1970s, cost efficiency and containment have become dominant across countries. With this in mind, examine the OECD's data on the total expenditure on health as a percentage of GDP (see Table 20.1) and answer the three questions below:

(Continued)

Table 20.1   *Total expenditure on health as percentage of GDP*

	1980	2003
Austria	7.4	7.5
France	7.1	10.1
Germany	8.7	11.1
Italy	7.7*	8.4
Netherlands	7.5	9.8
New Zealand	5.9	8.1
Spain	5.4	7.7
Sweden	9.1	9.4
United Kingdom	5.6	7.7
United States	8.7	15.0

*Figure for 1985.
Source: OECD Health Data 2005. Available at: http://www.oecd.org/dataoecd/60/28/35529791.xls

1 Looking at the figures for 2003, rank countries in order of the percentage of GDP spent on health care.

   • What is the difference in percentage points between the country at the top and the bottom of the list?
   • Are countries spread evenly or do they cluster into separate groups? Are there any clear outliers?

2 Looking at the development of health care expenditure between 1980 and 2003, rank countries in order of the relative increase in percentage of GDP spent on health care.

   • What is the difference in percentage points between the country at the top and the bottom of the list?
   • Are countries spread evenly or do they cluster into separate groups? Are there any clear outliers?

3 Using your analysis of OECD health expenditure data, list those observations you find particularly interesting, striking and/or surprising. Use this as a basis for formulating two or three research questions, which you feel require further comparative analysis.

(Continued)

(Continued)

Table 20.2 *The health care systems in Britain, Germany and Sweden*

	Germany	Britain	Sweden
Funding	• Access to health services on basis of social insurance membership • Funding through social insurance contributions raised by statutory, non-profit insurance funds • Allocation of funding based on decentralized contracts between insurance funds and providers; federal legislation as framework	• Access to health services on basis of social citizenship • Funding through general taxation raised by central government • Allocation of funding based on national global budget and through local budget allocations embedded in a central framework	• Access to health services on basis of social citizenship • Funding through income tax raised by regional governments • Allocation of funding based on regional global budget but through a variety of mechanisms
Provision	• Hospitals in public, non-profit or private ownership; service delivery based on decentralized contracts; control jointly by insurance funds and providers • Hospital doctors are salaried employees, office-based doctors work as independent contractors • Decisions about medical technology are part of decentralized budget negotiations between insurance funds and providers	• Hospitals are independent non-profit trusts; service delivery on basis of contracts, embedded in centralized structures with performance management and planning • Hospital doctors are public employees, GPs work as independent entrepreneurs in public primary care trusts • Decisions about medical technology by regional government agencies based on local applications	• Most hospitals are run by regional governments; service delivery subject to national framework and monitoring • Most hospital doctors and GPs (working in health centres) are public employees • Decisions on medical technology on a case-by-case basis by regional governments

With your questions for comparative research in mind, read the summaries in Table 20.2 of the health systems in Britain, Germany and Sweden. Based on the summaries, make a list of the factors relating to the organization of health care and the state, which facilitate and mitigate against successful cost containment respectively.

(Continued)

Designing a comparative study of cost containment policies: With your insight into the factors making for more/less successful health care cost containment in mind, reread the research questions you have formulated and address the following issues:

1   Which one research question do you think is most important and why?
2   Which two countries would it be most useful to compare to answer your research question and why? Consider the relative merits of drawing on either the 'most similar cases' or the 'most different cases' as a strategy.
3   What additional aspects of the institutional context for health care provision would you look at in each of the countries you have chosen, and why do you think these are important in answering your research question?

RECOMMENDED FURTHER READING

Blank, R.H. and Burau, V. (2004) *Comparative Health Policy*. Basingstoke: Palgrave Macmillan.
This introductory comparative text analyzes key issues in health policy from a research viewpoint and assesses how far policy problems and responses in different countries have common or diverse origins.

Burau, V. and Blank, R.H. (2006) 'Comparing health policy: an assessment of typologies of health systems', *Journal of Comparative Policy Analysis*, 8 (1): 63–76.
This recent article discusses the strengths and weaknesses of different approaches to understanding the country-specific contexts of health, health care and health policies.

Mabbett, D. and Bolderson, H. (1999) 'Theories and methods in comparative social policy', in J. Clasen (ed.), *Comparative Social Policy: Concepts, Theories and Methods*. Oxford: Blackwell.
This chapter discusses different approaches to comparative international research and the implications of the comparative approach for the research process.

REFERENCES

Blank, R.H. and Burau, V. (2004) *Comparative Health Policy*. Basingstoke: Palgrave Macmillan.
Burau, V. (1999a) 'Occupational governance and the dynamics of change – A comparative analysis of nursing in Britain and Germany'. PhD thesis, University of Edinburgh.

Burau, V. (1999b) 'The politics of internal boundaries: a comparative analysis of community nursing in Britain and Germany. Some preliminary observations', in I. Hellberg, M. Saks and C. Benoit (eds), *Professional Identities in Transition. Cross-cultural Dimensions*. Södertälje: Almqvist & Wiksell.

Burau, V. (2005) 'Comparing professions through actor-centred governance: community nursing in Britain and Germany', *Sociology of Health and Illness*, 27 (1): 114–37.

Burau, V. and Blank, R.H. (2006) 'Comparing health policy: an assessment of typologies of health systems', *Journal of Comparative Policy Analysis*, 8 (1): 63–76.

Chamberlayne, P. and King, A. (2000) *Cultures of Care: Biographies of Carers in Britain and the Two Germanies*. Bristol: Policy Press.

Clasen, J. (2004) 'Defining comparative social policy', in Patricia Kennett (ed.), *A Handbook of Comparative Social Policy*. Cheltenham: Edward Elgar.

Collins, R. (1990) 'Changing conceptions in the sociology of professions', in R. Torstendahl and M. Burrage (eds), *The Formation of Professions. Knowledge, State and Strategy*. London: Sage.

Dolowitz, D. and Marsh, D. (1996) 'Who learns what from whom: a review of the policy transfer literature', *Political Studies*, 44: 343–57.

Dunne, R. (2002) 'Will extra billions cure NHS ills?', *BBC News*. Available at: http://news.bbc.co.uk/1/hi/health/1935417.stm

Eyraud, C. (2001) 'Social policies in Europe and the issue of translation: the social construction of concepts', *International Journal of Social Research Methodology*, 4 (4): 279–85.

Freeman, R. (1999) 'Institutions, states and cultures: health policy and politics in Europe', in J. Clasen (ed.), *Comparative Social Policy: Concepts, Theories and Methods*. Oxford: Blackwell.

Freeman, R. (2000) *The Politics of Health in Europe*. Manchester: Manchester University Press.

Gibson, D. and Means, R. (2000) 'Policy convergence: restructuring long-term care in Australia and the UK', *Policy and Politics*, 29 (1): 43–58.

Glennerster, H. and Matsaganis, M. (1994) 'The English and Swedish health reforms', *International Journal of Health Services*, 24 (2): 231–51.

Haug, K. (1995) *Arbeitsteilung zwischen Ärzten und Pflegekräften in deutschen und englischen Krankenhäusern oder warum arbeiten doppelt so viel Krankenschwestern pro Arzt in englischen wie in deutschen Krankenhäusern?* Konstanz: Hartung-Gorre.

Hellberg, I., Saks, M. and Benoit, C. (eds) (1999) *Professional Identities in Transition. Cross-cultural Dimensions*. Södertälje: Almqvist & Wiksell.

Huber, M. (1999) 'Health care expenditure trends in OECD countries, 1970–1997', *Health Care Financing Review*, 21 (2): 99–117.

Jacobs, A. (1998) 'Seeing difference: market health reform in Europe', *Journal of Health Politics, Policy and Law*, 23 (1): 1–33.

Klein, R. (1997) 'Learning from others: shall the last be the first?', *Journal of Health Politics, Policy and Law*, 22 (5): 1267–78.

Lijphart, A. (1975) 'The comparable-bases strategy in comparative research', *Comparative Political Studies*, 8 (2): 158–77.

Mabbett, D. and Bolderson, H. (1999) 'Theories and methods in comparative social policy', in J. Clasen (ed.), *Comparative Social Policy: Concepts, Theories and Methods*. Oxford: Blackwell.

Mackie, T. and Marsh, D. (1995) 'The comparative method', in D. Marsh and G. Stoker (eds), *Theory and Methods in Political Science*. Basingstoke: Macmillan.

Moran, M. (1999) *Governing the Health Care State. A Comparative Study of the United Kingdom, the United States and Germany*. Manchester: Manchester University Press.

OECD (1987) *Financing and Delivering Health Care. A Comparative Analysis of OECD Countries*. Paris: OECD.

Øvretveit, J. (1998) *Comparative and Cross-cultural Health Research. A Practical Guide*. Abingdon: Radcliffe Medical Press.

Øyen, E. (2004) 'Living with imperfect comparisons', in P. Kennett (ed.), *A Handbook of Comparative Social Policy*. Cheltenham: Edward Elgar.

Peterson, M.A. (1997) 'The limits of social learning: translating analysis into action', *Journal of Health Politics, Policy and Law*, 22 (4): 1077–114.

Raffel, M.W. (ed.) (1997) *Health Care and Reform in Industrialized Countries*. University Park, PA: Pennsylvania State University Press.

Ranade, W. (ed.) (1998) *Markets in Health Care. A Comparative Analysis*. Harlow: Longman.

Rose, R. (2000) 'What can we learn from abroad?', *Parliamentary Affairs*, 53: 628–43.

World Health Organization (2000) *The World Health Report 2000. Health Systems: Improving Performance*. Geneva: WHO.

PART V
Disseminating Health Research

21

Writing Up Health Research and Getting Published

JUDITH ALLSOP AND MIKE SAKS

INTRODUCTION

This concluding chapter focuses on the challenge of writing up health research findings for both quantitative and qualitative studies and those employing mixed methods. However, to provide a platform for this discussion and to draw together some of the earlier threads of the volume, two points about undertaking health research are emphasized, irrespective of the particular methods used. First, and of fundamental importance, the research question should be framed appropriately and then the method(s) matched to the question. Second, in the contemporary context, the health researcher must be aware of ethical issues and other sensitivities in conducting research. These considerations are vital as, without a sound base, writing up the research and getting published are likely to run into problems. In this latter respect, the main part of this chapter goes on to note that conventions for writing up and publishing differ according to the method(s) used; the audience being addressed; and the publication outlet being considered. Despite the expansion of visual media, writing is still the main means of communication for scholarship in health research. A research degree will not normally be awarded without a written product and if research does not get published in some form, it will not inform other scholars or reach a wider audience. The opportunity to influence policy and practice may thus be lost.

THE FUNDAMENTALS OF DOING HEALTH RESEARCH

Developing and refining a research question

Despite the clear differences between health researchers using quantitative, qualitative or mixed methods, many authors see an essential first step as refining the research question. This applies whether this is in the form of a hypothesis to be tested or where the hypothesis, or identification and theorizing about themes, develops during the course of the research. As noted in Chapter 12 of this book, a question is likely to be answerable if it is explicit, focused and feasible.

For a health researcher, an interesting research question may initially arise from a personal life experience or from specialist knowledge of some kind. Curiosity about why things are as they are is a necessary attribute in a researcher. To develop an initial question into something that it is more explicit and focused, and therefore researchable, requires persistence in working through ideas, finding out what has already been written and talking through the issues with others. Chapter 3 on carrying out a literature review provides various techniques for finding out what data are available and what others have written. Most importantly, it argues, as do other contributors to the book, that it is vital to identify the theory that is implicit in a given question and the theories used by other scholars to investigate the topic. A decision on whether to adopt a quantitative or qualitative methodology linked to the positivist/interpretivist paradigms as outlined in Chapter 2 – and then on one or more specific methods – depends on the type of question posed. Chapters 4 to 14 in this volume provide a guide to the advantages and disadvantages of the various methods in the health field and give examples of the type of research questions that can be investigated through adopting a particular approach.

Having developed an explicit and focused question, the next step for a health researcher is to assess how feasible the research is within the resources available. This may be tested by sketching out the design for the project – that is, a plan for the method(s) that may be used to answer the research question, including an estimate of the time scale and costs. Much will depend on the secondary sources available and how much primary data will have to be collected. Researchers are often unaware that there are vast data sets in the Economic and Social Research Council archive held by Essex University; specialist archives in other universities; data sets held by the Office of National Statistics and other government departments as well as by market research organizations such as MORI. These data, which are both quantitative and qualitative, have often been under-analyzed and access may be negotiated. Researchers do not necessarily have to collect their own data in order to do good research.

Developing a research plan

Chapters 4 to 14 in this book provide guidance on what will be required from a planning viewpoint if a particular method is followed in the health field. A minimum structure for a research plan is set out in Box 21.1.

Box 21.1   *Elements of a research plan*

A research plan should include:

- Title
- Aims and objectives
- Background or context to the research question
- A brief review of the literature, including the theoretical approach and the key substantive studies — ideally identifying a gap in the literature
- Methods and rationale for the method and approach to data analysis
- The research timetable
- The resources required
- Dissemination strategy

The authors contributing to this book typically emphasize the importance of being explicit about the theories and concepts that underpin the research. Considering types of theoretical and conceptual frameworks that may explain findings is begun when refining a research question. A quantitative researcher is likely to argue for a very clear, simple primary question and a research method that will provide an answer or outcome. A qualitative researcher meanwhile will acknowledge that in more exploratory research, the question and indeed the theoretical framework for analysis may shift during the course of a study.

Whichever method is adopted, carrying out health research in practice will require both management and detective skills. It will also require resilience and imagination to overcome the problems that inevitably arise in the course of conducting a project. The difficulties encountered often provide opportunities for seeing things differently, particularly in qualitative research. It is also worth pointing out that most researchers will lack knowledge in certain areas. A novice researcher must be able to acknowledge where help is needed and seek out those with the necessary expertise. This is particularly the case in relation to obtaining statistical advice. It is also true of projects where a number of methods are being used, or people with different disciplinary backgrounds are working on a project. This makes it all the more important that the question addressed in each arm of the research is explicit and focused.

SHIFTS IN THE RESEARCH ENVIRONMENT

Ethical considerations

A number of the shifting sensitivities in the health research environment are covered in Chapters 15 to 20 in this volume. One key area to which these and other chapters refer is the heightened awareness that carrying out research often raises ethical issues. The ethical guidelines developed by funding bodies and institutions responsible for research and the greater scrutiny to which research proposals are now subjected are discussed most fully in the health context in Chapter 15. As part of their professional practice, health researchers should also develop sensitivity to possible ethical issues. Taking a proposal through an ethics committee is one part of the equation, but actually carrying out data collection and fieldwork is another. Here researchers are not so directly under scrutiny and must use their own judgement. A minimum requirement for the researcher is that they:

- Respect the autonomy of those who will take part in research by obtaining informed consent.
- Maintain confidentiality by keeping the information obtained and data collected secure and not disclose the identity of a participant either explicitly or implicitly without seeking their permission.

This brings us back to the importance of framing a research question explicitly and developing a written research proposal that research participants can be given to ensure that they are fully informed in giving consent in health and other fields of research.

The changing relationship between the researcher and the researched

Another related illustration of the increased sensitivity within the research environment is the changing relationship between the researcher and the researched in the health arena – including groups like patients, carers, the general public, communities, health professionals and health organizations. In this respect, there is a growing political emphasis on such groups being more fully involved in research, especially users of health services whose views were previously given all too little consideration. This shift in the research environment is reflected in the change in the language of researchers from objective terms such as patient, respondent, interviewee to the more inclusive term of research participant, who is engaged in the research process. In this volume a number of authors – such as in Chapters 5, 8, 15, 18 and 19 – refer to this changed relationship and suggest ways in which health researchers should now approach the research process.

Mixed and multidisciplinary methods

A range of contributors in the book also note that there is greater tolerance in the wider research environment towards using more than one method in a single project in health research and adopting multidisciplinary approaches – a theme which is covered most systematically in Chapter 16. While there are still quantitative researchers who firmly believe that qualitative methods do not create or add to knowledge and vice versa, the fact that all research proposals are likely to go through a common vetting process has increased understanding of other methods and disciplinary approaches – not least among the committee members concerned. This has also added to more rigorous scrutiny of research proposals in terms of the reliability, generalizability and validity of research proposals and findings. As discussed in various chapters of this book and in other publications (see, for example, Belgrave et al. 2002), this may be achieved in different ways in quantitative and qualitative research. The interrelated benefits of mixed and multidisciplinary methods to research in a specific area in this respect are highlighted in Chapter 17. The use of such methods poses real challenges, which are further extended in conducting health research in a comparative international context, as underlined in Chapter 20.

Tensions and dilemmas

It is vital that health researchers are responsive to the issues set out above in setting up and carrying out their research if they are to write up and publish their research effectively. They should be aware of differences of opinion and tensions in doing so. As a seeker of knowledge, the health researcher must maintain the position of a detached observer, and record phenomena and analyze results in a dispassionate and rigorous manner. Nonetheless, from an ethical viewpoint, the research community is divided on where knowledge creation should be given higher priority than the concerns of individual research participants – notwithstanding the safeguards of the system of ethical review. There will also always be differences of opinion on the methodological framework and methods best used for collecting and analyzing data. Moreover, all claims to knowledge gained are contingent on context, time and place. As such, researchers face dilemmas that they must resolve as they arise in practice in a principled way. In sum, carrying out health research is both an art and a skill. It involves learning from experience and acquiring techniques through research training (see Ramkalawan 2005).

The chapter now looks more specifically at the process of writing up research and disseminating research findings. There are hurdles to be overcome in both these areas, as well as ethical considerations about what to say and what not to say. Writing for the health and other fields is a time-consuming and often painful business. Moreover, turning research reports, dissertations or theses into publications can be a hit and miss affair, as a would-be author is in the hands of editors and publishers. Nonetheless, as well as luck, shrewd judgement and persistence are often rewarded. The remainder of the chapter aims to be of assistance in completing the research journey.

THE BENEFITS OF RESEARCH AND THE OBLIGATIONS OF HEALTH RESEARCHERS

As well as adding to the general body of knowledge about a particular area on which others can build, health research that is written up, disseminated and published brings a number of benefits. First, for the researcher there may be positive personal benefits in publication in terms of public prestige, further research funding and career development. Conversely, future funding may be jeopardized by poor outputs and a failure to publish. For funders, research consumes considerable resources in time and money. Researchers making a bid for funding are often now required to include proposals for dissemination, and to show they have considered the utility of the research and who will benefit from the findings and at what point in the process. Outputs are also subsequently audited.

Funding bodies themselves are monitored and audited as research grants are awarded by public bodies and charitable institutions, which are themselves accountable for ensuring value for money. Research funding bodies may specify interim reports or targets to be achieved during a project. For them, outputs signal a return from an investment and reporting on these is typically a requirement. The wider community of scholars, as well as professionals, policy makers and the general public, can benefit from research findings, but only if they are accessible.

In the case of health research, there is a further obligation, particularly on field researchers to publish findings even, and some would argue especially, if these are negative. Research subjects will have given their opinions, their time and sometimes access to their bodies for additional procedures, interventions and medications because they believe a project is worthwhile and may help others. Given that being a research participant may have emotional and physical costs, researchers have a moral obligation to carry out research as rigorously as they can, and then make the results available.

WRITING TEXTS: THE GENERAL AND THE SPECIFIC

Writing is about communication and giving an account of health research in a way that makes sense to the reader. In writing up a study, a researcher is engaged in a form of narrative, or 'story-telling' that will have a structure: at its most simple, a beginning, middle and end. An account of a research project should include a statement of purpose; how data were gathered and why; what the data consisted of; the interpretation of the data; and the conclusion. The aim of such writing is to convey to the reader as clearly, concisely and convincingly as possible the aims and outcome of the research – which may be helped by providing a brief summary that is separately available (Schober and Farrington 2000; Bowling 2002; Johnson 2004).

While this is a common denominator, there are different forms and conventions that vary between disciplines, including in the health field. The style of writing in terms of language and presentation will also vary according to the audience. Any would-be author should take time to find out, and think through, what is expected of them and tailor their account accordingly. After a period immersed in a research project, the minutiae of the findings and the task of interpretation, it is all too easy to forget that an account must be comprehensible to the reader. In some cases, knowledge of a technical language can be assumed, in other cases not. For example, in the case of many, if not most, clinical research proposals in the health area, the patient consent form requires rewriting to make what is involved comprehensible for the participant. Some tips are:

- The structure of a piece of writing is the key to achieving clarity.
- If in doubt, it is better to assume a lower level of knowledge.
- Reading aloud a piece you have written helps to establish rhythm and flow.
- Leaving your work aside for a while or getting someone else to read it through helps to create a more critical gaze.

TYPES OF NARRATIVE IN WRITING UP RESEARCH

In writing up research in health, there are two basic forms of narrative: the biomedical scientific or quantitative and the naturalistic or qualitative. Although each form of narrative is written within different conventions, increasingly there is cross-over in terms of audience. Health matters and so does scholarly research from whatever tradition and method. Some social experiments and randomized controlled trials are published in social science journals, while articles using qualitative methods are occasionally accepted by scientific journals. Recently, patient narratives, or patients' stories of their experience of health and illness, are seen to contribute to clinical practice. As previously noted, health researchers now employ increasingly a mix of quantitative and qualitative methods to study phenomena. This poses additional challenges for writing up results and integrating findings.

Biomedical scientific writing

Biomedical scientific writing on matters related to health tends to operate within a very strictly defined set of conventions, of which a subset would be scientific research using an experimental or quantitative method as shown in Box 21.2, as one paradigm type.

Box 21.2 *The structure of a scientific paper*

A scientific paper should contain:

- A descriptive title and author/s biographical details
- An abstract in 100–200 words (a summary of the research question, methods, findings, contribution to knowledge)
- Introduction: the research question being addressed and gaps in the research
- A review of the literature to put the research question in the context of existing knowledge
- The hypothesis or null hypothesis being addressed
- The type of study being done either primary (experiment, clinical trial or survey) or secondary (overview, guideline study, decision analysis or economic analysis)
- The study design such as a randomized controlled trial, a cohort study, a case-control study, a cross-sectional survey or a single case report. It should describe the population studied, the recruitment process, inclusion and exclusion criteria and how outcomes were measured
- The research results or findings
- A conclusion
- References
- A declaration of interests

Source: Adapted From Greenhalgh (1997a)

One characteristic of such writing is that the voice of the writer is absent from the text. The style adopted is to report the research as a series of facts. This serves to underline the scientific nature of the writing, although the author still structures, shapes and selects what is written, what constitutes evidence and how this is presented. The form has been constructed by scientists to structure knowledge in a particular way so as to draw on existing knowledge and to minimize the likelihood of bias and error. As Chapter 13 indicates, the preparatory work for the research is carried out prior to drawing up the research protocol and identifies the narrow and specific hypothesis that will be tested in the study. The structure of any scientific paper is reinforced by publication norms as adherence to a particular format is expected.

The nature of quantitative studies in the social sciences, such as economics, psychology and political science, varies according to the discipline. Typically papers are expected to define terms, set the research question in the context of existing theory, and present evidence in a way that addresses the research question. The assumptions underlying quantitative work should be stated. In such work, even what appear to be objective facts may need to be suitably contextualized, depending on the approach of the researcher.

Writing up qualitative research

Qualitative, descriptive or naturalistic research in health and other areas has been described as research that aims to study phenomena in their natural setting. The aim is to capture the meanings and understandings of people in everyday life. The authoritative voice of the author in terms of structuring the text and interpreting data tends to be more explicit in descriptive research as the data collected require analysis and interpretation. As Chapter 5 shows, for instance, although a qualitative study may begin with a theoretically based research question, themes and explanatory theories also develop from the data. A number of texts provide useful guides on writing up qualitative research (Lincoln and Guba 1985; Becker 1986; Strauss 1987; Richardson 1990; Woolcott 1990).

In writing up qualitative research, the role of the author in interpreting and constructing the account is more explicit and the author should be explicit about the methodological approach: why particular methods have been used and data have been analyzed and interpreted in a specific way. The researcher begins a project with some theory, research question or hypothesis in mind, and this will inform the choice of method for data collection through, amongst others, interview, observation or focus group. However, as analysis also occurs after data collection, further theoretically based analysis will be introduced during the course of the writing up. There is a zigzag between theory and data, during which themes arising from the data are identified (Strauss 1987; Denzin and Lincoln 2000). One consequence is that the final structure a work will take is less predictable; changes will occur during the writing process; and the period over which drafting takes place is typically longer than with a quantitative study.

The writing process should be continuous throughout the research. As Richardson (1990) comments, writing is an aid to thinking and part of the process of discovery and communication. As was seen in Chapter 3, writing usually begins with a literature review prior to data collection. It is likely that a short literature review will have been carried out at the proposal stage of a research project, thesis or conference paper. A more developed review can be written as the research progresses alongside data collection, and amplified in the light of issues that emerge from the data. Planning a structure for the final work may also be undertaken at an early stage and kept under continual revision. This can assist in maintaining a concept of the shape and structure of the research throughout the period in which the project is conducted.

Another useful strategy is to write extended memos on concepts and theories and on the themes as they develop during the data collection phase and the analysis. For example, a memo on a theme arising in early interviews can be identified, theorized and used to test robustness at a later stage in the research. Memos on the theories used in a conceptual framework, and decisions on how to manage data analysis, should also be recorded. Memos should be seen as resources or aids to writing final reports and working on publications. If a number of researchers are involved in a project, it is even more important to record not only decisions, but the reasons and rationale for a particular decision. It is particularly important when a number of people are concerned with identifying themes and coding data and it is necessary to cross-check for validity.

ISSUES OF AUTHORSHIP

It should also be noted that in health research projects where there is more than one researcher, issues of authorship – such as whose names should appear on publications and in what order – should be discussed openly. Ideally, this should be determined early on to avoid potential disputes at a later stage. In this respect, the conventions between scientific and social scientific disciplines differ. In the former, senior academics may be included in the list of authors even though they have had only a nominal part in a project. In this case, the current convention is that their name appears last. In social science research, however, distant help from supervisors or senior academics is more likely to simply be acknowledged in a footnote or elsewhere.

In a health research project when there are a number of authors, the lead author is generally the author who has played the major part in obtaining funding, in leading a project and in the analysis and writing. In writing with colleagues, one convention is that the lead author is the one who has produced the first draft. However, all the above are informal guidelines and the issue of designated authorship remains open to the influence of power and politics. Such influences may be particularly apparent when senior academics involved in research have particular career incentives to be first authors – and their interests are pursued at the expense of more junior researchers, whatever the ethics involved. At the other end of the spectrum, they also may be incentives when this increases opportunities for publication, especially in situations where the review process for articles and books is not blinded.

DEVELOPING A FINAL DRAFT

Preparing a final draft of a health research project usually involves an intensive period of thinking and writing and takes time, even for the most experienced writer. Experience suggests that around four to six drafts (or more) will be necessary and there are distinct phases. The first draft is the most difficult and it involves both thinking through structure and the physical act of writing. The final draft is about editing down, cutting out words, correcting typographical errors and shifting paragraphs. Writers do their writing in very different ways depending on personality, lifestyle and life stage. So, it is best to be aware of what works best for you – early mornings, late nights, short bursts or long sessions. Setting a word target or a time target is a possible strategy for getting work completed. Setting aside a period of time of days, weeks or months depending on the length probably works best. The shifting and sorting process often continues overnight. A problem that seems insurmountable in the evening may be resolved by the following morning.

A key aspect of writing up a health publication is to develop a clear structure. For a thesis, report, article or book certain elements will be standard. In a more scientifically oriented qualitative or quantitative paper, there will be an introduction, a review of the relevant literature to provide a context for the research question, a methods section, a substantive body of data, an analysis, discussion and conclusion. In a qualitative study, the discussion of methods would also typically include how the data were collected, coded and analyzed; any problems that arose during the research; and, particularly in a thesis, some form of auto-critique.

The quality of presentation and the succinctness of the writing are important and a number of drafts will be required to achieve clarity and intelligibility. The writer will need to persuade the reader that they have carried out the research in a thorough way and that their interpretation is well grounded in the data. As a narrative, a written output should aim to present a coherent and logical argument that runs through the work – whether a report, article or book. The introduction should be used to set up the argument. Although less predictable than the structure of a quantitative piece, the final product, whether in the form of a report, a thesis or paper, will require the elements shown in Box 21.3. The question of how to structure qualitative data is discussed further below.

Box 21.3 *The structure of a qualitative study*

The structure of a qualitative study should include:

- The title: This should be short, descriptive of the study and attract the reader
- Author: The name of the author with full biographical details
- Abstract and keywords: Abstracts may be published in an abstracting journal. Keywords are used for insertion in bibliographic indexes
- Introduction: Locates the topic; indicates why it is important; introduces controversies; states the research question, the aims and objectives and the gap the research fills
- The literature review: Locates the research in existing theoretical and empirical literature. It should draw only on material relevant to the research question. References to quantitative research should be included. For example, a qualitative study of the experiences of those living with HIV/AIDS might also refer to measures such as prevalence and incidence to indicate the impact and social predictors such as gender, ethnicity and socio-economic status
- The research strategy and process: The context of the study, for example the research site, the selection of respondents, method of data collection recording methods — in sum, sufficient detail to replicate the study
- The data and the interpretation of the data
- A concluding section and, in the case of reports, recommendations. These need to be geared to the particular audience
- References and appendices

Source: Adapted from Greenhalgh and Taylor (1997)

COMMON PROBLEMS AND USEFUL STRATEGIES

The voice of the author

In a qualitative study in health, the choice of the research question, the collection and selection of data and the interpretation of these data are more overtly subjective and in the control of the author than in quantitative work where objectivity is often emphasized. It is possible, for example, that another researcher would interpret the same data set differently. In acknowledging the presence of the author in the interpretation of naturalistic data, styles differ across social science disciplines and there are also cultural differences. For example, within sociology, research students in particular have been encouraged to be reflexive: to critique their own work and to reflect on how their own position and politics, in relation to matters such as gender, ethnicity and class, may affect their selection and interpretation of data. Some scholarly writers, particularly in American publications, emphasize the authorial presence stylistically by using the first person singular (I analyzed the data in the following way...) or plural (After completing the fieldwork, we developed a framework to code the data...). This indicates that the interpretation of data was their own.

Validating an analysis and structuring an argument

In relation to methodology and methods in the health area, theses, final reports or journal publications should provide sufficient detail of the methodological strategies employed to demonstrate to the reader how the research aims have been linked to the data analysis and the theoretical underpinning of the interpretation made. One difficulty in a qualitative study is selecting an effective way to illustrate this process – that is, to give a plausible account grounded in the data. Chapter 5, amongst others, discusses strategies for analysis. However, when writing up the research a researcher is faced with a range of choices about themes, the order of presentation and how to present data in order to convince the reader of the validity of their interpretation. The example set out in Box 21.4 illustrates the process of identifying a structure in accounts through coding, analyzing and interpreting using a single case.

Box 21.4   *Example: Complaints about doctors*

Theory: Attribution theory suggests untoward/adverse events are explained by allocation of blame in various ways (Antaki and Fielding 1981). Letters are also accounts written for a particular purpose and are structured in similar ways (see Chapter 4).

Data analysis: List technical allegations – for instance, the doctor failed to visit the patient, did not examine the patient, and did not diagnose the illness. List allegations of normative violations (behaviour) – for example, doctor was rude and did not listen.

Developing a coding frame:

I wish to make a complaint about Dr X to y *[the 'Trust' as the authoritative body]* ... my son Matthew (3 years old) *[complainant kin relationship to patient]* ... complained of earache ... he was holding both ears ... a severe headache and crying bitterly *[lay knowledge of mother that the child was ill]*. I tried to ... comfort him ... [he became] more upset and became hysterical *[good mother, limits of lay knowledge]*. He was ... rolling on the floor and holding his head and crying. I rang the surgery and Dr X was speaking on an answer phone service giving an emergency number, which I then rang *[competent lay action taken]*.

Later:

I took Matthew to Dr X's surgery *[lay action to seek medical help]* and Dr X was most annoyed *[allegation of poor social skills]* and said that I had cost him/her £24 by calling the emergency number three times ... *[not providing a service, breaking NHS norms]*. I asked him to examine Matthew but he refused saying there was no need *[lay action through request/allegation that help refused]*.

Structuring an empirical chapter in a qualitative study: Three devices were used to structure a coding framework that formed a basis for an empirical chapter. Complainants' allegations about a doctor's failure to provide a service (technical breaches) and the failure to meet professional norms of behaviour (normative breaches) were coded. Second, the strategies that complainants used to protect their identity as carers were identified. Frequencies and deviant cases were then calculated and both tables and selected quotations used to support the argument.

Source: Allsop (1998)

This example is based on a study of 100 complaints about general practitioners. Here, Judith Allsop linked quantitative data on who complained about what issues with a qualitative analysis of the complaint letters as accounts. Drawing on various theories, she argued that letters had a narrative structure designed (a) to make allegations against a doctor in terms of a failure to provide a service and unprofessional behaviour; and (b) to construct their identity as a competent lay actor in terms of their knowledge, skills and emotional commitment.

In essence, one argument is being made. In their account, complainants both defend themselves, and particularly their identity as carers, and also make allegations that the doctor has not provided a service, nor behaved as a doctor should – and do so in similar ways. In terms of structuring the argument, differences between complainants can be divided into subsets with illustrative quotations by who is making the complaint and their relationship with the patient and/or by what the complaint is about.

A further example of how to structure the analysis is used by Jane Lewis in a study of how couples making decisions about cohabitation and marriage think about trust and risk in making their decision. Lewis's main argument is that there are strong similarities whichever state is being contemplated. The risks considered are seen as the possibility of partnership breakdown, and matters related to housing, money and children. Whether married or cohabiting, couples say their decision to take a particulate course of action is ultimately based on trust (romantic love) in the prospective partner (Lewis 2006).

Approaching the subject selectively

A major problem for qualitative researchers in health and other fields is dealing with a large quantity of data. The example by Allsop (1998) above looked not only at complainants' letters, but also doctors' defences and tribunal decisions in over a hundred cases. The advantage was that the findings were well grounded. Disadvantages relate to the time taken to complete the study and the challenge of selecting illustrative material. The study by Lewis (2006) in contrast was based on a lesser number of 21 randomly selected interviews with both men and women. Although this is an adequate number for a qualitative study where both risk and trust have been well theorized, qualitative interview data are complex and still need careful selection.

Written outputs are, of course, of varying lengths. In a thesis, the methods chapter is a critical part of the work. In a report or article, a detailed explanation of methods may interrupt the flow of the narrative and findings, and may be of less interest to the reader. One device in a report or monograph is to give a short explanation in the main text, and add a methodological appendix. In an article or conference paper, a table or short footnote giving essential details may suffice. An account of methods should always be presented in a way that shows the approach as logical in relation to the research question. It should not normally focus on the actual process experienced by the researcher, which may include false starts and the pursuit of issues that were later abandoned.

A strategy for handling a large quantity of descriptive data has to be not only selective in identifying a hierarchy of themes as indicated above, but also to illustrate these with well-chosen, short quotations. A reader will tend to look for the argument in a text and skip over a quotation. The preceding text to a quotation should therefore always introduce the interpretation that the author intends. Data cannot be expected to speak for themselves. Quotations may also be edited down, unless they are absolutely necessary, as in the analysis of discourse. Authors are advised to inform themselves of contentious issues that relate to a particular discipline or method.

DISSEMINATION STRATEGIES FOR RESEARCH FINDINGS

The main outlets for publication in health research are books, monographs and reports, articles in scholarly, professional, popular journals and newspapers, and conference papers, the abstracts of which may be published in conference proceedings and may be available on the Internet. These are not mutually exclusive means of dissemination. For example, part of a research report can be published as a conference paper that may be turned into a journal article.

Having produced a dissertation, thesis or research report for a funding body, there is usually an expectation of further dissemination to reach a wider audience through publications or presentations. However, while researchers are typically required to publish, avenues to publication are controlled by a variety of producers who apply filters and can block access. Journal editors may apply restrictions on publication. Funding bodies may embargo research. Researchers should ensure that a funding contract includes the proviso that permission to publish must not be unreasonably withheld. As writing is a time-consuming process, researchers should plan their strategy carefully and be prepared to switch, if opportunities arise unexpectedly. For example, although publication in a high-ranking journal may be the ultimate objective, preparing a paper for a conference or giving a presentation to a group of professionals may be good preparation and offer opportunities for learning. Any form of presentation is better than none. If choices have to be made between competing offers, then ask the questions: Will this further my career? Does it pay well? Will I enjoy it? When two or more of these criteria apply, you may wish to choose this option concerned.

Offering to give a conference paper is a way of focusing on a particular aspect of a research project. It can allow for reflection and feedback on a paper that may later be refined as a book chapter or submitted to a journal. Care should be taken in writing a conference abstract, which is usually limited to around 200 words. This should fit with the conference theme and aim to make one major point. The abstract is important not only because it will need to pass through the conference filtering process, but because it may be published in the conference proceedings. Selected papers, or PowerPoint presentations, may also be published on the Web. However, it is as well to remember that such work, and the ideas, enter the public domain and may be used by others.

Presentations to policy makers and practitioners are particularly important for publicly funded policy research in health and indeed may be a requirement of funding. The costs of such presentations should be included in research proposals. Press releases, radio and television presentations may also be part of publicizing a research project. For all these forms of dissemination, the target audience must be considered carefully, any output carefully prepared and tailored to suit that audience. Generally, such presentations should also focus on one key theme – although flexibility is of course often required in responding to questions from the media, which may not always be predictable.

GETTING PUBLISHED

For a researcher in health, a book or monograph offers the best opportunity to present a full account of the research findings and reach a wide audience with a publisher bearing the costs of the publicity. However, there are some disadvantages, as even if a book is based on a research report, it is likely to take at least a further year to produce, and still longer to get into print. Moreover, although a book may make a researcher's reputation, under the United Kingdom's Research Assessment Exercise (the system for rating academics and distributing background research funding to their institutions) it has historically not been the most highly rated form of publication. This is the refereed article in high-impact journals in particular subject fields. There are also specific barriers to publication in both these potential outlets.

The process of book publication

Publishers are largely driven by market factors and will normally only publish books that have sufficient sales to make a profit, or at least cover their costs. It has in fact become increasingly difficult to obtain a publisher for research-based books as sales may be low. In the first instance, it is as well to discuss an idea for a book with a publisher to find out if an idea is attractive and has a fit with their publishing strategy. If there is a positive response, the researcher will be asked to write an outline of the book and its constituent chapters and indicate the likely market for the publication. The most significant sector is the student market and the optimum length is usually around 70–90,000 words. There may be a request for sample chapters as well. Typically, the proposal will be sent to one or more reviewers who will give their opinion, and the editorial team at the publishers will make a final decision. A rejection by a publisher should not necessarily be taken as an indication of the scholarly quality of the work as there are other factors, such as topicality and appeal to a wider audience, that a publisher will take into account in deciding whether to proceed.

As well as commercial publishers, there are a range of specialist academic and university-based publishers who provide outlets for more scholarly works, particularly for those with a connection with a university. Examples of these are the university presses of Cambridge, Manchester and Oxford in the United Kingdom and Cornell, Harvard and Yale in the United States. There are specialist university presses such as the Radcliffe Press for legal studies and the Policy Press for social policy monographs. A number of university departments also publish monographs or have occasional paper series, which have limited circulation. These tend to be shorter and may be an edited-down version of a research report for a funding body. While getting into print may be easier through this outlet, such publications may form part of the grey literature referred to in Chapter 3, especially in so far as they are not official publications and publicity and marketing is restricted.

A more recent form of outlet is Internet publishing through websites. This also has advantages and disadvantages. A wide range of organizations, such as scholarly and charitable foundations, government departments, university departments, research centres and professional associations, have websites that publish research reports and working papers. In the health field, this even includes elite research funding bodies such as the Economic and Social Research Council and the Medical Research Council in the United Kingdom. The advantage of publishing on the Web is that research becomes available quickly and at a low cost. One disadvantage is that, without publicity, the 'hit' rate of such sites may be low and publications may only be kept on websites for a limited period.

Publication in journals

Publication in a scholarly journal is, for most disciplines, the most highly rated form of research output in health and other areas. The requirements for publication are also relatively transparent. However, the filtering process, particularly in highly rated journals, is rigorous. Hargens (1988) estimated that between 50 and 80 per cent of articles submitted in the social sciences were rejected. Some journals give information on their rejection rate on their website. Box 21.5 shows the commonest reasons for rejection of quantitative and qualitative articles, the reasons for which are broadly similar.

Box 21.5   *Why papers were rejected by journals*

Quantitative research paper	Qualitative research paper
The study:	The study:
Did not address an important scientific issue	Did not address an important social scientific issue
Was not original	Was not original
Did not test the author's hypothesis	Did not test a research question
Research design was not appropriate for answering the research question	The method was not appropriate for answering the research question.
Was compromised by practical difficulties	Was compromised by practical difficulties
The sample size was too small	Had no rationale for numbers (interviews/observations/choice of sites etc.)
Was not adequately controlled	Had no rationale for the selection of respondents/groups
The statistical analysis was incorrect	The basis of the data analysis was not explained
Conclusions did not relate to the data	Conclusions did not relate to the data
Indicated a significant conflict of interest	Indicated a significant conflict of interest
Was incomprehensible due to poor writing and presentation	Was incomprehensible due to poor writing and presentation

Sources: Adapted from Greenhalgh (1997a); Belgrave et al. (2002)

In principle, any piece of research, from an undergraduate or postgraduate, as well as an employed scholar or researcher, may be suitable for journal submission if it is original, well written and has a clear conclusion. To be publishable, a paper should be based on sound and well-articulated methods and data analysis; generate appropriate data; and follow through an argument that is plausible. As journal articles are generally short, between 4,000 and 7,000 words, emphasis should be given to one main research question to drive the argument through the paper. Gilbert (1993) helpfully reconstructs an article from the *American Sociological Review* that explains the construction of a scholarly article. To indicate the openness of the process, a good example of one publication in a top international health journal, *Social Science and Medicine*, a study by Lovell (1983) of late miscarriage, stillbirth and perinatal death, began life as a Masters' dissertation.

Rigour is important, particularly when reporting health research, as publication in certain journals itself gives legitimacy to the research results and status to the author(s). This is of critical importance as, on the other side of the coin, poorly constructed or unethical research may risk damage to patients and can lead to setbacks in public policy. One example is the paper, now largely discredited, on the measles, mumps and rubella vaccine (MMR) published by the *Lancet* (Wakefield et al. 1998). The article was taken to suggest that there might be a link between this vaccine, bowel disease and autism. As this information was in tune with certain contemporary beliefs and attitudes, it had a significant effect on the numbers of children presenting for the vaccine – with a consequent impact on the level of population immunity. In this instance, the review process did not screen out the article and it was left to subsequent research to refute the claims.

Aspiring authors wishing to have a paper in the health field accepted for publication should identify the most appropriate journal early on. Each journal aims at a given audience and subject coverage and takes a particular line on methodological approaches. There will be specific requirements as to how a paper should be presented, which should be followed to the letter. When a paper is received it will generally be sent to two reviewers who will comment. Typically a reviewer, who will have some knowledge of the topic, but will not necessarily be an expert, will be asked whether the paper should be accepted (with minor amendments if necessary), returned for major revision, or rejected outright. A final decision is made by the editorial board. Editors and reviewers act as the final gatekeepers in this process.

In this respect, a rejection by one journal should not be taken as the end of an article, but an opportunity to revise and resubmit to the same or different academic journal with the benefits of comments from reviewers. External events such as the topicality of the content of the paper and academic contacts will play some part in its subsequent placement. An article may, for example, be published as a book chapter or adapted for a professional journal where the style necessarily is more accessible and applied. This also provides an indication of other outlets for health research. Publication does not just have to be in high-level academic journals, it can also separately, or at the same time, include the presentations for health care practitioners or other groups as well as articles for popular magazines or newspapers.

THE DOWNSIDE OF RESEARCH DISSEMINATION

Finally, it should be noted that the dissemination of research findings in the health field may not be an unequivocal benefit. Once in the public domain, a work can take on a life of its own. It can be misinterpreted, misquoted or misapplied. There is little the researcher can do to prevent this. There is also the question of the ownership of ideas and attribution to be considered. It is true that publication in a scholarly journal or book for fellow scholars who understand the conventions of citation and attribution may limit circulation, but safeguard ownership. However, Morse (2000) comments from personal experience that, having placed a presentation on the Web, her ideas were very rapidly colonized and distorted in a way that she did not intend. Perhaps the message is that the dissemination of ideas operates within a free market. The best that a health researcher can do is to aim for the more secure forms of dissemination or, alternatively, accept that their ideas and research will percolate down and influence the thinking of others – even if it is in unintended fashion.

CONCLUSION

In this concluding chapter, we initially commented on some of the common issues emerging for the various chapters of the book in relation to the setting up and conduct of health research projects. It is vital that this task is undertaken on a sound basis, if a strong platform for dissemination is to be established. We have also drawn on the advice given by those who have written about writing up research results and getting work published, which, from our own experience in the health field, we have found useful. Given the strong emphasis on dissemination and publication, it is perhaps surprising that there is relatively little guidance on how to write for scientific or social scientific audiences, but some suggestions for further reading are given below.

We have highlighted the importance of writing up and disseminating research findings in the health field. We have also pointed out the hurdles to publication. Having said this, the dissemination of health research can also be a most rewarding process. Writing up research and getting published are exciting for researchers as they have the potential to make an impression on the wider community – whether from a scholarly or applied perspective. Although there is no guarantee of results being implemented, there is a real opportunity – assuming that the research findings are accessed by appropriate sections of the community – of making an impact on thinking, policy and practice in the health field. To be sure, in the promotion of change, dissemination may need to be complemented by other associated interventions, such as education, audit, interpersonal contact from respected people, pressure from consumers and financial incentives (Bowling 2002). However, whatever the outcome, the expertise contained in the previous chapters of this edited collection will not be fully utilized unless the reader is prepared to face the challenge of publicizing the work being conducted. Therein perhaps lies the ultimate fulfilment for those involved in the fascinating task of researching health.

RECOMMENDED FURTHER READING

Becker, H.S. (1986) *Writing for Social Scientists: How to Start and Finish Your Thesis, Book, or Article*. Chicago: University of Chicago Press.
In this book, Becker, a master of research and pioneer in qualitative methods, provides a readable and stimulating account of the writing process based on long experience of teaching doctoral students at universities in the United States.

Johnson, M. (2004) *Effective Writing for Health Professionals: A Practical Guide to Getting Published*. London: Routledge.
This book provides insights and strategies for publishing and has the advantage of being specifically directed towards a health professional audience.

Schober, J. and Farrington, A. (2000) 'Presenting and disseminating research', in M. Saks, M. Williams and B. Hancock (eds), *Developing Research in Primary Care*. Abingdon: Radcliffe Medical Press.
This chapter provides concisely expressed advice on writing up a research project, as well as on presenting and disseminating research in the health field.

REFERENCES

Allsop, J. (1998) 'Complaints and disputes in the family practitioner committee setting: an empirical and theoretical analysis', PhD dissertation, University of London.

Antaki, C. and Fielding, G. (1981) 'Research on ordinary explanations', in C. Antaki (ed.), *The Psychology of Ordinary Explanations in Social Behaviour*. London: Academic Press.

Becker, H.S. (1986) *Writing for Social Scientists: How to Start and Finish Your Thesis, Book, or Article*, Chicago: University of Chicago Press.

Belgrave, L., Zablotsky, D. and Guadango, M.A. (2002) 'How do we talk to each other? Writing qualitative research for quantitative readers', *Qualitative Health Research*, 12 (10): 1427–39.

Bowling, A. (2002) *Research Methods in Health: Investigating Health and Health Services*, 2nd edition. Buckingham: Open University Press.

Denzin, N. and Lincoln, Y.S. (eds) (2000) *Handbook of Qualitative Research*, 2nd edition. Thousand Oak. CA: Sage.

Gilbert, N. (1993) 'Writing about social research', in N. Gilbert (ed.), *Researching Social Life*. London: Sage.

Greenhalgh, T. (1997a) 'How to read a paper: getting your bearings (deciding what the paper is about)', *British Medical Journal*, 315: 243–46.

Greenhalgh, T. (1997b) 'How to read a paper: assessing the methodological quality of published papers', *British Medical Journal*, 315: 305–308.

Greenhalgh, T. and Taylor, R. (1997) 'How to read a qualitative paper: papers that go beyond numbers (qualitative research)', *British Medical Journal*, 315: 740–43.

Hargens, L.L. (1988) 'Scholarly consensus and rejection rates', *American Sociological Review*, 53: 139–51.

Johnson, M. (2004) *Effective Writing for Health Professionals*: *A Practical Guide to Getting Published*. London: Routledge.

Lewis, J. (2006) 'Perceptions of risk in intimate relationships: the implications for social provision', *Journal of Social Policy*, 35 (1): 39–48.

Lincoln, Y.S. and Guba, E.G (1985) *Naturalistic Inquiry*. Newbury Park, CA: Sage.

Lovell, A. (1983) 'Some questions of identity: late miscarriage, stillbirth and perinatal loss', *Social Science and Medicine*, 17 (11): 755–61.

Morse, J. (2000) 'The downside of dissemination', *Qualitative Health Research*, 10 (3): 291–92.

Ramkalawan, T. (2005) 'Training for research', in A. Bowling and S. Ebrahim (eds), *Handbook of Health Research Methods: Investigation, Measurement and Analysis*. Maidenhead: Open University Press.

Richardson, L. (1990) *Writing Strategies: Reaching Diverse Audiences*. London: Sage.

Schober, J. and Farrington, A. (2000) 'Presenting and disseminating research', in M. Saks, M. Williams and B. Hancock (eds), *Developing Research in Primary Care*. Abingdon: Radcliffe Medical Press.

Strauss, A.L. (1987) *Qualitative Analysis for Social Scientists*. Cambridge: Cambridge University Press.

Wakefield, A.J., Murch, S.H., Anthony, A., Linnell, J., Casson, D.M., Malik, M., Berelowitz, M., Dhillon, A.P., Thomson, M.A., Harvey, P., Valentine, A., Davies, S.E. and Walker-Smith, J.A. (1998) 'Ileal-lymphoid-modular hyperplasia, non-specific colitis and pervasive developmental disorder in children', *Lancet*, 351: 637–41.

Woolcott, H.F. (1990) *Writing Up Qualitative Research*. London: Sage.

Glossary

This glossary briefly sets out the meaning of selected key research-related terms used in the text.

Action research is a participative method of research that aims both to gain more knowledge and to change people's circumstances for the better by engaging them in the research process.

Bivariate analysis addresses the possible relationship between two variables. To facilitate this form of analysis, devices are employed such as the *stacked bar chart* and the *bivariate table* (see also measures of association and correlation).

Case–control studies use a descriptive method to compare the characteristics of a particular phenomenon or group of interest to a control or reference group.

Case study is the selection of one or more examples of a phenomenon that are taken as illustrative of a wider process or structure.

Cochrane Collaboration is an international non-profit and independent organization set up in 1993 to ensure that up-to-date, accurate information about the effects of health care interventions is readily available worldwide. Systematic reviews, which contribute to practice through assessments of the efficacy of particular interventions, are published in the *Cochrane Library* on the Internet.

Cohort studies are where particular populations are studied over time to investigate the effect of a particular variable.

Comparative research examines a specific unit of analysis across countries (or other entity). *Exploratory comparative research* investigates the same phenomenon in different countries, asking questions about why differences and similarities have occurred.

Concept is an abstract summary of a set of behaviours, attitudes and characteristics which have something in common.

Confounding occurs when the outcome of an intervention is affected as a consequence of an unknown factor or intervening variable.

Content analysis refers to all forms of textual analysis, but can also apply more narrowly to the identification of specific information such as recurring themes.

Covert research refers to research that takes place without the participant/subject's knowledge or consent.

Critical reflection by an individual or group refers to the process of identifying and examining the assumptions that underpin daily activity, and asking whether, and how, ideologies and attitudes influence interpretation and practice.

Data analysis refers to what is done with qualitative and quantitative research information once it has been gathered.

Descriptive statistics are the numerical, graphical and tabular techniques for organizing, analyzing and presenting data.

Documentary research is based on records relating to individuals or groups that have been generated in the course of their daily life.

Epistemology refers to the nature of knowledge or how we come to know certain things about the world. Different research methods draw on different traditions and produce different understandings of the world and different forms of knowledge.

Equipoise refers to a situation where there is an equal belief (or disbelief) on the part of a research participant and the researcher about the likely outcome of, or benefit from, one or more interventions associated with a health care research study.

Ethical guidelines address questions of justice, respect, harm and benefit. *Principles of ethics* are based on respect for autonomy, justice, doing no harm and using resources fairly and efficiently. *Rights* provide for basic needs with the best available service; protect people from harm, abuse, neglect and discrimination; respect their freedoms, of information, expression, thought and conscience; and promote social inclusion and self-determination.

Ethical outcomes aim to avoid or reduce harm and costs and to promote benefits.

Ethnography is an approach to research that includes methods such as observation, the ethnographic interview and the analysis of cultural artefacts.

Experimental methods include a wide variety of techniques, which are used to maintain scientific rigour in situations where it is not possible to set up controls. In an experiment, the relationship between two (or more) things is investigated by deliberately producing a change in one of them and examining the change in the other. Experiments test hypotheses as opposed to the strength of associations between variables, and may be randomized or non-randomized. *Pre-experimental designs* are non-randomized experiments where a particular outcome of interest is measured only in the intervention group. *Quasi-experimental designs* include the non-randomized control group before and after study, and the interrupted time series design.

Explanatory trials are used to discover which specific component of an intervention produces the outcome, by examining factors such as time, the active intervention and the setting.

Focus groups involve a researcher bringing together a group to discuss a topic in a focused way. This may be either a group of strangers or a group of people who already know each other.

Frequency tables enable a more precise understanding of data than can be gleaned from a chart – providing a detailed breakdown of a distribution by tallying the number of times each value of a variable appears. *Relative frequencies* express the number of cases within each value of a variable as a percentage or proportion of the total number of cases. *Cumulative frequencies* and *cumulative relative frequencies* are represented by columns on a frequency table indicating the number and/or percentage of cases that fall above or below a certain point on the scale. *Class intervals* that group together a range of values for presentation and analysis are used to construct *frequency distributions,* which are employed if the range of values that appears in the distribution is so large that this is difficult.

Generalization is the extrapolation of findings from a smaller to a larger population. In quantitative studies, generalization is based on statistical techniques to extrapolate from a sample to a larger population. *Theoretical generalization* refers to studies ranging from those designed to replicate previous research to those designed to disconfirm, or support, the theoretical propositions generated by earlier case studies. In qualitative research, theoretical or conceptual generalizations about perceptions, beliefs and experiences in everyday life are usually based on a smaller number of informants, but are indicators of larger socio-cultural features or generic social processes.

Graphs (or charts) are the simplest method for describing data. A *pie graph* presents the distribution of cases in the form of a circle, in which the relative size of each slice of the pie is equal to the proportion of cases within the category represented by the slice. *Bar graphs* and *histograms* emphasize the frequency of cases in each category relative to each other. Along one axis of bar graphs are the categories or values of the scale and along the other are the frequencies. The main difference between bar graphs and histograms is that the former are constructed for discrete variables, which are usually measured on a nominal or ordinal scale.

Grounded theory (or analytical induction) refers to a method of analysis used in qualitative research. Researchers begin their research with a general orientation towards the research topic rather than a hypothesis to be tested. In the initial phase of data collection, relevant problems and concepts are identified, and theoretical propositions for further investigation formulated. Analysis goes on as data are collected and further data collection takes its direction from the provisional analysis to generate theory.

Hypothesis is a proposition to be tested. A *null hypothesis* is a proposition that suggests that statistically it is unlikely that the intervention will be shown to have an effect. A *hypothesis of cause* is when one variable (the independent variable) may lead to a corresponding change, or effect, in another (the dependent) variable.

Ideal type is a construct based on identifying the basic variants of a particular phenomenon and can be used in research as a tool to look for similarity and difference (see also typology).

Inclusion and exclusion criteria are based on the definition of the boundaries of the group or phenomenon to be studied.

Interpretivist/constructivist paradigm enables the researcher to understand people's lives, experiences and their subjective meanings through an inductive process of data gathering, which then draws on theory to establish shared patterns of meaning. The assumption is that realities are constructed rather than 'set in stone'. These are sought out by the researcher and are not seen as objectively measurable.

Measures of association and correlation are used to assess the strength of a relationship.

Measures of central tendency indicate the typical or average value for a distribution. There are three common measures of central tendency: mode, mean and median. The *mode* is the value in a distribution that has the highest frequency. The *mean* is the sum of all scores in a distribution divided by the total number of cases. An alternative measure of central tendency is the *median*, which is the score in the middle of a given sequence of numbers.

Measures of dispersion are descriptive statistics that indicate the spread or variety of scores in a distribution. The simplest measure of dispersion is the *range*, which is the difference between the lowest score and highest score. The *inter-quartile range* is the range for the middle 50 per cent of cases in a rank-ordered series, ignoring the extreme ends of the distribution. The *standard deviation* is a more complex measure of spread, the value of which captures the average distance each score is away from the mean.

Methodology relates to the broader principles and philosophies governing research.

Methods are the means of gathering and analyzing qualitative and quantitative research data.

Mixed methods are increasingly being used in research based on data collected through different methods, which often involves the application of multidisciplinary perspectives (see also triangulation).

Narrative analysis identifies the ways in which the narrator or author of a text structures and uses a particular narrative and the devices they employ.

Narrative literature review places emphasis on identifying the key concepts or specific terms used in the literature about a topic and the theoretical approaches adopted by different authors.

Naturalistic setting refers to events or discussions as they happen in everyday life.

Open coding refers to the process of breaking down, examining, comparing, conceptualizing and categorizing data.

Paradigm is an overarching philosophical or ideological framework – a system of beliefs about the nature of the world, or, in a research setting, the assumptive base from which researchers go about producing knowledge.

Participant observation involves gathering data through observing, interacting with and listening to the human subjects under study.

Participants/subjects/informants/respondents are terms used to refer to those taking part in research programmes.

Placebo is a dummy intervention used so that research participants, and ideally the researchers, do not know who is receiving the active and inactive ingredient or procedure.

Positivist paradigm is based on a deductive, quantitative approach and involves the researcher testing an existing theory or hypothesis. A positivist assumes that reality is concrete and objectivity is achievable; the researcher can collect and interpret social facts objectively; and can produce laws and models of behaviour from social facts to predict future outcomes.

Pragmatic trials study the policy context in which an intervention will be used and raise the question of whether it will work in everyday practice.

Protocol is a proposal required for research. It provides a road map or process for a trial setting out such aspects as the aims and rationale, a detailed methods section covering recruitment, the process of the research over time, the end points for measurement, any risks to participants, the statistical advice received and concludes with a consent form for the subjects of research.

Randomized controlled trial evaluates the effects of a particular intervention or management strategy in a population where it is introduced, by comparing the outcome with a control group where no intervention has been made. It is based on the analysis of dependent and independent variables. Randomization controls for anticipated and unknown intervening variables. When the population is well defined, carefully selected and the trial is double blinded this traditionally ranks very high in the hierarchy of evidence. A *double-blind trial* is where both the investigating researchers and the trial participants are unaware whether they are receiving or delivering active or placebo intervention, thus removing expectations of outcome and bias. A *single-blind trial* is where the person delivering the intervention knows which is the placebo and which is the active treatment, but the subject thinks that both interventions are equally likely to be effective. A *cross-over study* is where an intervention is introduced in a first phase, followed by a washout period with no intervention, and then a second randomized intervention occurs with a control group in a further phase. Every individual takes part in both phases, but the order of interventions is randomized.

Regression analysis seeks to depict the relationship between an independent variable and one or more dependent variables in the form of a regression equation. Regression analysis can be extended to take into account even more complex relationships involving three or more variables.

Reliability refers to the extent to which research instruments yield a measurement that does not vary in quantitative or qualitative research. In the former, *test–retest reliability* measures show the same result when repeated after a short interval. *Internal reliability* relates to the degree of rigour or consistency in a measure. In the latter, *synchronic reliability* refers to the similarity of observations within the same time period – thus in an unstructured interview, for example, the words informants use may vary, but the concepts employed are consistent.

Replication refers to a study or experimental procedure that can be completely duplicated by any other interested and trained researcher.

Sampling is the practice of selecting information from populations in a manner that allows defensible inferences to be drawn from the data. *Sampling error* relates to situations where the overall sample statistics are different from those researchers would have obtained if they studied the whole population. This is addressed through inferential statistics, including significance tests and confidence intervals. *Quota sampling* involves selecting a sample according to a predetermined distribution across certain defined categories. *Convenience sampling* is where selection is based on the ease of recruitment. *Snowball sampling* is when the convenience method is used, but there are criteria for the inclusion of an initial group who help to recruit others with similar characteristics. *Purposive sampling* increases the deliberative or judgement element by selecting the entire sample according to defined criteria. *Theoretic or theoretical sampling* is a method of selection in qualitative research where the researcher collects, codes and analyzes data, and decides what data to collect next to develop theory (see grounded theory).

Scales come in various forms and are used as a level of measurement. A *nominal scale* classifies cases into categories that have no quantitative ordering. An *ordinal scale* enables cases to be ranked according to their quantity or intensity. An *interval/ratio scale* (sometimes called a *metric scale*) allows the differences (or intervals) between cases to be measured.

Stratification is a technique used to structure the population of interest in advance in the design of the sample.

Structural analysis is a method that involves identifying the structure of each text; the similarities and differences between the structures of the text; an explanation of why a particular structure exists; and how this is used to create a form of social reality.

Survey is a method for collecting data based on a set of characteristics, analyzing the similarities and differences and, in certain circumstances, identifying the causal factors to explain the findings.

Theoretic saturation is achieved in qualitative research when no new information is generated by subsequent interviews.

Triangulation is a navigational term based on using two bearings to locate an object. The parallel aggregation of data from different sources in research has been used to validate particular accounts or findings. Similarly, different methods have been used to gain a greater understanding and/or a more rounded picture of particular phenomena from a number of perspectives.

Typology is an abstraction drawn from the real world that simplifies, but helps to clarify, complexity.

Univariate analysis refers to the methods used for describing the distribution of a single variable.

Validity refers to the 'truthfulness' or accuracy of research findings. *Face validity* refers to the relevance of the outcome measure or finding to the study questions. *Content validity* is the outcome measure or finding that includes the range of issues considered important by participants and experts in the field. *Construct validity* is the outcome measure or finding that has been confirmed in previous studies. *Criterion validity* is the outcome measure that is congruent with accepted best research practice in the field.

Index